Abdominal Wall Reconstruction

Editor

MICHAEL J. ROSEN

SURGICAL CLINICS
OF NORTH AMERICA

www.surgical.theclinics.com

Consulting Editor
RONALD F. MARTIN

October 2013 • Volume 93 • Number 5

ELSEVIER

1600 John F. Kennedy Boulevard • Suite 1800 • Philadelphia, Pennsylvania, 19103-2899
http://www.surgical.theclinics.com

SURGICAL CLINICS OF NORTH AMERICA Volume 93, Number 5
October 2013 ISSN 0039–6109, ISBN-13: 978-0-323-22742-1

Editor: John Vassallo, j.vassallo@elsevier.com
Developmental Editor: Susan Showalter

Surgical Clinics of North America (ISSN 0039–6109) is published bimonthly by Elsevier Inc., 360 Park Avenue South, New York, NY 10010-1710. Months of publication are February, April, June, August, October, and December. Business and Editorial Offices: 1600 John F. Kennedy Blvd., Suite 1800, Philadelphia, PA 19103-2899. Periodicals postage paid at New York, NY and additional mailing offices. Subscription prices are $353.00 per year for US individuals, $598.00 per year for US institutions, $173.00 per year for US students and residents, $432.00 per year for Canadian individuals, $741.00 per year for Canadian institutions, $487.00 for international individuals, $741.00 per year for international institutions and $238.00 per year for Canadian and foreign students/residents. To receive student/resident rate, orders must be accompanied by name of affiliated institution, date of term, and the *signature* of program/residency coordinator on institution letterhead. Orders will be billed at individual rate until proof of status is received. Foreign air speed delivery is included in all *Clinics* subscription prices. All prices are subject to change without notice. POSTMASTER: Send address changes to *Surgical Clinics*, Elsevier Health Sciences Division, Subscription Customer Service, 3251 Riverport Lane, Maryland Heights, MO 63043. **Customer Service (orders, claims, online, change of address): Telephone: 1-800-654-2452 (U.S. and Canada); 314-447-8871 (outside U.S. and Canada). Fax: 314-447-8029. E-mail: journalscustomerservice-usa@elsevier.com (for print support); journalsonline support-usa@elsevier.com (for online support).**

Reprints. For copies of 100 or more, of articles in this publication, please contact the Commercial Reprints Department, Elsevier Inc., 360 Park Avenue South, New York, New York 10010-1710. Tel. 212-633-3874, Fax: 212-633-3820, e-mail: reprints@elsevier.com.

The *Surgical Clinics of North America* is also published in Spanish by McGraw-Hill Interamericana Editores S.A., P.O. Box 5-237 06500 Mexico D.F. Mexico; and in Portuguese by Interlivros Edicoes Ltda., Rua Comandante Coelho 1085, CEP 21250, Rio de Janeiro, Brazil; and in Greek by Paschalidis Medical Publications, Athens Greece.

The *Surgical Clinics of North America* is covered in *MEDLINE/PubMed (Index Medicus), EMBASE/Excerpta Medica, Current Contents/Clinical Medicine, Current Contents/Life Sciences, Science Citation Index,* and *ISI/BIOMED.*

Printed and bound by CPI Group (UK) Ltd, Croydon, CR0 4YY

Transferred to digital print 2012

Contributors

CONSULTING EDITOR

RONALD F. MARTIN, MD, FACS
Staff Surgeon, Department of Surgery, Marshfield Clinic, Marshfield, Wisconsin; Clinical Associate Professor, University of Wisconsin School of Medicine and Public Health, Madison, Wisconsin; Colonel, Medical Corps, United States Army Reserve

EDITOR

MICHAEL J. ROSEN, MD, FACS
Co-Director, Case Acute Intestinal Failure Unit; Associate Professor of Surgery; Chief, Division of GI and General Surgery, Department of Surgery; Director, Case Comprehensive Hernia Center, Case Medical Center, University Hospitals of Cleveland, Case Western Reserve University, Cleveland, Ohio

AUTHORS

ANDREA MARIAH ALEXANDER, MD
MIS Fellow/Clinical Instructor, Department of Surgery, Southwestern Center for Minimally Invasive Surgery, University of Texas Southwestern Medical Center, Dallas, Texas

DONALD P. BAUMANN, MD, FACS
Associate Professor, Department of Plastic Surgery, The University of Texas MD Anderson Cancer Center, Houston, Texas

CURTIS BOWER, MD
Instructor of Surgery, Section of Gastrointestinal and Minimally Invasive Surgery, Division of General Surgery, A. B. Chandler Medical Center, University of Kentucky, Lexington, Kentucky

CHARLES E. BUTLER, MD, FACS
Professor with Tenure, Director, Graduate Medical Education Programs, Department of Plastic Surgery, The University of Texas MD Anderson Cancer Center, Houston, Texas

ALFREDO M. CARBONELL, DO, FACS, FACOS
Associate Professor of Surgery, Chief, Division of Minimal Access and Bariatric Surgery, Co-director, Hernia Center, Greenville Health System, University of South Carolina School of Medicine – Greenville, Greenville, South Carolina

GORDON LAWRENCE CARLSON, BSc, MD, FRCS
Professor, Department of Surgery, National Intestinal Failure Centre, Salford Royal NHS Foundation Trust, Salford, Manchester, United Kingdom

LEANDRO TOTTI CAVAZZOLA, MD, PhD
Assistant Professor, Department of Surgery, Universidade Federal do Rio Grande do Sul, Bairro Petrópolis, Porto Alegre, Rio Grande do Sul, Brazil

WILLIAM S. COBB, MD, FACS
Associate Professor of Surgery, Vice Chair of Clinical Affairs, Department of Surgery, Co-director, Hernia Center, Greenville Health System, University of South Carolina School of Medicine - Greenville, Greenville, South Carolina

RANDALL O. CRAFT, MD
Plastic and Reconstructive Surgery, Division of Surgery, Banner MD Anderson Cancer Center, Gilbert, Arizona

CLIFFORD W. DEVENEY, MD
Professor, Department of Surgery, Oregon Health and Science University, Portland, Oregon

DAVID B. EARLE, MD, FACS
Director of Minimally Invasive Surgery and Esophageal Physiology Lab, Department of Surgery, Baystate Medical Center, Springfield; Associate Professor of Surgery, Tufts University School of Medicine, Boston, Massachusetts

KRISTI L. HAROLD, MD
Associate Professor, Department of Surgery, Mayo Clinic Hospital, Phoenix, Arizona

HOBART W. HARRIS, MD, MPH
J. Englebert Dunphy Chair in Surgery, Professor and Chief, Division of General Surgery, Department of Surgery, UCSF, San Francisco, California

W. BORDEN HOOKS III, MD
Assistant Professor, Department of Surgery, New Hanover Regional Medical Center, South East Area Health Education Center, University of North Carolina-Chapel Hill, Wilmington, North Carolina

WILLIAM W. HOPE, MD
Assistant Professor, Department of Surgery, New Hanover Regional Medical Center, South East Area Health Education Center, University of North Carolina-Chapel Hill, Wilmington, North Carolina

LEIF A. ISRAELSSON, MD, PhD
Associate Professor, Department of Surgery and Perioperative Science, Umeå University, Umeå; Department of Surgery, Sundsvall Hospital, Sundsvall, Sweden

KATHERINE B. KELLY, MD
Division of Pediatric Surgery, Pediatric Surgery Center, Akron Children's Hospital, Akron, Ohio

ROBERT G. MARTINDALE, MD, PhD
Professor and Chief, Division of General Surgery, Oregon Health and Science University, Portland, Oregon

JENNIFER A. MCLELLAN, MD
Minimally Invasive Surgery Fellow, Department of Surgery, Baystate Medical Center, Springfield, Massachusetts

DANIEL MILLBOURN, MD, PhD
Department of Surgery, Sundsvall Hospital, Sundsvall, Sweden

YURI W. NOVITSKY, MD
Director, Surgical Research, Associate Professor of Surgery, Department of Surgery,
Co-Director, Case Comprehensive Hernia Center, University Hospitals Case Medical
Center, Case Western Reserve University, Cleveland, Ohio

ERIC M. PAULI, MD
Department of Surgery, Penn State Hershey Medical Center, Hershey, Pennsylvania

TODD A. PONSKY, MD, FACS
Associate Professor of Surgery and Pediatrics, Division of Pediatric Surgery, Pediatric
Surgery Center, Akron Children's Hospital, Akron, Ohio

MICHAEL J. ROSEN, MD, FACS
Co-Director, Case Acute Intestinal Failure Unit; Associate Professor of Surgery;
Chief, Division of GI and General Surgery, Department of Surgery; Director, Case
Comprehensive Hernia Center, Case Medical Center, University Hospitals of Cleveland,
Case Western Reserve University, Cleveland, Ohio

J. SCOTT ROTH, MD
Professor of Surgery, Section Head, Section of Gastrointestinal and Minimally Invasive
Surgery, Division of General Surgery, A. B. Chandler Medical Center, University of
Kentucky, Lexington, Kentucky

DANIEL J. SCOTT, MD, FACS
Professor, Department of Surgery, Frank H. Kidd Jr, MD Distinguished Professorship in
Surgery, Director, Southwestern Center for Minimally Invasive Surgery, University of
Texas Southwestern Medical Center, Dallas, Texas

NILAY R. SHAH, MD, MS
Surgery Resident, Department of Surgery, Mayo Clinic Hospital, Phoenix, Arizona

DOMINIC ALEXANDER JAMES SLADE, MB ChB, FRCS
Department of Surgery, National Intestinal Failure Centre, Salford Royal NHS Foundation
Trust, Salford, Manchester, United Kingdom

Contents

Foreword: Abdominal Wall Reconstruction   xiii

Ronald F. Martin

Preface: Abdominal Wall Reconstruction   xvii

Michael J. Rosen

Prevention of Incisional Hernias: How to Close a Midline Incision   1027

Leif A. Israelsson and Daniel Millbourn

The development of wound complications is closely related to the surgical technique at wound closure. The risk of the suture technique affecting the development of wound dehiscence and incisional hernia can be monitored through the suture length to wound length ratio. Midline incisions should be closed in one layer by a continuous-suture technique using a monofilament suture material tied with self-locking knots. Excessive tension should not be placed on the suture. Closure must always be with a suture length to wound length ratio higher than 4.

Preoperative Risk Reduction: Strategies to Optimize Outcomes   1041

Robert G. Martindale and Clifford W. Deveney

The success of hernia repair is measured by absence of recurrence, appearance of the surgical scar, and perioperative morbidity. Perioperative surgical site occurrence (SSO), defined as infection, seroma, wound ischemia, and dehiscence, increases the risk of recurrent hernia by at least 3-fold. The surgeon should optimize all measures that promote healing, reduce infection, and enhance early postoperative recovery. In the population with ventral hernia, the most common complication in the immediate perioperative period is surgical site infection. This article reviews several preoperative measures that have been reported to decrease SSOs and shorten length of hospital stay.

Repair of Umbilical and Epigastric Hernias   1057

David B. Earle and Jennifer A. McLellan

Umbilical and epigastric hernias are primary midline defects that are present in up to 50% of the population. In the United States, only about 1% of the population carries this specific diagnosis, and only about 11% of these are repaired. Repair is aimed at symptoms relief or prevention, and the patient's goals and expectations should be explicitly identified and aligned with the health care team. This article details some relevant and interesting anatomic issues, reviews existing data, and highlights some common and important surgical techniques. Emphasis is placed on a patient-centered approach to the repair of umbilical and epigastric hernias.

Laparoscopic Ventral Hernia Repair   **1091**

Andrea Mariah Alexander and Daniel J. Scott

Laparoscopic ventral hernia repair (LVHR) has established itself as a well-accepted option in the treatment of hernias. Clear benefits have been established regarding the superiority of LVHR in terms of fewer wound infections compared with open repairs. Meticulous technique and appropriate patient selection are critical to obtain the reported results.

Open Ventral Hernia Repair with Component Separation   **1111**

Eric M. Pauli and Michael J. Rosen

In this article, the authors describe their current operative technique for open ventral hernia repair using component separation. Although methods of anterior component separation are described, in their current practice, the authors primarily use posterior component separation with transversus abdominis release to permit dissection beyond the retrorectus space. This method adheres to the literature-supported principles of a tension-free midline fascial closure with wide mesh overlap of mesh positioned in a sublay position. The authors' experience with this method supports a low recurrence rate and reduced wound morbidity.

Atypical Hernias: Suprapubic, Subxiphoid, and Flank   **1135**

William W. Hope and W. Borden Hooks III

Thorough knowledge of anatomy, appropriate preoperative planning, and reliance on the principles of hernia repair ensure successful outcomes. There are many options for repair, including technique and mesh choice. The hernia surgeon should be well versed in the open and laparoscopic approaches and apply them based on the individual clinical presentation. Long-term outcomes related to suprapubic, subxiphoid, and lateral hernia repairs are limited; however, open and laparoscopic repairs using wide mesh overlap and adequate fixation have acceptable outcomes and recurrence rates. Future research will likely focus on comparative studies based on patient factors, techniques, mesh, and cost.

**Takedown of Enterocutaneous Fistula and Complex Abdominal Wall
Reconstruction**   **1163**

Dominic Alexander James Slade and Gordon Lawrence Carlson

Key steps in managing patients with enterocutaneous fistulation and an abdominal wall defect include dealing effectively with abdominal sepsis and providing safe and effective nutritional support and skin care, then assessing intestinal and abdominal anatomy, before undertaking reconstructive surgery. The complexity, cost, and morbidity associated with such cases justifies creation of specialized centers in which gastroenterologic, hernia, and plastic surgical expertise, as well as experienced wound and stoma nursing and nutritional and psychological support, can be made available for patients with these challenging problems.

Parastomal Hernia Repair   **1185**

Nilay R. Shah, Randall O. Craft, and Kristi L. Harold

Occurrence of parastomal hernia is considered a near inevitable consequence of stoma formation, making their management a common clinical dilemma. This article reviews the outcomes of different surgical approaches for hernia repair and describes in detail the laparoscopic Sugarbaker technique, which has been shown to have lower recurrence rates than other methods. Also reviewed is the current literature on the impact of prophylactic mesh placement during ostomy formation.

Soft Tissue Coverage in Abdominal Wall Reconstruction

1199

Donald P. Baumann and Charles E. Butler

Abdominal wall defects requiring soft tissue coverage can be either partial-thickness defects or full-thickness composite defects. Soft tissue flap reconstruction offers significant advantages in defects that cannot be closed primarily. Flap reconstruction is performed in a single-stage procedure obviating chronic wound management. If the defect size exceeds the availability of local soft tissue for coverage, regional pedicled flaps can be delivered into the abdominal wall while maintaining blood supply from their donor site. Microsurgical free tissue transfer increases the capacity to provide soft tissue coverage for abdominal wall defects that are not amenable to either local or regional flap coverage.

Biology of Biological Meshes Used in Hernia Repair

1211

Yuri W. Novitsky

Successful repair of most hernias requires the use of a prosthetic implant for reinforcement of the defect. Because of the need for prosthetic implants to resist infections as well to support repairs in contaminated or potentially contaminated fields, biological meshes have been developed to take the place of nondegradable synthetic meshes in cases where mesh infection is of high concern. The ideal is a biological matrix that resists infection while providing durable reinforcement of a hernia repair. This article reviews the validity of assumptions that support the purported notion of the biological behavior of biological meshes.

Clinical Outcomes of Biologic Mesh: Where Do We Stand?

1217

Hobart W. Harris

After review and evaluation of current clinical data, including significant wound complications, a noteworthy failure rate at 1 year, and high product costs, it is difficult to support the continued use of biologic meshes in incisional hernia repair outside of well-designed and rigorously conducted clinical trials. An industry-sponsored, publicly available registry of biologic prosthetic use for ventral hernia repairs is needed. This straightforward mandate, if properly constructed and implemented, would significantly expand knowledge regarding how these intriguing biomaterials are used and their overall clinical efficacy, thus yielding a more robust basis for the continued use of biologic prosthetics in hernia repair than is currently available.

Safety of Prosthetic Mesh Hernia Repair in Contaminated Fields

1227

Alfredo M. Carbonell and William S. Cobb

For years, surgical dictum has posited that permanent synthetic mesh is contraindicated in the repair of a hernia in a contaminated field. Numerous investigators, however, have demonstrated the acceptably low morbidity associated with the use of heavy-weight polypropylene mesh in clean-contaminated and contaminated fields. Recently, experience utilizing more modern, light-weight polypropylene mesh constructs in contaminated fields has grown considerably. The time has come to critically reevaluate the unfounded fear of utilizing permanent synthetic mesh in contaminated fields, as we will review the data speaking to the safety of mesh in these contaminated fields.

Economics of Abdominal Wall Reconstruction   1241

Curtis Bower and J. Scott Roth

The economic aspects of abdominal wall reconstruction are frequently overlooked, although understandings of the financial implications are essential in providing cost-efficient health care. Ventral hernia repairs are frequently performed surgical procedures with significant economic ramifications for employers, insurers, providers, and patients because of the volume of procedures, complication rates, the significant rate of recurrence, and escalating costs. Because biological mesh materials add significant expense to the costs of treating complex abdominal wall hernias, the role of such costly materials needs to be better defined to ensure the most cost-efficient and effective treatments for ventral abdominal wall hernias.

Pediatric Abdominal Wall Defects   1255

Katherine B. Kelly and Todd A. Ponsky

This article reviews the incidence, presentation, anatomy, and surgical management of abdominal wall defects found in the pediatric population. Defects such as inguinal hernia and umbilical hernia are common and are encountered frequently by the pediatric surgeon. Recently developed techniques for repairing these hernias are aimed at improving cosmesis and decreasing pain while maintaining acceptably low recurrence rates. Less common conditions such as femoral hernia, Spigelian hernia, epigastric hernia, lumbar hernia, gastroschisis, and omphalocele are also discussed. The surgical treatment of gastroschisis and omphalocele has undergone some advancement with the use of various silos and meshes.

Laparoscopic Versus Open Inguinal Hernia Repair   1269

Leandro Totti Cavazzola and Michael J. Rosen

The laparoscopic approach to inguinal hernia surgery is safe and reliable. It has a similar recurrence rate as open tension-free mesh repair. Because the laparoscopic approach has less chronic postoperative pain and numbness, fast return to normal activities, and decreased incidence of wound infection and hematoma, it should be considered an appropriate approach for inguinal hernia surgery. These results can be achieved if a surgeon is proficient in the technique, has a clear understanding of the anatomy, and performs it on a regular basis. This article focuses on questions related to laparoscopic inguinal hernia surgery and provides answers based on published literature.

Index   1281

SURGICAL CLINICS
OF NORTH AMERICA

FORTHCOMING ISSUES

December 2013
Current Topics in Transplantation
A. Osama Gaber, MD, *Editor*

February 2014
Acute Care Surgery
George C. Velmahos, MD, *Editor*

April 2014
Biliary Tract Surgery
Jessica A. Wernberg, MD, *Editor*

RECENT ISSUES

August 2013
Vascular Surgery and Endovascular Therapy
Girma Tefera, MD, *Editor*

June 2013
Modern Concepts in Pancreatic Surgery
Stephen W. Behrman, MD, FACS, and
Ronald F. Martin, MD, FACS, *Editors*

April 2013
Multidisciplinary Breast Management
George M. Fuhrman, MD, and
Tari A. King, MD, *Editors*

February 2013
**Complications, Considerations and
Consequences of Colorectal Surgery**
Scott R. Steele, MD, *Editor*

ISSUE OF RELATED INTEREST

Emergency Medicine Clinics May 2011 (Vol. 29, Issue 2)
Gastrointestinal Emergencies
Angela M. Millis, MD, and Anthony J. Dean, MD, *Editors*

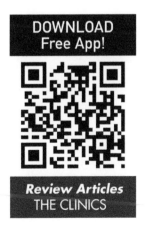

Foreword
Abdominal Wall Reconstruction

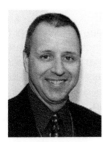

Ronald F. Martin, MD, FACS
Consulting Editor

Perhaps the most important thing we strive to achieve with the *Surgical Clinics of North America* series is to find very capable people who can effectively summarize a vast amount of material, some or much of it conflicting, and put that material into context. In essence, we ask our contributors to not only drink from the fire hydrant that has become our source of information but to give you a report on the quality of the water and suggest how you can use it to your patients' advantage. One of the concepts we always try to particularly consider is whether the ideas that we sometimes cling to most fervently are actually correct—frequently, they are not.

When I was in my residency, which seems like a long time ago to my current residents and a short time ago to me, people would refer to appendectomies and hernia repairs as "intern cases." I would like to submit that in that regard we were dead wrong. We were wrong then and we are far more wrong now when we make that assertion. We were wrong then because we assumed, perhaps arrogantly, that all hernia repairs were "easy." They are not, even if one is referring solely to inguinal hernias, still not easy. We were also wrong then because that assumption that each patient presents without variations that may markedly increase the complexity of repair is intellectually flawed. We are more wrong today if we claim that these are "intern cases" for multiple reasons: changes in training, changes in trainees, changes in technology, and changes in technique.

The training changes are among the most significant. In 2003 the Institute of Medicine released its "To Err is Human" report that formed the basis for a major and unprecedented impact on resident work hours regulation. Of course, this was followed in 2011 by the more significant changes to not only further reduce work hours,

Surg Clin N Am 93 (2013) xiii–xv
http://dx.doi.org/10.1016/j.suc.2013.07.002
0039-6109/13/$ – see front matter © 2013 Elsevier Inc. All rights reserved.

for some residents more than others, but also alter on a PGY-specific basis the degree and type of resident supervision. Without commenting on the merits of these changes, the net result of this for most programs was a marked decrease of exposure to patients for all residents to some degree but even more impactful on PGY-1 residents. Also lost substantially, but perhaps less often written about, was the decreased ability (because of work hour constraints, not other regulations) for a senior resident to serve as "teaching assistants," a role that most certainly focuses the mind of many surgeons.

The trainees have changed as well. Unless one has been working as a member of a medical student faculty or a resident training faculty, it might not be as apparent. Having the opportunity to work in both of those roles, I would suggest that the changes to medical student education, particularly in regard to ability to assume responsibility and participate significantly in patient care, have been more dramatic than the changes in resident education. This has led to a concerted effort to create "surgical boot camps" and led in part to the diminution of the PGY-1 resident role by the ACGME. Whether one agrees or disagrees with the changes, one fact remains incontrovertible: some things that used to be learned by most students in medical school now have to be taught in residency. And we have less time in residency to cover the same, or more, ground than we used to.

Technology has changed on multiple fronts, although this is certainly not news. In particular regard to hernia repair, the advent of videoscopic techniques, the emergence and perhaps decline of biological substrates, and changes in physical characteristics of synthetic mesh materials have all altered the landscape. Many of these changes have significantly changed our approaches to hernia repair in elective, urgent, primary, reoperative, and even contaminated clinical situations.

Last, at least for this discussion, changes in techniques have played a major role. Very few of us are left who routinely had to choose between the various eponymous repairs of Bassini, Shouldice, MacVeigh, or others. Asking a surgical resident today to describe the benefits or pitfalls of various primary repairs usually elicits a pretty brief response. It would probably be somewhat amusing to poll a few hundred residents to see how they would describe relaxing incisions. I have heard some pretty creative ideas in response to that question. Yet perhaps none of it matters so much. The concept of the tension-free repair, the changes in material sciences alluded to above, the ability to insert material by small incision, using either open technique or videoscopic technique, all to some degree or another mute the importance of some many of the "primary" repairs.

Hernia repairs can be performed easily but they can also strain the patience and skill of very seasoned surgeons. Add into the conversation the more complicated ventral hernias and one can really send chills up the spines of those who have "been there and done that." I have met very few senior surgeons who would not admit privately if not publicly that they never felt like they began to understand hernia repairs until they were a senior resident. Furthermore, most will admit that until they had performed a fair number as a staff surgeon they had not established a comfort level with the procedures. Also, almost all will confess that the more hernia repairs they performed, the more respect they developed for the potential, although thankfully rare, complications of these "intern cases."

As always, the best way to shorten the learning curve and to minimize the likelihood of creating potentially avoidable complications is to start by learning what others have learned. This issue, compiled by Dr Rosen and his colleagues, is an outstanding review and, perhaps for some, introduction to what one must know to safely advise patients on when and how their hernias may be treated. We are deeply indebted to the contributors for producing a truly exceptional review of these complicated topics.

Ronald F. Martin, MD, FACS
Department of Surgery
Marshfield Clinic
1000 North Oak Avenue
Marshfield, WI 54449, USA

E-mail address:
martin.ronald@marshfieldclinic.org

Preface

Abdominal Wall Reconstruction

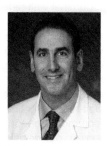

Michael J. Rosen, MD, FACS
Editor

The field of abdominal wall reconstruction has seen significant innovations and contributions over the past decade. With a renewed scientific and clinical interest, the old adage "it's just a hernia" is no longer true. The complexity of defect characteristics, patient comorbidities, surgical approaches, and prosthetics available to the reconstructive surgeon has grown at exponential rates. One of the advantages of this renewed interest in this very common disease process is the fostering of a multidisciplinary team approach. This team often consists of a nutritionist, general surgeon, plastic surgeon, trauma surgeon, and a herniologist. This issue of the *Surgical Clinics of North America* highlights the collaborative efforts of each of the members of this reconstructive team.

While this issue focuses on many technical details to repair a ventral hernia, it also evaluates the most appropriate technique to close a midline laparotomy to prevent the problem. This compelling article should challenge every surgeon to take the time to accurately and precisely close the midline fascia with the appropriate suture-to-wound ratio. Likely, if these methods are followed, many of the challenging problems we all face could be avoided. However, once a hernia develops, it often will require surgery. This issue also describes appropriate preoperative optimization of patients to maximize results. Understanding the benefits of glucose control, nutritional supplementation, smoking cessation, and obesity management not only will improve results in abdominal wall reconstruction but also will be valuable to any surgical patient.

The surgical approach to abdominal wall reconstruction has evolved from simply patching a defect to rebuilding the abdominal wall to its original structure. With this foundation, several innovative approaches have been described to achieve this goal. Several articles describe key components of abdominal wall anatomy, muscular releases that can be performed to gain midline closure, and unique mesh deployment techniques. Several leaders in the field have described approaches to relatively routine hernias up to very complex situations such as parastomal hernias, atypical lateral

Surg Clin N Am 93 (2013) xvii–xviii
http://dx.doi.org/10.1016/j.suc.2013.07.001
0039-6109/13/$ – see front matter © 2013 Published by Elsevier Inc.

defects, dealing with large defects in the setting of an enterocutaneous fistula, and the use of myocutaneous flaps during abdominal wall reconstruction. Perhaps most importantly, a careful description of how to approach relatively "simple" hernias such as epigastric or umbilical hernias has been presented. Likely, if these methods are followed during the first repair, many of the advanced repair techniques will not be necessary for future failures.

No doubt the multitude of surgical approaches to repair an abdominal wall defect can be overwhelming to any reconstructive surgeon, but the dizzying array of mesh materials on the market can confuse even the most seasoned surgeon. Several articles in this issue are dedicated to understanding the advantages and limitations of the current products available on the market. Likewise, the potential advantage of newer, cost-effective large-pore polypropylene materials, even in the setting of contamination, is under investigation. With the growing pressures to provide excellent care in a cost-effective manner, the economics of abdominal wall reconstruction is critically evaluated. With ventral hernias being one of the most common procedures performed by general surgeons, the financial implications of many of our decisions is now coming under careful scrutiny. It is important for all surgeons to understand the financial impact on the decisions they make in the operating room, to both improve patients' outcomes and provide cost effective care.

The old saying in surgery that if there is more than one way to perform an operation, there is often no one right way, likely will never hold true for hernia surgery. In fact, this wide spectrum of disease process is one of the most exciting and fascinating aspects of caring for patients with hernias. Any surgeon dealing with abdominal wall defects must familiarize themselves with all aspects of the preoperative, intraoperative, and postoperative care of these very challenging but rewarding patients. Despite the clinical strides made over the past decade in dealing with these challenging problems, there remains much room for innovations and improvements. I hope that this issue of the *Surgical Clinics of North America* will provide the practicing surgeon with a useful foundation to improve the outcomes of their patients undergoing abdominal wall reconstruction.

Michael J. Rosen, MD, FACS
Division of GI and General Surgery
Case Western Reserve University
University Hospitals of Cleveland
11100 Euclid Avenue
Cleveland, OH 44106, USA

E-mail address:
Michael.Rosen@UHhospitals.org

Prevention of Incisional Hernias
How to Close a Midline Incision

Leif A. Israelsson, MD, PhD[a,b,*], Daniel Millbourn, MD, PhD[b]

KEYWORDS

- Wound closure techniques • Postoperative complications • Surgical wound infection
- Surgical wound dehiscence • Hernia

KEY POINTS

- To minimize the rate of wound complications in midline abdominal incision, it is recommended to:
  - Use a monofilament suture material, USP 2/0, slowly absorbable or nonabsorbable, mounted on a small needle
  - Use self-locking anchor knots
  - Use a continuous-suture technique and close the incision in one layer, avoiding high tension on the suture, adapting but not compressing wound edges
- Place the stitches:
  - In the aponeurosis only
  - 5 to 8 mm from the wound edge
  - 4 to 5 mm apart
- Measure the length of the wound and the suture remnants for calculation and documentation of the suture length to wound length ratio.
- Do not accept closure with a suture length to wound length ratio lower than 4.

INTRODUCTION

Access to the abdominal cavity is often gained through a midline incision. An incision through the midline can be made rapidly and, because no major anatomic structures are crossing the midline, it causes minimal damage to muscles, nerves, and blood supply of the abdominal wall. Postoperative wound complications, such as surgical-site infection (SSI), wound dehiscence, and incisional hernia cause patients much suffering and generate costs for the welfare system.[1-3] In the United States the

Disclosures: The authors have no conflicts of interest.
[a] Department of Surgery and Perioperative Science, Umeå University, SE-901 87 Umeå, Sweden;
[b] Department of Surgery, Sundsvall Hospital, SE-851 86 Sundsvall, Sweden
* Corresponding author.
E-mail address: leif.israelsson@lvn.se

magnitude of the problem is illustrated by more than 2 million laparotomies annually being made for benign conditions alone,[4] with approximately 100,000 patients undergoing incisional hernia repair.[3,5]

Patient and operative factors important for the subsequent rate of wound complications may be given by the circumstances, for example, patient age or overweight, urgency of surgery, and the degree of contamination. Other important factors can, however, be totally controlled by the surgeon, for example, the choice of suture material, the method of wound closure, and the quality of the suture technique.

Numerous experimental and clinical studies are available showing that the quality of the suture technique is of utmost importance for the subsequent development of wound complications in midline incisions. As the surgical technique is within the surgeon's total control, adherence to the recommendations deriving from these studies offers a way of substantially reducing the rate of wound complications.

THE CHOICE OF INCISION

Alternatives to the midline incision are a paramedian (medial or lateral), a transverse, an oblique, or a muscle-splitting incision. All incisions except the midline incision may compromise the placement of an ostomy, which is of importance in colorectal surgery and in emergent bowel surgery.

There are studies reporting a lower rate of incisional hernia with lateral paramedian incisions than with midline incisions,[6–8] but also studies that have failed to detect any difference.[9,10] Opening and closing a paramedian incision is time consuming, and later reentry may be difficult.[7,8]

For procedures in the lower abdomen muscle, splitting incisions such as the gridiron incision and the Pfannenstiel incision are alternatives often held to be associated with a low rate of wound complications.[6,11] However, the rate of wound dehiscence is similar with Pfannenstiel and midline incisions.[12] In a Swedish survey, incisional hernia repair after muscle-splitting incisions was frequent.[13] These incisions provide limited access to the abdomen and are associated with a risk of nerve injury.[11,14]

In a Cochrane review comparing transverse (including oblique) and midline incisions, it was concluded that no differences in infection rates could be detected, but that the likelihood of wound dehiscence and incisional hernia appeared to be lower with transverse incisions.[15] None of the included studies individually report any significant difference regarding wound dehiscence. There are only 3 studies available concerning incisional hernia with a follow-up of more than 1 year,[16–18] only 1 of which reports a monitored suture technique.[18]

WOUND HEALING

The healing of a midline incision follows the general principles of tissue healing.[19,20] Wound healing is similar in all tissues, but the time needed for its completion differs.[21] Aponeurotic tissue needs a considerably longer time to heal than, for example, skin and mucosa.

The inflammatory phase starts immediately after the incision is made and lasts for about 4 days. Inflammation is seen within a zone up to 15 mm from the wound edge.[22] During this phase the wound has no intrinsic strength, and its integrity depends entirely on the suture and the suture-holding capacity of the tissues.[20,21,23]

A proliferative phase follows the inflammatory phase, and lasts for approximately 3 weeks.[20,24] The collagen deposition leads to an increase in the strength of the wound, but at the end of this phase the strength is still only 15% to 20% of the unaffected abdominal wall.[19,21,25]

The following maturation phase may continue for more than 12 months.[25] It is characterized by cross-linking and remodeling of collagen fibers.[19,21] Up to the second postoperative month there is a rapid gain in wound strength.[21] After 1 month, 40% to 60% of normal wound strength can be expected, after 2 months 60% to 80%, and after 1 year 60% to 90%.[21,26] A normally healed wound has gained 50% of its original strength after approximately 6 weeks.[27] After an incision, the aponeurosis will never completely regain its original strength.[21]

Suture Technique in Relation to Surgical-Site Infection

SSI is defined as purulent discharge from the wound, irrespective of the presence of positive bacteriologic cultures.[28] After major surgery through a midline incision, the rate of SSI may be as high as 15%.[29,30] SSI increases the risk for the development of both wound dehiscence and incisional hernia.[9,31–33]

The choice of suture material affects the rate of SSI, and generally a monofilament suture material should always be chosen. The rate of SSI is higher with multifilament suture materials,[34] probably because bacteria escape phagocytosis within the filament interstitials.[35] It is more difficult to form secure knots with a monofilament suture than with a braided suture.[36] This drawback can be completely overcome by using self-locking knots for the anchor knots in a continuous suture line (**Fig. 1**). Self-locking knots cannot slip and are smaller than conventional knots.[37] With conventional knots the strength of the suture is reduced by at least 40%, whereas with self-locking knots the strength is lessened by only 5% to 10%.[37]

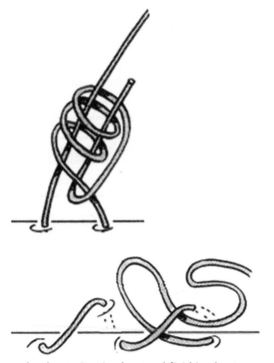

Fig. 1. Self-locking anchor knots. Starting knot and finishing knot.

The degree of bacterial contamination in the wound affects the risk of developing an SSI,[19] and a high rate is often reported in gastrointestinal surgery and emergency surgery, and with long operation times.[38,39] The amount of necrotic tissue in the wound, constituting a nidus for bacterial growth, also seems to be very important for the risk of developing an SSI.[19] Qualities of the suture technique may affect the amount of necrotic tissue in the wound and, hence, the rate of SSI. One example is that with high tension on the suture line the rate of SSI is higher than with low tension,[40] probably because the soft tissues included in a tight stitch are compressed and devitalized to a larger extent than with low tension. It is difficult to standardize the tension applied on the suture in the clinical setting. The clinical recommendation is that wound edges should be adapted but not compressed. If in a closed midline incision the individual stitches are not visible because they are deeply embedded in soft tissue, the tension placed on the suture line is probably too high.

An association with an increased rate of SSI has also been found when closure is with large stitches.[41,42] It has been demonstrated that with large stitches, more soft tissue is compressed or cut through than with small stitches (**Fig. 2**).[43,44] In a randomized clinical trial, midline incisions were closed continuously with a suture length to wound length (SL to WL) ratio of more than 4 and was allocated to suture with either large stitches, placed more than 10 mm from the wound edge, or smaller stitches. With large stitches the rate of SSI was 10.2% and with small stitches it was 5.2% (**Table 1**). Thus, closing midline incisions with small stitches placed 5 to 8 mm from the wound edge reduced the rate of SSI significantly compared with stitches placed more than 10 mm from the edge (see **Table 1**).[45]

Thus several factors that can be completely controlled by the surgeon are important in minimizing the rate of SSI. A monofilament suture should be used, high tension on the suture line should be avoided, and wounds should be closed with small stitches at close intervals, placed 5 to 8 mm from the wound edge (**Table 2**).

Risk Factors for Wound Dehiscence and Incisional Hernia

The mechanisms causing a wound dehiscence and an incisional hernia are similar, as are the identified risk factors. Overweight, male sex, abdominal distension, and

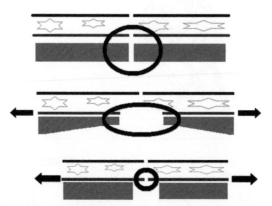

Fig. 2. A large stitch incorporating the aponeurosis (*blue*) as well as subcuticular fat (*yellow*) and muscle (*red*). When traction is applied on a large stitch, it compresses or cuts through subcuticular fat and muscle. Then the stitch slackens and aponeurotic edges separate. When traction is applied on a small stitch, no soft tissues are compressed and the aponeurotic edges do not separate.

Table 1
Wound complications related to the size of stitches in a randomized trial

	Small Stitches	Large Stitches
Wound dehiscence	0% (0 of 356)	0.3% (1 of 381)
Surgical-site infection	5.2% (17 of 326)	10.2% (35 of 343)
Incisional hernia	5.6% (14 of 250)	18.0% (49 of 272)

Fisher's exact test.
Data from Millbourn D, Cengiz Y, Israelsson LA. Effect of stitch length on wound complications after closure of midline incisions: a randomized controlled trial. Arch Surg 2009;144(11):1056–9.

postoperative respiratory failure increase the tension on the suture line, and have been associated with a greater risk of dehiscence and incisional hernia.[9,46–48] Abdominal distension that elongates the wound and increases the pull on the suture line increases the risk of the suture breaking, the knots slipping, or the suture cutting through suture-holding tissues and causing a wound dehiscence.[49] Soft tissue held in the suture may be compressed, causing necrosis and inflammation, weakening the wound, and augmenting the risk of the suture cutting through the tissues.[43] Separation of wound edges leading to an incisional hernia may be a result of an incomplete early wound dehiscence. A raised risk of incisional hernia arises after multiple operations through the same scar and after wound dehiscence.[50,51]

Smoking is a risk factor for incisional hernia.[52] Old age, diabetes mellitus, malignant disease, malnutrition, jaundice, the use of glucocorticosteroids, among others, are factors that may delay wound healing and have been suggested to be associated with wound dehiscence and incisional hernia.[6,9,46,47,50] In patients operated on for abdominal aortic aneurysm (AAA), the rate of incisional hernia has been reported to be high,[16,53] but when taking the quality of the suture technique into account the rate has been similar in patients with AAA and in patients operated on for other diagnoses.[54]

An SSI may delay or even reverse the normal wound-healing process[20] and increases the risk for the development of both wound dehiscence and incisional hernia.[9,31–33] A severe necrotizing infection may disintegrate the aponeurosis, and the sutures placed in this tissue can then no longer support the wound.

During the early period the wound is entirely dependent on the suture line for its integrity,[20,21,23] and there is strong evidence that the suture technique is important for the prevention of a dehiscence or an incisional hernia.[32,47,49]

Suture Technique in Relation to Wound Dehiscence

Wound dehiscence is a complete disruption of the sutured wound with evisceration, demanding emergent reoperation. Dehiscence usually happens within the first

Table 2
Measurements necessary for calculating the suture length to wound length ratio in a continuously sutured wound

Original length of the suture	A
Length of suture remnants at the starting knot	B
Length of suture remnants at the finishing knot	C
Length of the skin incision	D

The suture length to wound length ratio is calculated as (A − (B + C))/D.

10 days[31] after wound closure, as the integrity of the wound is then entirely dependent on the suture and the suture-holding capacity of the tissues.[20] The main mechanism is the suture cutting through the suture-holding tissues.[31,43,47] A rate of wound dehiscence of less than 1% is often regarded as acceptable, although rates of 4% or higher continue to be reported.[30,33] Wound dehiscence is associated with a mortality rate as high as 35%[55] and with considerable morbidity, including a high rate of subsequent incisional hernia.[47]

A necrotizing infection may disintegrate the suture-holding tissues and reduce suture-holding capacity, and greatly increases the risk of wound dehiscence occurring. Dehiscence caused by a necrotizing infection may often occur relatively late, 7 to 10 days after wound closure, as a major infection takes some time to develop. However, this type of wound dehiscence does not seem to happen very often. In 1760 midline closures, wound dehiscence associated with a severe SSI occurred in only 2 (0.1%) patients.[45,46]

A wound dehiscence probably often occurs because the quality of the suture technique at wound closure was such that the suture-holding capacity of the normal tissues was exceeded. The SL to WL ratio achieved at wound closure is therefore crucial, and the strength of the sutured wound increases with a higher ratio.[56] In congruence, wound dehiscence seems to be a rare event when wound closure is with an SL to WL ratio higher than 4.[32,45] In 1760 patients, wound dehiscence occurred in a total of 6 (0.3%). In 2 patients (0.1%) this was in association with a severe wound infection, in 1 the suture broke, and in the other 4 the SL to WL ratio was very much lower than 4.[45,46] The size of stitches does not seem to be important; provided that the SL to WL ratio was higher than 4, similar rates of wound dehiscence were produced with small and large stitches (see **Table 1**).[45] In clinical practice the size of the suture material used is, in view of the experimental findings concerning the forces acting on the wound, often much larger than necessary.[57] In accordance, USP 2/0 was sufficiently strong to achieve a zero rate of wound dehiscence in 356 midline incisions (see **Table 1**).[45]

A continuous-suture technique produces a stronger wound than an interrupted technique[56] and is also more rapid.[30,33] Closing the wound in a single layer has produced lower rates of wound dehiscence than closure with several layers.[9] Including the peritoneum in the suture line does not contribute to the tensile strength[58] of the wound but may contribute to the formation of postoperative adhesions.[59]

It is very difficult to counter a wound dehiscence that occurs because the suture-holding tissues are disintegrated by a severe infection. Wound dehiscence related to the quality of the suture technique, however, can to a large extent be avoided if wounds are closed continuously in one layer with an SL to WL ratio higher than 4 (**Box 1**).

Suture Technique in Relation to Wound Dehiscence

There is no definite information available on how to close the wound when a wound dehiscence has occurred. The situation is characterized by wound edges being severed by the suture cutting through the tissues, by inflammation distorting of the anatomy of the wound edges, and by weakening of the tissues by inflammation or a concomitant infection. Placing stitches in strong suture-holding tissue thus implies that sutures are placed at a fairly large distance from the wound edge, and often a distance of 3 cm is necessary. The stitch should include all layers of the abdominal wall except the skin, as a classic mass-closure stitch. Placing stitches at an interval of 4 to 5 mm means that the tension is distributed on a large volume of tissue, decreasing the risk of the suture cutting through the tissues. This goal may be accomplished if the

---

Box 1

Recommendations on how to close a midline incision to minimize the rate of surgical-site infection

Use a monofilament suture material

Avoid high tension on the suture; adapt but do not compress wound edges

Place stitches:

    In the aponeurosis only

    5 to 8 mm from the wound edge

    4 to 5 mm apart

---

length of the suture used for wound closure is 10 to 15 times longer than the sutured wound (**Box 2**). This method has been used at the authors' department for decades, and the authors have not encountered any instance of re-dehiscence of the wound or, strangely enough, a higher rate of incisional hernias. Although it has been possible to close all dehisced wounds with this technique, there are of course wounds that should be left open and handled according to the principles of the treatment of an abdominal compartment syndrome.

Suture Technique in Relation to Incisional Hernia

Incisional hernia should be defined as any abdominal wall defect, with or without a bulge, in the area of a postoperative scar perceptible or palpable by clinical examination or imaging.[60] The definition used at follow-up affects the rate of incisional hernia reported. If any palpable defect or protrusion detected in the wound is regarded as an incisional hernia, higher rates will be reported than if only large visible bulges are regarded as a hernia.

An initially small defect in the wound may gradually develop into a protrusion and, eventually, a visible bulge, so the definition used at follow-up also affects the time at which an incisional hernia is detected.[61] Thus, if any palpable defect or protrusion in the wound is regarded as a hernia, less than 10% appear late, that is, after 5 to 10 years; if a palpable defect with a bulge is regarded as a hernia, 30% appear late; and if hernia is defined as a visible bulge at follow-up, more than 50% appear late.

Most incisional hernias probably develop during the early postoperative period, the main mechanism being early separation of aponeurotic edges.[62] In clinical studies an incisional hernia always develops if wound edges become separated more than

---

Box 2

Recommendations on how to close a midline incision to minimize the rate of wound dehiscence

Close the wound in one layer

Use a continuous-suture technique

Use self-locking anchor knots

Measure the length of the wound and the suture remnants for calculation of the SL to WL ratio

Document the SL to WL ratio

Do not accept closure with an SL to WL ratio lower than 4

---

12 mm during the first postoperative month.[63] As the regenerative power of the aponeurosis is limited, a defect larger than 12 mm cannot be bridged over. The ability of the suture line to hold wound edges into apposition during the early postoperative period is therefore very important for the subsequent development of incisional hernia. For midline incisions, there is considerable experimental and clinical evidence available concerning how this is to be achieved.

The suture material must contribute to the strength of the wound during a sufficiently long period and, as the aponeurosis heals rather slowly, it needs support of the suture for at least 6 weeks.[27] Nonabsorbable monofilament suture materials and slowly absorbable materials, supporting the wound for at least 6 weeks, produce similar rates of incisional hernia.[64–66] At present, polydioxanone is the only slowly absorbable monofilament suture material that has been evaluated in comparison with a nonabsorbable suture a randomized trial also monitoring the quality of the suture technique.[66] With quickly absorbable materials contributing to the strength of the wound for a shorter time than 6 weeks, the rate of incisional hernia is considerably higher than with slowly absorbable or nonabsorbable sutures.[29,30] In trials comparing sutures, monitoring the quality of the suture technique is vital because the introduction of a new suture material affects the surgeon, and wound closure is achieved with a more meticulous suture technique using the new material.[67]

The quality of the suture technique is easily monitored through the SL to WL ratio (**Box 3**), which correlates strongly with the subsequent rate of incisional hernia.[32,45,68] A low rate of incisional hernia is achieved when the SL to WL ratio is 4 or more,[32] and with a lower ratio the rate of incisional hernia is 4 times higher.[45,46,68] Measuring the ratio is easy and can be used as a means of a continuous quality control (see **Box 3**). Suturing with a high SL to WL ratio prolongs the operation by a few minutes, but is cost effective because the expense of subsequent incisional hernias is lower.[1]

A high SL to WL ratio can be accomplished with large stitches or with small stitches placed at closer intervals. Based entirely on experimental studies,[24,57,69] it has long been recommended to place large stitches at least 1 cm from the wound edge.[6,70,71] A clinical report actually pointed in the opposite direction and indicated a higher rate of incisional hernia with large stitches.[48] Recent experimental studies accounting also for the SL to WL ratio revealed that placing stitches close to the wound edge does not have any deleterious effects on wound strength.[44,72] After 4 days, a wound closed with an SL to WL ratio of 4 is stronger with stitches placed 3 mm

---

Box 3
Recommendations on how to close a midline incision to minimize the rate of incisional hernia

Use a slowly absorbable or nonabsorbable suture material

Use a suture USP 2/0 mounted on a small needle

Place stitches:

    In the aponeurosis only

    5 to 8 mm from the wound edge

    4 to 5 mm apart

Measure the wound length and the suture remnants for calculation of the SL to WL ratio

Document the SL to WL ratio

Do not accept closure with an SL to WL ratio lower than 4

from the wound edge than with stitches placed 10 mm from the edge (**Fig. 3**).[72] This finding supports that a high ratio should be accomplished with many small stitches placed at short intervals rather than with fewer large stitches. A large stitch being related to the development of incisional hernia is probably due to the suture cutting through or compressing soft tissue such as muscle and subcuticular fat included in the stitch. As soft tissue gives way under the suture the stitch then slackens, allowing the aponeurotic edges to become separated more than 12 mm, and consequently an incisional hernia develops (see **Fig. 2**).[43,44]

The SL to WL ratio depends on the number of stitches, the size of the stitches, and the tension on the suture line. The tensile strength is higher in wounds approximated with low tension than in wounds closed with high tension.[24,56]

In a randomized trial including 737 patients, the effect on the rate of incisional hernia was studied with small stitches in comparison with large stitches. Closure with small stitches was made with a polydioxanone suture USP 2/0 mounted on a needle so small that stitches could not be placed more than 5 to 8 mm from the wound edge, only incorporating the aponeurosis. The rate of incisional hernia was 5.6% with small stitches, and was 3 times higher with large stitches placed more than 10 mm from the wound edge (see **Table 1**).[45] Closing wounds with many small stitches at close intervals prolonged each operation by about 4 minutes, but was cost effective owing to the reduced cost for subsequent hernia repairs.[45,73]

In this trial, closure was often with an SL to WL ratio very much higher than 4, and several patients had their wounds closed with a ratio of up to 12. With small stitches, increasing the SL to WL ratio very much above 4 had no deleterious effect on the rate of wound complications.[74] In fact, with small stitches an effect of classic risk factors, such as overweight and SSI, on the rate of herniation was not detected (**Box 4**).[74]

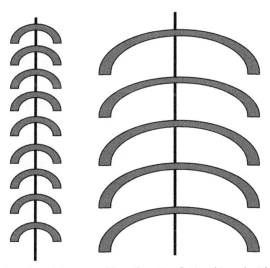

Fig. 3. (*Right*) a suture length to wound length ratio of 4 is achieved with large stitches. To achieve the same ratio with small stitches (*left*), the number of stitches placed in the wound must be increased. In an experimental study it was clear that 4 days after wound closure, the tensile strength of wounds closed with many small stitches was higher than with that with large stitches. (*Data from* Cengiz Y, Blomquist P, Israelsson LA. Small tissue bites and wound strength: an experimental study. Arch Surg 2001;136(3):272–5.)

Box 4
Recommendations on how to resuture a dehisced midline incision

Use a monofilament suture material, slowly absorbable or nonabsorbable

Use a suture USP 0 mounted on a large needle

Use a continuous-suture technique and self-locking anchor knots

Close the wound in one layer

Avoid high tension on the suture; adapt but do not compress wound edges

Place stitches:

    As mass closure stitches including all layers of the abdominal wall except the skin

    30 mm from the wound edge

    4 to 5 mm apart

Measure the wound length and the suture remnants for calculation of the SL to WL ratio

Document the SL to WL ratio

An SL to WL ratio of 10 to 15 should be achieved

Discussion

There is considerable accumulated evidence concerning how to close a midline incision to achieve a low rate of wound complications. Similar evidence is largely lacking regarding other abdominal incisions such as various transverse or muscle-splitting incisions, which constitutes a problem, especially as incisional hernia repair, to a surprisingly large extent, is performed after incisions not generally regarded to be associated with a substantial rate of herniation. Thus, during 1 year in Sweden 25% of all incisional hernia repairs performed were after muscle-splitting incisions in the right lower quadrant, laparoscopic ports, subcostal incisions, and Pfannenstiel incisions.[13]

Patients operated on because of an AAA have for a long time been held to be prone to develop incisional hernias. Several reports have shown, however, that with an adequate suture technique they do not develop incisional hernia to any larger extent than others.[54,68]

The choice to adhere to the experimental and clinical evidence accrued concerning the effect on the rate of wound complications of the closure technique and the quality of the suture technique is totally within the hands of the surgeon. The recommendations are easy to follow, and the effect on the subsequent rate of wound complications makes it cost effective. The only way to ascertain that the wound is closed with an adequate SL to WL ratio is to always measure, calculate, and document the ratio at every midline incision.

To the significance of a high SL to WL ratio must now be added the importance of closing wounds with small stitches. Thus, methods must be found to implement an adequate suture technique regarding both these factors. To achieve this, it is probably wise to focus on surgeons in training and teach them a proper technique during the early period of their education. In Sweden, the British Basic Surgical Skills Course has been adopted and slightly modified to be compatible with Swedish conditions. During this mandatory course, all Swedish residents in surgery are taught the principles outlined in this article.

Changing the technique to using small stitches is probably an easier task than implementing the SL to WL ratio. Having ensured a ratio greater than 4, wound closure with small stitches is easily achieved by providing surgeons with a suture mounted on a needle so small that only small stitches can be accomplished.

Cost savings are generated and patient suffering is reduced if the basic principles of suturing with small stitches and an SL to WL ratio greater than 4 are followed. Suturing with small stitches and a high ratio can easily be achieved by individual surgeons, but the choice to do so cannot be left to each individual. An effective implementation is probably only possible if professionals in charge on a local, or even national level, direct this change.

REFERENCES

1. Israelsson LA, Wimo A. Cost minimisation analysis of change in closure technique of midline incisions. Eur J Surg 2000;166(8):642–6.
2. de Lissovoy G, Fraeman K, Hutchins V, et al. Surgical site infection: incidence and impact on hospital utilization and treatment costs. Am J Infect Control 2009;37(5):387–97.
3. Poulose BK, Shelton J, Phillips S, et al. Epidemiology and cost of ventral hernia repair: making the case for hernia research. Hernia 2012;16(2):179–83.
4. DeFrances CJ, Hall MJ. 2002 National Hospital Discharge Survey. Adv Data 2004;(342):1–29.
5. Rutkow IM. Demographic and socioeconomic aspects of hernia repair in the United States in 2003. Surg Clin North Am 2003;83(5):1045–51, v–vi.
6. Ellis H, Bucknall TE, Cox PJ. Abdominal incisions and their closure. Curr Probl Surg 1985;22(4):1–51.
7. Cox PJ, Ausobsky JR, Ellis H, et al. Towards no incisional hernias: lateral paramedian versus midline incisions. J R Soc Med 1986;79(12):711–2.
8. Kendall SW, Brennan TG, Guillou PJ. Suture length to wound length ratio and the integrity of midline and lateral paramedian incisions. Br J Surg 1991;78(6):705–7.
9. Bucknall TE, Cox PJ, Ellis H. Burst abdomen and incisional hernia: a prospective study of 1129 major laparotomies. Br Med J (Clin Res Ed) 1982;284(6320):931–3.
10. Sahlin S, Ahlberg J, Granström L, et al. Monofilament versus multifilament absorbable sutures for abdominal closure. Br J Surg 1993;80:322–4.
11. Luijendijk RW, Jeekel J, Storm RK, et al. The low transverse Pfannenstiel incision and the prevalence of incisional hernia and nerve entrapment. Ann Surg 1997;225(4):365–9.
12. Hendrix SL, Schimp V, Martin J, et al. The legendary superior strength of the Pfannenstiel incision: a myth? Am J Obstet Gynecol 2000;182(6):1446–51.
13. Israelsson LA, Smedberg S, Montgomery A, et al. Incisional hernia repair in Sweden 2002. Hernia 2006;10:258–61.
14. Loos MJ, Scheltinga MR, Mulders LG, et al. The Pfannenstiel incision as a source of chronic pain. Obstet Gynecol 2008;111(4):839–46.
15. Brown Steven R, Tiernan J. Transverse verses midline incisions for abdominal surgery. Cochrane Database Syst Rev 2005;(4):CD005199.
16. Fassiadis N, Roidl M, Hennig M, et al. Randomized clinical trial of vertical or transverse laparotomy for abdominal aortic aneurysm repair. Br J Surg 2005;92(10):1208–11.
17. Halm JA, Lip H, Schmitz PI, et al. Incisional hernia after upper abdominal surgery: a randomised controlled trial of midline versus transverse incision. Hernia 2009;13(3):275–80.

18. Seiler CM, Deckert A, Diener MK, et al. Midline versus transverse incision in major abdominal surgery: a randomized, double-blind equivalence trial (POVATI: ISRCTN60734227). Ann Surg 2009;249(6):913–20.

19. Peacock EE, van Winkle W. Wound repair. 3rd edition. Philadelphia: W.B. Saunders; 1984.

20. Rath AM, Chevrel JP. The healing of laparotomies: review of the literature. Part 1. Physiologic and pathologic aspects. Hernia 1998;2:145–9.

21. Douglas DM. The healing of aponeurotic incisions. Br J Surg 1952;40:79–84.

22. Adamsons RJ, Musco F, Enquist IF. The chemical dimensions of a healing incision. Surg Gynecol Obstet 1966;123:515–21.

23. Hogstrom H, Haglund U, Zederfeldt B. Suture technique and early breaking strength of intestinal anastomoses and laparotomy wounds. Acta Chir Scand 1985;151(5):441–3.

24. Sanders RJ, DiClementi D, Ireland K. Principles of abdominal wound closure. Arch Surg 1977;112:1184–7.

25. Hardy MA. The biology of scar formation. Phys Ther 1989;69(12):1014–24.

26. Nilsson T. The relative rate of wound healing in longitudinal and transverse laparotomy incisions. Animal experiments. Acta Chir Scand 1982;148(3):251–6.

27. Carlson MA, Chakkalakal D. Tensile properties of the murine ventral vertical midline incision. PLoS One 2011;6(9):e24212.

28. Horan TC, Gaynes RP, Martone WJ, et al. CDC definitions of nosocomial surgical site infections, 1992: a modification of CDC definitions of surgical wound infections. Infect Control Hosp Epidemiol 1992;13(10):606–8.

29. Diener MK, Voss S, Jensen K, et al. Elective midline laparotomy closure: the INLINE systematic review and meta-analysis. Ann Surg 2010;251(5):843–56.

30. van 't Riet M, Steyerberg EW, Nellensteyn J, et al. Meta-analysis of techniques for closure of midline abdominal incisions. Br J Surg 2002;89(11):1350–6.

31. Gislason H, Gronbech JE, Soreide O. Burst abdomen and incisional hernia after major gastrointestinal operations—comparison of 3 closure techniques. Eur J Surg 1995;161(5):349–54.

32. Israelsson LA, Jonsson T. Suture length to wound length ratio and healing of midline laparotomy incisions. Br J Surg 1993;80(10):1284–6.

33. Seiler CM, Bruckner T, Diener MK, et al. Interrupted or continuous slowly absorbable sutures for closure of primary elective midline abdominal incisions: a multicenter randomized trial (INSECT: ISRCTN24023541). Ann Surg 2009; 249(4):576–82.

34. Osther PJ, Gjode P, Mortensen BB, et al. Randomized comparison of polyglycolic acid and polyglyconate sutures for abdominal fascial closure after laparotomy in patients with suspected impaired wound healing. Br J Surg 1995;82(8):1080–2.

35. Osterberg B. Enclosure of bacteria within capillary multifilament sutures as protection against leukocytes. Acta Chir Scand 1983;149(7):663–8.

36. Trimbos JB, Booster M, Peters AA. Mechanical knot performance of a new generation polydioxanon suture (PDS-2). Acta Obstet Gynecol Scand 1991;70(2): 157–9.

37. Israelsson LA, Jonsson T. Physical properties of self locking and conventional surgical knots. Eur J Surg 1994;160(6–7):323–7.

38. Bremmelgaard A, Raahave D, Beier-Holgersen R, et al. Computer-aided surveillance of surgical infections and identification of risk factors. J Hosp Infect 1989; 13:1–18.

39. Raahave D. Wound contamination and postoperative infection. Dan Med Bull 1991;38:481–5.

40. Mayer AD, Ausobsky JR, Evans M, et al. Compression suture of the abdominal wall: a controlled trial in 302 major laparotomies. Br J Surg 1981;68:632–4.
41. Israelsson LA, Jonsson T, Knutsson A. Suture technique and wound healing in midline laparotomy incisions. Eur J Surg 1996;162(8):605–9.
42. Millbourn D, Israelsson LA. Wound complications and stitch length. Hernia 2004;8(1):39–41.
43. Cengiz Y, Gislason H, Svanes K, et al. Mass closure technique: an experimental study on separation of wound edge. Eur J Surg 2001;167(1):60–3.
44. Harlaar JJ, van Ramshorst GH, Nieuwenhuizen J, et al. Small stitches with small suture distances increase laparotomy closure strength. Am J Surg 2009;198(3):392–5.
45. Millbourn D, Cengiz Y, Israelsson LA. Effect of stitch length on wound complications after closure of midline incisions: a randomized controlled trial. Arch Surg 2009;144(11):1056–9.
46. Israelsson LA, Jonsson T. Overweight and healing of midline incisions: the importance of suture technique. Eur J Surg 1997;163(3):175–80.
47. Carlson MA. Acute wound failure. Surg Clin North Am 1997;77(3):607–36.
48. Pollock AV, Greenall MJ, Evans M. Single-layer mass closure of major laparotomies by continuous suturing. J R Soc Med 1979;72(12):889–93.
49. Jenkins TP. The burst abdominal wound: a mechanical approach. Br J Surg 1976;63(11):873–6.
50. Lamont PM, Ellis H. Incisional hernia in re-opened abdominal incisions: an overlooked risk factor. Br J Surg 1988;75(4):374–6.
51. Carlson MA, Ludwig KA, Condon RE. Ventral hernia and other complications of 1,000 midline incisions. South Med J 1995;88(4):450–3.
52. Sorensen LT, Hemmingsen UB, Kirkeby LT, et al. Smoking is a risk factor for incisional hernia. Arch Surg 2005;140(2):119–23.
53. Takagi H, Sugimoto M, Kato T, et al. Postoperative incision hernia in patients with abdominal aortic aneurysm and aortoiliac occlusive disease: a systematic review. Eur J Vasc Endovasc Surg 2007;33(2):177–81.
54. Israelsson LA. Incisional hernias in patients with aortic aneurysmal disease: the importance of suture technique. Eur J Vasc Endovasc Surg 1999;17(2):133–5.
55. Niggebrugge AH, Trimbos JB, Hermans J, et al. Influence of abdominal-wound closure technique on complications after surgery: a randomised study. Lancet 1999;353(9164):1563–7.
56. Hoer J, Klinge U, Schachtrupp A, et al. Influence of suture technique on laparotomy wound healing: an experimental study in the rat. Langenbecks Arch Surg 2001;386(3):218–23.
57. Campbell JA, Temple WJ, Frank CB, et al. A biomechanical study of suture pull-out in linea alba. Surgery 1989;106(5):888–92.
58. Hugh TB, Nankivell C, Meagher AP, et al. Is closure of the peritoneal layer necessary in the repair of midline surgical abdominal wounds? World J Surg 1990;14(2):231–3 [discussion: 3–4].
59. Pearl ML, Rayburn WF. Choosing abdominal incision and closure techniques: a review. J Reprod Med 2004;49(8):662–70.
60. Muysoms FE, Miserez M, Berrevoet F, et al. Classification of primary and incisional abdominal wall hernias. Hernia 2009;13(4):407–14.
61. Cengiz Y, Israelsson LA. Incisional hernias in midline incisions: an eight-year follow up. Hernia 1998;2:175–7.
62. Burger JW, Lange JF, Halm JA, et al. Incisional hernia: early complication of abdominal surgery. World J Surg 2005;29(12):1608–13.

63. Pollock AV, Evans M. Early prediction of late incisional hernias. Br J Surg 1989; 76:953–4.

64. Bloemen A, van Dooren P, Huizinga BF, et al. Randomized clinical trial comparing polypropylene or polydioxanone for midline abdominal wall closure. Br J Surg 2011;98(5):633–9.

65. Carlson MA, Condon RE. Polyglyconate (Maxon) versus nylon suture in midline abdominal incision closure: a prospective randomized trial. Am Surg 1995; 61(11):980–3.

66. Israelsson LA, Jonsson T. Closure of midline laparotomy incisions with polydioxanone and nylon: the importance of suture technique. Br J Surg 1994;81(11): 1606–8.

67. Israelsson LA. Bias in clinical trials: the importance of suture technique. Eur J Surg 1999;165(1):3–7.

68. Gruppo M, Mazzalai F, Lorenzetti R, et al. Midline abdominal wall incisional hernia after aortic reconstructive surgery: a prospective study. Surgery 2012; 151(6):882–8.

69. Tera H, Aberg C. Tissue strength of structures involved in musculo-aponeurotic layer sutures in laparotomy incisions. Acta Chir Scand 1976;142(5):349–55.

70. Hunt TK, Dunphy JE. Fundamentals of wound management. New York: Appleton-Century-Crofts; 1979.

71. Rath AM, Chevrel JP. The healing of laparotomies: a bibliographic study. Part two: technical aspects. Hernia 2000;4:41–8.

72. Cengiz Y, Blomquist P, Israelsson LA. Small tissue bites and wound strength: an experimental study. Arch Surg 2001;136(3):272–5.

73. Millbourn D. Closure of midline abdominal incisions with small stitches. Studies on wound complications and health economy [Doctoral Thesis]. Umeå (Sweden): Umeå University; 2012.

74. Millbourn D, Cengiz Y, Israelsson LA. Risk factors for wound complications in midline abdominal incisions related to the size of stitches. Hernia 2011;15(3): 261–6.

Preoperative Risk Reduction
Strategies to Optimize Outcomes

Robert G. Martindale, MD, PhD[a],*, Clifford W. Deveney, MD[b]

KEYWORDS

- Hernia repair • Perioperative morbidity • Surgical site infection • Obesity
- Intervention

KEY POINTS

- The success of hernia repair is measured by absence of recurrence, appearance of the surgical scar, and perioperative morbidity.
- Smoking cessation, glucose control, and nutritional support can all be achieved over a short time to promote wound healing, but obesity is a more significant problem.
- Each segment of the patient's surgical journey should be addressed and optimized when possible.
- The interventions performed in the immediate perioperative period, such as appropriate choice and timing of prophylactic antibiotics, metabolic preparation with specific nutrients or carbohydrate loading, and choice of alcohol-containing skin preparations are reasonable interventions that minimize perioperative morbidity.

INTRODUCTION

The success of hernia repair is measured not only by absence of recurrence and appearance of the surgical scar but also by perioperative morbidity. Although the recurrence rate after ventral hernia repair varies widely between the numerous studies, ranging from 10% to 63%, the risk of recurrence essentially lasts for a lifetime.[1] Perioperative surgical site occurrence (SSO) defined as infection, seroma, wound ischemia, and dehiscence, increases the risk of recurrent hernia by at least 3-fold.[2] Therefore, the surgeon should optimize any and all measures that promote healing, reduce infection, and enhance early postoperative recovery. In the population with ventral hernia, the most common complication in the immediate perioperative period

Disclosures: The authors have nothing to disclose related to this topic.
[a] Division of General Surgery, Department of Surgery, Oregon Health & Science University, 3181 Southwest Sam Jackson Park Road, L223A, Portland, OR 97239, USA; [b] Department of Surgery, Oregon Health & Science University, 3181 Southwest Sam Jackson Park Road, Portland, OR 97239, USA
* Corresponding author.
E-mail address: martindr@ohsu.edu

is surgical site infection (SSI).[3] This article reviews several preoperative measures that have been reported to decrease SSOs and shorten length of hospital stay.

Several factors such as smoking, obesity, poor glycemic control, malnutrition, and surgical site contamination are all detrimental to wound healing and should be optimized before surgery. Wound healing or a propensity for postoperative infections is the primary target, both of which increase the incidence of hernia recurrence, and there are some management options that improve wound healing. Obesity and smoking have been shown to be independent risk factors associated with increased recurrence of abdominal hernia and SSO. Poor glycemic control in the remote preoperative period (30–60 days), immediate perioperative and intraoperative period, and postoperative periods has been repeatedly shown to lead to an increase in superficial and deep tissue infections. Malnourished patients have significant alterations in wound healing and immune function and consequently have an increased incidence of postoperative hernia recurrence and SSI. In many cases, patients have several of these detrimental issues at the time of hernia repair; for the sake of clarity, they are reviewed individually.

Many of the things that surgeons do that are said to decrease infections and wound complications are steeped in tradition, have few if any randomized prospective trials, and are not evidence based. Examples including using shoe covers, scrubs not leaving the operating theater, and even wearing surgical masks have limited or no significant data to support them; one large prospective randomized clinical trial of performing surgery with and without surgical masks showed that it made no difference.[4]

This article discusses several of the interventions that have adequate studies to evaluate their effectiveness.

SMOKING

Smoking reduces both blood and tissue oxygen tension, as well as the deposition of collagen in healing wounds.[5–7] Both of these effects adversely influence healing of surgical wounds. Numerous animal and human models have studied the deleterious physiologic effects of smoking and have compared wound complications in smokers versus nonsmokers. Many of the initial studies involved orthopedics (tendon and fascial healing) and plastic surgery (flap viability).[8,9] In a study of 4855 patients undergoing elective open gastrointestinal surgery,[10] smoking was associated with significantly increased postoperative complications. Several investigators have examined the effect of smoking on postoperative wound infection and have found wound infection after repair of ventral hernias to be increased in smokers.[11–13] Smoking is also a risk factor for developing an incisional hernia after abdominal surgery.[13]

Attention has subsequently focused on the effect of smoking cessation on reduction of postoperative complications. Lindstrom and colleagues[14] prospectively studied 117 patients undergoing primary hernia repair, hip or knee prosthesis, or laparoscopic cholecystectomy. Half of the patients were treated with smoking cessation therapy and nicotine patches. This therapy was started 4 weeks before surgery and continued for 4 weeks after surgery. The control group was allowed to smoke as they were preoperatively. The group with smoking cessation and nicotine therapy had a total postoperative complication rate of 21%, whereas the smokers had a total postoperative complication rate of 41%. This study clearly showed the adverse effects of smoking; however, the study focused on total complications, and the difference in wound complications did not achieve significance. The other 2 findings from this study were that this reduction in complications occurred after 4 weeks cessation, and the reduction in

SSO was noted in patients using the nicotine patch. This study confirms another landmark study by this group in which volunteers were divided into 4 groups: smokers, nonsmokers, those who quit smoking for 30 days preoperatively, and those who quit smoking and had a nicotine patch placed. Four full-thickness dermal incisions were made on each volunteer for a total of 228 incisions. The nonsmoking group had a wound site occurrence at a rate of 2%, whereas the smoking group had a 12% occurrence. The group who quit smoking and those who quit smoking and had the nicotine patch had a wound occurrence rate of 2.3%, which indicates that smoking cessation for 30 days allows for the deleterious effects of smoking to be alleviated; the nicotine patch did not alter the beneficial influence of cessation.[15] Thus, 4 weeks may be an effective time of abstinence to reverse the complications associated with smoking.[15] The other interesting and unexpected phenomenon is that nicotine patches did not have a deleterious effect on complications. This fact suggests that it is not nicotine but something else in the cigarette smoke that is deleterious. In a randomized clinical trial examining the effect of the nicotine patch on wound infection, the patients with placebo patches compared with patients wearing nicotine patches had similar wound infection rates.[15] It is now believed that nicotine in low concentration may promote wound healing.[16,17] Others have observed similar reduction of postoperative complications comparing patients who had quit smoking from 3 to 6 weeks preoperatively with those who continued to smoke.[18–20] A recent meta-analysis and systematic review of the literature[21] reviews the influence of smoking on postoperative complications and the benefits of smoking cessation.

Because of well-substantiated association of smoking with wound infections and dehiscences, at Oregon Health and Science University, we require patients undergoing elective ventral incisional hernia to be smoke-free for at least 4 weeks before surgery for difficult abdominal wall hernias.[22] We allow the use of nicotine patches whenever the patient asks, because there are reasonably good data indicating that nicotine is not a factor in cigarette smoke that causes problems with wound healing. The patient cannot be tested for nicotine levels when the patch is used.

NUTRITION AND METABOLIC CONTROL

In an era of evidence-based surgical and medical practice, recommendations for nutrition therapy for the surgical patient are supported by abundant large observational studies, more than 40 randomized controlled trials (RCTs), and numerous meta-analyses and systematic reviews. Every surgical patient has a highly variable metabolic/immune response to major surgery, regardless of preexisting nutritional state. Suboptimal outcome is clearly associated with malnutrition.[23] This association was shown in the large Preoperative Risk Assessment Study performed by the US Department of Veterans Affairs. This prospective trial included more than 87,000 patients from 44 separate medical centers; investigators collected 67 variables on each patient. This study reported that the single most valuable predictor of poor outcome and increased morbidity was a serum albumin level less than 3.0 g/dL.[24] Kudsk and colleagues[25] confirmed that albumin, although not a marker of nutritional status, is a good surrogate marker for poor surgical outcome. However, not all patients with ventral hernia or abdominal wall reconstruction (AWR) derive the same benefit from nutrition therapy intervention either preoperatively or postoperatively. Previously well-nourished patients with minor surgery and who are expected to be discharged home after surgery or who have only a short stay in hospital derive little benefit from early nutrition therapy. On the other hand, most patients undergoing major AWR with an expected extended stay in hospital and intensive care unit at moderate to severe nutrition risk appreciate significant outcome benefits from early attention to nutrition. Although this has not been shown definitively in hernia surgery, it has been well shown for major visceral surgical procedures.[26] In patients undergoing emergent or urgent AWR secondary to obstruction or infection who are preoperatively malnourished, these benefits of attention to nutrition are even greater.[27] Whether a benefit from nutrition therapy is realized depends on factors such as route and timing of delivery, content of nutrient substrate, and efforts to promote patient mobility. Recent data support a preoperative assessment and nutritional intervention if the patient meets high-risk criteria.[27] Several nutritional scoring systems have recently been proposed, with only 1 (Nutrition Risk Score 2002) being validated in a surgical population.[28]

PREOPERATIVE METABOLIC PREPARATION FOR SURGICAL INTERVENTION

The concept of preoperative preparation of the patient with specific metabolic and immune active nutrients acquired a clinical application after several landmark studies by Gianotti and colleagues.[29–31] These investigations showed benefit in decreasing perioperative complications by adding the amino acid arginine and omega-3 fatty acids, docosahexaenoic acid, and eicosapentaenoic acid for 5 days preoperatively. The investigators reported that major morbidity could be reduced by approximately 50% in patients undergoing major foregut surgery, including esophageal, stomach, or pancreas procedures. This benefit was noted in both well-nourished and malnourished patient populations.[29,32] The revelation that even well-nourished patients would benefit was a paradigm shift from the notion that correction of malnutrition alone was the only important factor.[29,31] In these studies, the patients consumed 750 mL to 1 L per day of the metabolic-modulating formula in addition to their regular diet. The formula used by Gianotti and Braga contained additional arginine, omega-3 fatty acids, and nucleic acids, and resulted in significant decreases in infectious morbidity, length of hospital stay, and hospital-related expenses.[29–31] In a recent meta-analysis and systematic review of the evidence including 35 articles, Drover and colleagues[33] reported that these arginine-containing nutritional supplements yielded a significant benefit in decreasing infectious complications across the several surgical specialties included. This meta-analysis also reported a signal for a decrease in length of hospital stay. The mechanisms of the active ingredients are yet to be elucidated. It has been shown that the fish oils have multiple mechanisms, including attenuating the metabolic response to stress, altering gene expression to minimize the proinflammatory cytokine production, beneficially modifying the T helper type 1 to T helper type 2 lymphocyte population to decrease the inflammatory response, increasing production of the anti-inflammatory lipid compounds resolvins and protectins, and regulating bowel motility via vagal efferents.[34–39] Arginine has been reported to have a multitude of potential benefits in the surgical populations. These benefits include improved wound healing, optimizing lymphocyte proliferation, and enhancing blood flow via the nitric oxide vasodilation effects.[40,41] The influence of the RNA found in these preoperative formulas has theoretic benefits that have still to be elucidated in mammalian trials.[41]

Another area of metabolic manipulation of growing interest is preoperative carbohydrate loading.[42] This metabolic strategy uses an isotonic carbohydrate solution given at midnight on the night before surgery, then 3 hours preoperatively, to maximally load the tissues with glycogen before the surgical stress.[43] In most Western surgical settings, the routine is for the patient to fast after dinner the night before surgery and remain nil by mouth after midnight before surgery in the morning. Essentially, following this routine, glycogen stores are nearly depleted before the surgical insult. Soop and colleagues,[44] Fearon and colleagues,[45] and more recently Awad[46,47] have shown the beneficial effects of carbohydrate loading in several animal and clinical studies. Caution with direct cause-and-effect conclusions is needed because most large human studies dealing with carbohydrate loading were performed as part of several preoperative interventions, with the experimental groups receiving multimodality treatment, including avoidance of drains, controlled perioperative sodium and fluid administration, epidural anesthesia, and early mobilization in addition to the carbohydrate loading.[42] These carbohydrate loading studies have consistently reported several metabolic benefits, including significantly reduced insulin resistance, decreased postoperative nitrogen loss, and better retention of muscle function.[44,45]

Several other micronutrients, supplements, or anabolic medications have occasionally been reported to benefit in reducing metabolic response to stress, enhancing lean body tissue, or preserving antioxidant capacity. None of these has shown consistent outcome benefits or had adequate prospective randomized trials to support routine use. Some of these agents are amino acid leucine and glutamine, antioxidants, the trace minerals selenium and zinc, and vitamins E and C. Anabolic agents such as oxandrolone and human recombinant growth hormone have essentially no prospective data in the preoperative setting to support use other than in experimental protocols.[48]

SSI

There is evidence that wound infection after incisional hernia repair is higher than that noted with other cases designated as clean cases. If the index case from which the hernia developed had a wound infection, then subsequent incisional hernia repair has a higher level of infection than would be expected from a clean case.[49]

Virtually all incisional hernias greater than 4 to 6 cm require mesh for optimal repair, and if the mesh is synthetic and becomes infected, it is not possible to sterilize it and completely eradicate the infection without removing the mesh. Synthetic mesh clearance rates after mesh-related wound infections are reported between 10% and 70% and depend on the type of mesh involved. Polytetrafluoroethylene is the most difficult and is virtually impossible to clear, whereas porous polypropylene yields the best chance of clearance.[50,51] The clearance rates are dependent on the type of mesh used, location of mesh placement, and the extent of contamination, as well as the viability of the tissue and host defenses.[2,50] In addition, infected mesh is associated with costly morbidities such as enterocutaneous fistulae and recurrent hernia. These complications can be severe and expose the patient to significant morbidity and even mortality. Treating the complications of infected mesh is also expensive[51]; therefore, all reasonable measures should be taken to prevent wound or mesh infection.

PERIOPERATIVE ANTIBIOTICS

Rios and colleagues[52] reported a decrease in wound infection after the use of prophylactic antibiotics in patients undergoing incisional hernia repair. This group experienced a wound infection rate of 26.3% in 76 control patients compared with 13.6% in 140 patients receiving prophylactic antibiotics. According to guidelines that were developed jointly by the American Society of Health-System Pharmacists, the Infectious Diseases Society of America, the Surgical Infection Society, and the Society for Healthcare Epidemiology of America, patients undergoing routine ventral hernia repair should be given prophylactic antibiotics using a first-generation cephalosporin.[53] The antibiotics should be given with adequate time to allow for levels in the tissue to reach a level higher than the minimum inhibitory concentration for the bacteria that is to be inhibited; usually, this is at least 30 minutes before incision.[54]

Antibiotics should be redosed, if necessary, during the operation as indicated based on duration of surgery, half-life of antibiotic being used, blood loss, and use of cell saver. Antibiotics are not given postoperatively because several randomized trials have shown no benefit of dosing prophylactic antibiotics after the skin has been closed.[55–59] These outcomes have been similar across several surgical disciplines. Most hospitals have preoperative protocols; in large surveys, more than 90% of procedures use the correct antibiotic for prophylaxis, according to published guidelines, and the patient receives their antibiotics in a timely fashion. Prophylaxis is commonly inadequate in patients with a body mass index (BMI, calculated as weight in kilograms divided by the square of height in meters) of more than 30. In a recent large survey, only 66% of patients received prophylactic dosing to reach adequate serum levels when BMI was more than 30.[60] If the patient has a BMI more than 30, it is recommended to consider increasing the dose. When cephazolin is used, a 2-g dose should be given for patients with BMI more than 30 to establish adequate serum levels. For patients with BMI >50, consider an even higher dose of prophylactic antibiotics.

Many investigators believe that a previous wound infection that subsequently healed increases the risk of subsequent wound infection in this group of patients.[61,62] Others have not observed an increase in wound infections after repair of incisional hernias when the initial incision was infected.[63] We consider a previous wound infection to increase the risk of subsequent wound infections. We attempt to use appropriate prophylactic antibiotics when culture results of the initial infection are available. If the patient has had methicillin-resistant *Staphylococcus aureus* (MRSA), we use vancomycin. In these patients, we also prefer biomesh as our reinforcing agent.[64] This preference is especially important in patients who have had previous infections with MRSA involving synthetic, mesh even when no overt signs of infection have been present for up to 10 years. The foreign body yields the substrate for the biofilm to form on and to allow the bacteria to flourish. Once this process occurs, the bacteria have adequate numbers for quorum sensing. Within the bacterial colony, intracellular signals allow some bacterial cells in the colony to change phenotypically, with some becoming dormant, some actively dividing, and some becoming planktonic.[65] Several studies have speculated that if previous mesh infection was present, the patient should no longer be treated with prophylaxis but should be treated empirically with a full course of antibiotics.[65] One must be cautious of overusing vancomycin prophylaxis without adequate indications, because several studies have now shown a higher risk of methicillin-sensitive *S aureus* (MSSA) when vancomycin is used over a β-lactam antibiotic.[66]

For those patients with ongoing wound infections, infected mesh, and active fistulas, we debride all infected tissue before repair; and in some instances in which the bioburden of bacteria is high, we stage the repair with a wound VAC or close with Vicryl mesh and perform a subsequent repair, with a acellular dermal matrix as a future repair depending on the patient's condition and the amount of contamination.[67]

PERIOPERATIVE BLOOD GLUCOSE MANAGEMENT

Glycemic control in the perioperative period should be considered in 3 distinct periods. In elective patients, glucose control in the 30 to 60 days before surgery is beneficial in decreasing perioperative complications. Dronge and colleagues,[68] evaluating patients from Veterans Administration hospitals, found that SSIs were reduced in patients whose HbA1c was less than 7% and recommended that HbA1c less than 7% is a preoperative target to aim for.

In the immediate perioperative period, the first 24 hours postoperatively seem to be especially important, because hyperglycemia results in nonfunctional or poorly functional neutrophils. Hyperglycemia has been shown to alter chemotaxis, pseudopod formation, phagocytosis, and oxidative burst, which prevent the early killing of bacteria that entered the wound during surgery.[69]

Postoperative glycemic control was initially shown to be of benefit in preventing complications in a large study of primarily cardiac patients.[70] In the early 2000s, meticulous glucose control (80–110 mg/dL) was popular in the surgical patients in the intensive care unit. This popularity was stimulated by a large RCT showing a significant decrease in mortality when this strict glucose control protocol was instituted.[70] This finding has subsequently been shown not to be the case, because the risk of hypoglycemia and its complications outweigh the risk of meticulous glycemic control.[71] Postoperative hyperglycemia has been shown to be a strong predictor of postoperative SSI. Ramos and colleagues,[72] in a retrospective study of 995 patients, correlated postoperative infections with postoperative hypoglycemia, which was a strong indicator of the probability of postoperative infection in a multivariate regression model. In this study, every 40-point increase from 110 mg/dL serum glucose increased the risk of infection by 30%. Ata and colleagues[73] examined the records of 1561 patients undergoing general or vascular surgery and found that a postoperative glucose level of greater than 140 mg/L was the only significant predictor of SSIs. The target for the immediate perioperative period seems optimal in the 140-mg/dL to 160-mg/dL range.

OBESITY

Obesity is a major factor, perhaps the most important factor, in the causation and recurrence of incisional hernias. The propensity for obese patients to develop incisional hernias was noted early on by surgeons performing bariatric procedures.[74] The incidence of postoperative incisional hernia occurred in up to 40% of patients after open gastric bypass.[75] The reduction of postoperative incisional hernias after laparoscopic gastric bypass was one of the major reasons for performing the bypass laparoscopically.

Increased recurrence rates are also seen in the obese after repair of incisional hernias.[64,76] The rate of recurrence may be related to BMI; that is, as BMI increases, so does the recurrence rate. We have found that in patients with BMI of 50 or higher, the rate is prohibitively high, and we no longer perform elective herniorrhaphies in these patients.

Obesity is difficult to modify or lessen, short of performing a bariatric procedure. If we are performing a bariatric procedure in a patient with an incisional hernia, we attempt to perform the bariatric procedure without repairing the hernia and wait until the patient has lost weight before we attempt repair. If the bariatric procedure is performed open and the hernia is in the epigastric area, the hernia has to be repaired during the initial operation to close the abdomen.

PREOPERATIVE AXIAL IMAGING

The use of preoperative axial imaging clearly adds to preoperative planning in the patient with multiple recurrences, for evaluation of vasculature, tissue planes, and possibility of other smaller hernias not noted on examination. The loss of anterior wall blood from previous abdominal wall surgery has been directly linked to postoperative wound complications.[77] If renal compromise is an issue, noncontrast computed tomography is usually adequate to evaluate abdominal wall defects. This imaging becomes of critical importance in the morbidly obese, because additional abdominal wall defects are often not palpable.[78]

SKIN PREPARATION AND DECOLONIZATION PROTOCOLS

The data on choice of skin preparations immediately before incision are clear. Two major trials have recently been published; the first from a surgical iodine group in Virginia. Swenson and colleagues[79] reported in a prospective trial of more than 3200 patients that iodine skin preparations were superior to chlorhexidine preparations. Soon after the study by Swenson and colleagues was published, a prospective randomized clinical trial with intention-to-treat analysis in more than 800 patients was published, reporting that chlorhexidine was superior to iodine preparations.[80] Swenson and Sawyer[81] reanalyzed the data from both studies. This analysis revealed that the key to decreased infections was the alcohol in the preparations, that Duraprep and Cloraprep had equivalent surgical infection risk, and that the iodine preparation with no alcohol was most commonly associated with infections. It has been the standard of care for several years that clippers rather than razor be used to clear the surgical site hair that would interfere with the surgical site.[82] Surgical site barriers and skin sealants have not been studied in ventral hernia repair. The data on these applications are widely variable, with reports from beneficial to detrimental. The data on skin sealants and surgical site barriers are too inconsistent to make any recommendation for their use in ventral hernia repair or AWR. The use of preoperative showers with antiseptic soaps to decrease SSIs has been inconsistent. Showering with antiseptic agents such as chlorhexidine or Betadine when compared with showering with soap has no proven benefit.[83] Most studies are underpowered or were studied in a widely heterogeneous population, which makes consistent results nearly impossible. Many of the early studies do report a decrease in skin bacterial colonization at time of surgery but have not shown a consistent decrease in SSI. Few of the smaller studies have shown benefit of preoperative chlorhexidine shower in reducing SSI, but these are few.[84] This inconsistency in the literature led to the Cochrane analysis in 2012 that concluded that preoperative showers with antiseptics have no significant benefit.[83,85] Preoperative clearance of MSSA has gained significant popularity in the last several months after a landmark study published in 2010 by Bode and colleagues[86] in the *New England Journal of Medicine*. This study was closely followed by a second study by Kim and colleagues[87] supporting the concept of *Staphylococcus* clearance preoperatively to decrease postoperative wound infections. In the study by Bode and colleagues, 6771 patients were screened on admission, with approximately 1200 being positive for *S aureus*. The investigators then prospectively randomized, with an intention-to-treat analysis, the patients carrying *S aureus* to twice-daily mupirocin applied to the nostrils with a once-daily chlorhexidine shower versus placebo. The investigators reported a 42% decrease in *S aureus* postoperative infections in the treated group. The logistics of screening then treating those positive is cumbersome and requires consistency and patient compliance, but when performed according to protocol, it is clearly cost-effective.

Hair removal has been addressed and shown to reduce wound complications only when performed immediately before surgery and to have optimal outcome when clippers rather than razors are used.[88]

MISCELLANEOUS TECHNIQUES AND TREATMENTS TO REDUCE RISK

Additional measures reported to decrease postoperative infectious complications include antibiotic-impregnated suture, perioperative patient warming, and intraoperative and postoperative hyperoxygenation. Antibiotic-impregnated sutures have limited support in the literature.[89] Only one prospective randomized trial has reported that using triclosan-impregnated suture reduced infection risk in a routine midline closure.

With only this single industry-sponsored study, it seems that routine use of antibiotic-impregnated suture cannot be justified in ventral hernia repair, although it does seem safe.

Intraoperative wound protectors are designed to protect from desiccation, contamination, and mechanical trauma. They have also been reported to decrease wound infections. No data on wound protectors in hernia surgery are available. At least six randomized clinical trials have been performed. Four reported no benefit in decreasing SSI and two showed benefit. When weighing the quality of the studies and using the grade system to evaluate studies, the evidence points toward no benefit.[90,91]

The concept of patient warming to prevent SSI has received significant attention in the past 10 years, and now most operating rooms have patient warming as part of the protocol to minimize SSI. Several observational studies reported a significant correlation between hypothermia and SSI. The theoretic belief is that euthermia helps maintain better perfusion to skin and that better oxygen tension at the skin level decreases SSI.[92] Hypothermia has also been associated with adverse influence on the immune function, T-cell–mediated antibody production, and decrease in both oxidative and nonoxidative killing of bacteria by neutrophils.[93] These concepts were supported by two moderate-sized RCTs both showing that hypothermia was significantly associated with increase SSI. A large, nested, case-controlled study performed using the National Surgery Quality Improvement Program database does not seem to have confirmed these earlier findings.[94]

Supplemental perioperative oxygenation (hyperoxia) has been investigated, but not in hernia surgery. The concept that adequate oxygenation is required for neutrophil and macrophage killing of bacteria and the association that surgical wounds have a lower partial pressure of oxygen than normal tissue make this an attractive hypothesis for decreasing SSI.[95] Two landmark studies in patients who have had colorectal surgery that showed benefit in reducing SSI led to multiple protocols of using supplemental oxygenation.[96,97] This finding led to a large study of 1400 patients, with governmental funding, showing no benefit.[98] A more recent meta-analysis favored supplemental oxygen protocols in the higher-risk population, such as patients undergoing colorectal surgery.[99] Although no direct studies have been performed in AWR, this population has a risk for SSI similar to patients undergoing colorectal surgery.

Perioperative antibiotic use commonly results in antibiotic-associated diarrhea (AAD) in an estimated 20% of patients, with perioperative use of antibiotics being a major source for AAD and *Clostridium difficile* diarrhea.[100,101] Numerous recent prospective trials have shown that appropriate selection and supplementation of probiotics (live viable bacteria when given in adequate amounts show benefit in the host) are safe and can significantly decrease both AAD and *C difficile* diarrhea.[100–102]

Several other factors can be addressed in the intraoperative period and postoperative period that can optimize patient outcome and minimize SSO, but these are beyond the scope of this article. One concept that is rapidly gaining credence in major surgery is the idea that a preoperative routine scheduled physical activity program can decrease length of stay and decrease total complications associated with major surgery.[103]

SUMMARY

Smoking cessation, glucose control, and nutritional support can all be achieved over a short time (1–5 weeks), but obesity is a weightier problem. It takes months for a patient to lose significant weight, even after a bariatric operation. If the surgeon has the luxury of waiting (minimally or nonsymptomatic reducible hernia), they should wait until the

---

Table 1
Interventions performed in the immediate perioperative period

Solid data to support use	Good preliminary data: awaiting confirmation
Smoking cessation	
Attention to nutrition	Bowel preparations
Preoperative and postoperative	Patient warming
Consider specific nutrients	Perioperative hyperoxygenation
Glucose control	Statins
Preoperative–intraoperative–postoperative	Carbohydrate loading
Antibiotic prophylaxis	Prehabilitation
Choice of drug	
First generation in most	
Vancomycin in high-risk populations	
Duration of therapy	
Should stop when last suture placed	
Redosing	
Consider half-life of antibiotic being used	
Alcohol-containing skin preparation	

---

patient has lost considerable weight. For those hernias that are symptomatic or incarcerated, the surgeon does not have the advantage of waiting. Each segment of the patient's surgical journey should be addressed and optimized when possible (**Table 1**). Preoperative and perioperative minor interventions have been shown to be safe and even cost-effective in most cases. Interventions performed in the immediate perioperative period, like appropriate choice and timing of prophylactic antibiotics, metabolic preparation with specific nutrients or carbohydrate loading, choice of alcohol-containing skin preparations, and preoperative decolonization of MRSA and MSSA from the nostrils and skin, are reasonable interventions that when implemented, minimize perioperative morbidity.

REFERENCES

1. Flum DR, Horvath K, Koepsell T. Have outcomes of incisional hernia repair improved with time? A population-based analysis. Ann Surg 2003;237(1): 129–35.
2. Sanchez VM, Abi-Haidar YE, Itani KM. Mesh infection in ventral incisional hernia repair: incidence, contributing factors, and treatment. Surg Infect (Larchmt) 2011;12(3):205–10.
3. Hawn MT, Gray SH, Snyder CW, et al. Predictors of mesh explantation after incisional hernia repair. Am J Surg 2011;202(1):28–33.
4. Eisen DB. Surgeon's garb and infection control: what's the evidence? J Am Acad Dermatol 2011;64(5):960.e1–20.
5. Jensen JA, Goodson WH, Hopf HW, et al. Cigarette smoking decreases tissue oxygen. Arch Surg 1991;126(9):1131–4.
6. Knuutinen A, Kokkonen N, Risteli J, et al. Smoking affects collagen synthesis and extracellular matrix turnover in human skin. Br J Dermatol 2002;146(4):588–94.
7. Sorensen LT, Toft BG, Rygaard J, et al. Effect of smoking, smoking cessation, and nicotine patch on wound dimension, vitamin C, and systemic markers of collagen metabolism. Surgery 2010;148(5):982–90.
8. Chang DW, Reece GP, Wang B, et al. Effect of smoking on complications in patients undergoing free TRAM flap breast reconstruction. Plast Reconstr Surg 2000;105(7):2374–80.

9. Mallon WJ, Misamore G, Snead DS, et al. The impact of preoperative smoking habits on the results of rotator cuff repair. J Shoulder Elbow Surg 2004;13(2): 129–32.

10. Sorensen LT, Hemmingsen U, Kallehave F, et al. Risk factors for tissue and wound complications in gastrointestinal surgery. Ann Surg 2005;241(4):654–8.

11. Sorensen LT, Horby J, Friis E, et al. Smoking as a risk factor for wound healing and infection in breast cancer surgery. Eur J Surg Oncol 2002;28(8):815–20.

12. Finan KR, Vick CC, Kiefe CI, et al. Predictors of wound infection in ventral hernia repair. Am J Surg 2005;190(5):676–81.

13. Yang GP, Longaker MT. Abstinence from smoking reduces incisional wound infection: a randomized, controlled trial. Ann Surg 2003;238(1):6–8.

14. Lindstrom D, Sadr Azodi O, Wladis A, et al. Effects of a perioperative smoking cessation intervention on postoperative complications: a randomized trial. Ann Surg 2008;248(5):739–45.

15. Sorensen LT, Karlsmark T, Gottrup F. Abstinence from smoking reduces incisional wound infection: a randomized controlled trial. Ann Surg 2003;238(1):1–5.

16. Morimoto N, Takemoto S, Kawazoe T, et al. Nicotine at a low concentration promotes wound healing. J Surg Res 2008;145(2):199–204.

17. Sorensen LT, Jorgensen LN, Zillmer R, et al. Transdermal nicotine patch enhances type I collagen synthesis in abstinent smokers. Wound Repair Regen 2006;14(3):247–51.

18. Moller AM, Villebro N, Pedersen T, et al. Effect of preoperative smoking intervention on postoperative complications: a randomised clinical trial. Lancet 2002; 359(9301):114–7.

19. Kuri M, Nakagawa M, Tanaka H, et al. Determination of the duration of preoperative smoking cessation to improve wound healing after head and neck surgery. Anesthesiology 2005;102(5):892–6.

20. Manchio JV, Litchfield CR, Sati S, et al. Duration of smoking cessation and its impact on skin flap survival. Plast Reconstr Surg 2009;124(4):1105–17.

21. Mills E, Eyawo O, Lockhart I, et al. Smoking cessation reduces postoperative complications: a systematic review and meta-analysis. Am J Med 2011; 124(2):144–154.e8.

22. Sorensen LT, Hemmingsen UB, Kirkeby LT, et al. Smoking is a risk factor for incisional hernia. Arch Surg 2005;140(2):119–23.

23. Martindale RG, McClave SA, Vanek VW, et al. Guidelines for the provision and assessment of nutrition support therapy in the adult critically ill patient: Society of Critical Care Medicine and American Society for Parenteral and Enteral Nutrition: executive summary. Crit Care Med 2009;37(5):1757–61.

24. Daley J, Khuri SF, Henderson W, et al. Risk adjustment of the postoperative morbidity rate for the comparative assessment of the quality of surgical care: results of the national veterans affairs surgical risk study. J Am Coll Surg 1997;185(4):328–40.

25. Kudsk KA, Tolley EA, DeWitt RC, et al. Preoperative albumin and surgical site identify surgical risk for major postoperative complications. JPEN J Parenter Enteral Nutr 2003;27(1):1–9.

26. Munroe C, Frantz D, Martindale RG, et al. The optimal lipid formulation in enteral feeding in critical illness: clinical update and review of the literature. Curr Gastroenterol Rep 2011;13(4):368–75.

27. Jie B, Jiang ZM, Nolan MT, et al. Impact of preoperative nutritional support on clinical outcome in abdominal surgical patients at nutritional risk. Nutrition 2012;28(10):1022–7.

28. Kondrup J, Rasmussen HH, Hamberg O, et al. Nutritional risk screening (NRS 2002): a new method based on an analysis of controlled clinical trials. Clin Nutr 2003;22(3):321–36.

29. Gianotti L, Braga M, Nespoli L, et al. A randomized controlled trial of preoperative oral supplementation with a specialized diet in patients with gastrointestinal cancer. Gastroenterology 2002;122(7):1763–70.

30. Braga M, Gianotti L, Vignali A, et al. Hospital resources consumed for surgical morbidity: effects of preoperative arginine and omega-3 fatty acid supplementation on costs. Nutrition 2005;21(11–12):1078–86.

31. Braga M, Gianotti L, Nespoli L, et al. Nutritional approach in malnourished surgical patients: a prospective randomized study. Arch Surg 2002;137(2):174–80.

32. Braga M. Perioperative immunonutrition and gut function. Curr Opin Clin Nutr Metab Care 2012;15(5):485–8.

33. Drover JW, Dhaliwal R, Weitzel L, et al. Perioperative use of arginine-supplemented diets: a systematic review of the evidence. J Am Coll Surg 2011;212(3):385–99, 399.e1.

34. Pluess TT, Hayoz D, Berger MM, et al. Intravenous fish oil blunts the physiological response to endotoxin in healthy subjects. Intensive Care Med 2007;33(5):789–97.

35. Calder PC. Fatty acids and inflammation: the cutting edge between food and pharma. Eur J Pharmacol 2011;668(Suppl 1):S50–8.

36. Calder PC. Omega-3 polyunsaturated fatty acids and inflammatory processes: nutrition or pharmacology? Br J Clin Pharmacol 2013;75(3):645–62.

37. Lee HN, Surh YJ. Therapeutic potential of resolvins in the prevention and treatment of inflammatory disorders. Biochem Pharmacol 2012;84(10):1340–50.

38. Calder PC. Mechanisms of action of (n-3) fatty acids. J Nutr 2012;142(3):592S–9S.

39. Spite M, Norling LV, Summers L, et al. Resolvin D2 is a potent regulator of leukocytes and controls microbial sepsis. Nature 2009;461(7268):1287–91.

40. Marik PE, Flemmer M. The immune response to surgery and trauma: implications for treatment. J Trauma Acute Care Surg 2012;73(4):801–8.

41. Rudolph FB, Van Buren CT. The metabolic effects of enterally administered ribonucleic acids. Curr Opin Clin Nutr Metab Care 1998;1(6):527–30.

42. Burden S, Todd C, Hill J, et al. Pre-operative nutrition support in patients undergoing gastrointestinal surgery. Cochrane Database Syst Rev 2012;(11):CD008879.

43. Svanfeldt M, Thorell A, Hausel J, et al. Effect of "preoperative" oral carbohydrate treatment on insulin action–a randomised cross-over unblinded study in healthy subjects. Clin Nutr 2005;24(5):815–21.

44. Soop M, Nygren J, Myrenfors P, et al. Preoperative oral carbohydrate treatment attenuates immediate postoperative insulin resistance. Am J Physiol Endocrinol Metab 2001;280(4):E576–83.

45. Fearon KC, Ljungqvist O, Von Meyenfeldt M, et al. Enhanced recovery after surgery: a consensus review of clinical care for patients undergoing colonic resection. Clin Nutr 2005;24(3):466–77.

46. Awad S, Constantin-Teodosiu D, Constantin D, et al. Cellular mechanisms underlying the protective effects of preoperative feeding: a randomized study investigating muscle and liver glycogen content, mitochondrial function, gene and protein expression. Ann Surg 2010;252(2):247–53.

47. Awad S, Fearon KC, Macdonald IA, et al. A randomized cross-over study of the metabolic and hormonal responses following two preoperative conditioning drinks. Nutrition 2011;27(9):938–42.

48. Maung AA, Davis KA. Perioperative nutritional support: immunonutrition, probiotics, and anabolic steroids. Surg Clin North Am 2012;92(2):273–83, viii.
49. Houck JP, Rypins EB, Sarfeh IJ, et al. Repair of incisional hernia. Surg Gynecol Obstet 1989;169(5):397–9.
50. Cevasco M, Itani KM. Ventral hernia repair with synthetic, composite, and biologic mesh: characteristics, indications, and infection profile. Surg Infect (Larchmt) 2012;13(4):209–15.
51. Le D, Deveney CW, Martindale RG, et al. Mesh choice in ventral hernia repair. Am J Surg 2013;205(5):602–7.
52. Rios A, Rodriguez JM, Munitiz V, et al. Antibiotic prophylaxis in incisional hernia repair using a prosthesis. Hernia 2001;5(3):148–52.
53. Bratzler DW, Dellinger EP, Olsen KM, et al. Clinical practice guidelines for antimicrobial prophylaxis in surgery. Surg Infect (Larchmt) 2013;14(1):73–156.
54. Junker T, Mujagic E, Hoffmann H, et al. Prevention and control of surgical site infections: review of the Basel Cohort Study. Swiss Med Wkly 2012;142:w13616.
55. Enzler MJ, Berbari E, Osmon DR. Antimicrobial prophylaxis in adults. Mayo Clin Proc 2011;86(7):686–701.
56. Berbari EF, Osmon DR, Lahr B, et al. The Mayo Prosthetic Joint Infection Risk Score: implication for surgical site infection reporting and risk stratification. Infect Control Hosp Epidemiol 2012;33(8):774–81.
57. Bratzler DW, Houck PM, Surgical Infection Prevention Guidelines Writers Workgroup, et al. Antimicrobial prophylaxis for surgery: an advisory statement from the National Surgical Infection Prevention Project. Clin Infect Dis 2004;38(12):1706–15.
58. Suehiro T, Hirashita T, Araki S, et al. Prolonged antibiotic prophylaxis longer than 24 hours does not decrease surgical site infection after elective gastric and colorectal surgery. Hepatogatsroenterology 2008;55(86–87):1636–9.
59. Fonseca SN, Kunzle SR, Junqueira MJ, et al. Implementing 1-dose antibiotic prophylaxis for prevention of surgical site infection. Arch Surg 2006;141(11): 1109–13 [discussion: 1114].
60. Hanley MJ, Abernethy DR, Greenblatt DJ. Effect of obesity on the pharmacokinetics of drugs in humans. Clin Pharmacokinet 2010;49(2):71–87.
61. Ventral Hernia Working Group, Breuing K, Butler CE, et al. Incisional ventral hernias: review of the literature and recommendations regarding the grading and technique of repair. Surgery 2010;148(3):544–58.
62. Dunne JR, Malone DL, Tracy JK, et al. Abdominal wall hernias: risk factors for infection and resource utilization. J Surg Res 2003;111(1):78–84.
63. Blatnik JA, Krpata DM, Novitsky YW, et al. Does a history of wound infection predict postoperative surgical site infection after ventral hernia repair? Am J Surg 2012;203(3):370–4 [discussion: 374].
64. Lin HJ, Spoerke N, Deveney C, et al. Reconstruction of complex abdominal wall hernias using acellular human dermal matrix: a single institution experience. Am J Surg 2009;197(5):599–603 [discussion: 603].
65. Kiedrowski MR, Horswill AR. New approaches for treating staphylococcal biofilm infections. Ann N Y Acad Sci 2011;1241:104–21.
66. Bull AL, Worth LJ, Richards MJ. Impact of vancomycin surgical antibiotic prophylaxis on the development of methicillin-sensitive *Staphylococcus aureus* surgical site infections: report from Australian surveillance data (VICNISS). Ann Surg 2012;256(6):1089–92.
67. Diaz JJ Jr, Conquest AM, Ferzoco SJ, et al. Multi-institutional experience using human acellular dermal matrix for ventral hernia repair in a compromised surgical field. Arch Surg 2009;144(3):209–15.

68. Dronge AS, Perkal MF, Kancir S, et al. Long-term glycemic control and postoperative infectious complications. Arch Surg 2006;141(4):375–80 [discussion: 380].

69. Turina M, Fry DE, Polk HC Jr. Acute hyperglycemia and the innate immune system: clinical, cellular, and molecular aspects. Crit Care Med 2005;33(7):1624–33.

70. van den Berghe G, Wouters P, Weekers F, et al. Intensive insulin therapy in critically ill patients. N Engl J Med 2001;345(19):1359–67.

71. NICE-SUGAR Study Investigators, Finfer S, Liu B, et al. Hypoglycemia and risk of death in critically ill patients. N Engl J Med 2012;367(12):1108–18.

72. Ramos M, Khalpey Z, Lipsitz S, et al. Relationship of perioperative hyperglycemia and postoperative infections in patients who undergo general and vascular surgery. Ann Surg 2008;248(4):585–91.

73. Ata A, Lee J, Bestle SL, et al. Postoperative hyperglycemia and surgical site infection in general surgery patients. Arch Surg 2010;145(9):858–64.

74. Sugerman HJ, Kellum JM, Reines HD, et al. Greater risk of incisional hernia with morbidly obese than steroid-dependent patients and low recurrence with prefascial polypropylene mesh. Am J Surg 1996;171:80–4.

75. Puzziferri N, Austrheim-Smith I, Wolfe B, et al. Three-year follow-up of a prospective randomized trial comparing laparoscopic versus open gastric bypass. Ann Surg 2006;243(2):181–8.

76. Sauerland S, Korenkov M, Kleinen T. Obesity is a risk factor for recurrence after incisional hernia repair. Hernia 2004;8:42–6.

77. Rickard RF, Hudson DA. Influence of vascular delay on abdominal wall complications in unipedicled TRAM flap breast reconstruction. Ann Plast Surg 2003; 50(2):138–42.

78. Beck WC, Holzman MD, Sharp KW, et al. Comparative effectiveness of dynamic abdominal sonography for hernia vs computed tomography in the diagnosis of incisional hernia. J Am Coll Surg 2013;216(3):447–53 [quiz: 510–1].

79. Swenson BR, Hedrick TL, Metzger R, et al. Effects of preoperative skin preparation on postoperative wound infection rates: a prospective study of 3 skin preparation protocols. Infect Control Hosp Epidemiol 2009;30(10):964–71.

80. Darouiche RO, Wall MJ Jr, Itani KM, et al. Chlorhexidine-alcohol versus povidone-iodine for surgical-site antisepsis. N Engl J Med 2010;362(1):18–26.

81. Swenson BR, Sawyer RG. Importance of alcohol in skin preparation protocols. Infect Control Hosp Epidemiol 2010;31(9):977.

82. Tanner J, Norrie P, Melen K. Preoperative hair removal to reduce surgical site infection. Cochrane Database Syst Rev 2011;(11):CD004122.

83. Dumville JC, McFarlane E, Edwards P, et al. Preoperative skin antiseptics for preventing surgical wound infections after clean surgery. Cochrane Database Syst Rev 2013;(3):CD003949.

84. Edmiston CE Jr, Okoli O, Graham MB, et al. Evidence for using chlorhexidine gluconate preoperative cleansing to reduce the risk of surgical site infection. AORN J 2010;92(5):509–18.

85. Chlebicki MP, Safdar N, O'Horo JC, et al. Preoperative chlorhexidine shower or bath for prevention of surgical site infection: a meta-analysis. Am J Infect Control 2013;41(2):167–73.

86. Bode LG, Kluytmans JA, Wertheim HF, et al. Preventing surgical-site infections in nasal carriers of *Staphylococcus aureus*. N Engl J Med 2010;362(1):9–17.

87. Kim DH, Spencer M, Davidson SM, et al. Institutional prescreening for detection and eradication of methicillin-resistant *Staphylococcus aureus* in patients undergoing elective orthopaedic surgery. J Bone Joint Surg Am 2010;92(9):1820–6.

88. Jose B, Dignon A. Is there a relationship between preoperative shaving (hair removal) and surgical site infection? J Perioper Pract 2013;23(1–2):22–5.
89. Justinger C, Moussavian MR, Schlueter C, et al. Antibacterial [corrected] coating of abdominal closure sutures and wound infection. Surgery 2009; 145(3):330–4.
90. Reid K, Pockney P, Draganic B, et al. Barrier wound protection decreases surgical site infection in open elective colorectal surgery: a randomized clinical trial. Dis Colon Rectum 2010;53(10):1374–80.
91. Horiuchi T, Tanishima H, Tamagawa K, et al. Randomized, controlled investigation of the anti-infective properties of the Alexis retractor/protector of incision sites. J Trauma 2007;62(1):212–5.
92. Flores-Maldonado A, Medina-Escobedo CE, Rios-Rodriguez HM, et al. Mild perioperative hypothermia and the risk of wound infection. Arch Med Res 2001;32(3):227–31.
93. Qadan M, Gardner SA, Vitale DS, et al. Hypothermia and surgery: immunologic mechanisms for current practice. Ann Surg 2009;250(1):134–40.
94. Lehtinen SJ, Onicescu G, Kuhn KM, et al. Normothermia to prevent surgical site infections after gastrointestinal surgery: holy grail or false idol? Ann Surg 2010; 252(4):696–704.
95. Fakhry SM, Montgomery SC. Peri-operative oxygen and the risk of surgical infection. Surg Infect (Larchmt) 2012;13(4):228–33.
96. Greif R, Akca O, Horn EP, et al, Outcomes Research Group. Supplemental perioperative oxygen to reduce the incidence of surgical-wound infection. N Engl J Med 2000;342(3):161–7.
97. Belda FJ, Aguilera L, Garcia de la Asuncion J, et al. Supplemental perioperative oxygen and the risk of surgical wound infection: a randomized controlled trial. JAMA 2005;294(16):2035–42.
98. Meyhoff CS, Wetterslev J, Jorgensen LN, et al. Effect of high perioperative oxygen fraction on surgical site infection and pulmonary complications after abdominal surgery: the PROXI randomized clinical trial. JAMA 2009;302(14): 1543–50.
99. Al-Niaimi A, Safdar N. Supplemental perioperative oxygen for reducing surgical site infection: a meta-analysis. J Eval Clin Pract 2009;15(2):360–5.
100. Hempel S, Newberry SJ, Maher AR, et al. Probiotics for the prevention and treatment of antibiotic-associated diarrhea: a systematic review and meta-analysis. JAMA 2012;307(18):1959–69.
101. Johnston BC, Ma SS, Goldenberg JZ, et al. Probiotics for the prevention of Clostridium difficile-associated diarrhea: a systematic review and meta-analysis. Ann Intern Med 2012;157(12):878–88.
102. Goldenberg JZ, Ma SS, Saxton JD, et al. Probiotics for the prevention of Clostridium difficile-associated diarrhea in adults and children. Cochrane Database Syst Rev 2013;(5):CD006095.
103. Valkenet K, van de Port IG, Dronkers JJ, et al. The effects of preoperative exercise therapy on postoperative outcome: a systematic review. Clin Rehabil 2011; 25(2):99–111.

Repair of Umbilical and Epigastric Hernias

David B. Earle, MD[a,b,]*, Jennifer A. McLellan, MD[a]

KEYWORDS

- Umbilical hernia • Epigastric hernia • Abdominal wall • Incisional hernia • Mesh

KEY POINTS

- Explicitly identify and document the goals and objectives of hernia repair for each patient.
- Align the patient's goals with the entire surgical team.
- Choose a technique that best fits the goals in the context of the clinical scenario and the anatomy of the hernia.
- Choose a technique and prosthetic that best fits the patient's history, physical examination, and is most likely to best achieve the patient's goals.
- Make your prosthetic choice based on raw material and architecture of the prosthetic, keeping in mind the patient's goals, clinical scenario, and proposed beneficial features of the prosthetic.

"It is unwise to be too sure of one's own wisdom. It is healthy to be reminded that the strongest might weaken and the wisest might err."

—*Mahatma Gandhi*

INTRODUCTION

Hernias in general are frequently misunderstood and underestimated in terms of complexity by both patients and doctors.[1–3] Umbilical and epigastric hernias are no exception, and all hernia specialists have cared for patients with unanticipated

Disclosures: Atrium Medical, consulting fee/consulting; Bard/Davol, consulting fee and honoraria/consulting and speaking; Covidien, grant support/fellowship, honoraria/speaking/teaching, consulting fee/consulting; Endosphere, stock/scientific advisory board; Kensey-Nash, consulting fee/consulting; RTI Biologics, consulting fee/consulting; Surgiquest, honoraria/stock/scientific advisory board; Via Surgical, stock/scientific advisory board (D.B. Earle). Atrium Medical and Covidien, consulting (J.A. McLellan).

[a] Department of Surgery, Baystate Medical Center, Springfield, MA 01199, USA; [b] Tufts University School of Medicine, Boston, MA, USA
* Corresponding author. Department of Surgery, Baystate Medical Center, Springfield, MA 01199.
E-mail address: david.earle@baystatehealth.org

Surg Clin N Am 93 (2013) 1057–1089
http://dx.doi.org/10.1016/j.suc.2013.06.017   surgical.theclinics.com
0039-6109/13/$ – see front matter © 2013 Elsevier Inc. All rights reserved.

complications that arose from a "simple" hernia repair, often unbeknownst to the original surgeon. Because the overall complication rate is low, and frequently not temporally adjacent to the operation itself, some surgeons perceive that complications, such as recurrence, are nonexistent in their hands. Furthermore, some complications are catastrophic, and can be directly related to the technical aspects of the hernia repair itself, emphasizing the need to keep updated with the continuously changing knowledge base related to hernia repair. Additionally, aligning goals and expectations between the health care team and the patient can help many minor problems that may even be part of the normal postoperative course pass without fanfare, rather than become a source of consternation.

The presentation as an elective, urgent, or emergent problem will lay the foundation for the planning and performance of the repair. This will necessarily include details of the medical and surgical history, anatomic details of the hernia, and how they relate to the goals of operation. Although neither patients nor surgeons can predict the future, thoughtful discussion about future issues, such as pregnancy, promote a mutual sense of confidence and thoughtfulness that may have an impact on the psychological well-being of everyone involved, and could lead to improved clinical outcomes and patient satisfaction.[4–7]

This article details some relevant and interesting anatomic issues, reviews existing data, and highlights some common and important surgical techniques. Emphasis is placed on a patient-centered approach to the repair of umbilical and epigastric hernias, although this concept could be extrapolated to any hernia repair, and potentially any other disease.

ANATOMY
Embryology of the Abdominal Wall

The ventral body wall first begins to form during the third week of development. This process begins with the differentiation of the mesoderm, located between the ectoderm and endoderm. At this stage, the embryo is a flat disc, the circumference of which will eventually become the umbilical ring. The embryo begins folding during the fourth week of development, characterized by proliferation of the neuroectoderm and mesoderm, but at the same time, cell death and subsequent growth arrest occurs at the umbilical ring.[8] At the fifth week, the umbilical vessels (2 arteries and 1 vein), the allantois, the yolk stalk, and the canal connecting the intraembryonic and extraembryonic cavities pass through the umbilical ring.[9] This is also the period when there is rapid growth and expansion of the liver, which temporarily makes the abdominal cavity too small to contain all of the intestinal loops, which then enter the extraembryonic cavity through the umbilical ring, referred to as the physiologic umbilical herniation, during the sixth week of development. The intestines remain herniated until the 10th week, when they begin returning to the abdominal cavity. Abnormalities in this process can lead to congenital defects of the abdominal wall.

The umbilical ring remains located at the center of the abdomen and is a transition zone between the body wall and the amnion. By the 10th week, the epithelial tissues have fused in the midline of the embryo, leaving only the umbilical vessels in the region of the umbilical ring.[8] At this time, the umbilical cord has formed. The cord contains 2 umbilical arteries, 1 umbilical vein, and the remnants of the allantois, which is referred to as the urachus after it becomes obliterated.[9] These structures all have remnants in the adult abdominal wall and can be used as surgical landmarks (**Fig. 1**).

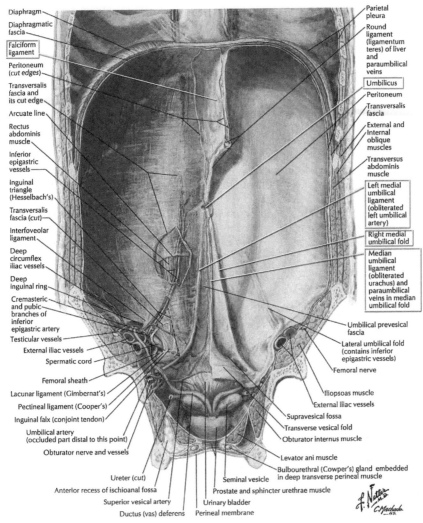

Fig. 1. Adult anatomical remnants of the umbilical ring and its contents. (Netter illustration from www.netterimages.com. © Elsevier Inc. All rights reserved.)

Anatomy of the Adult Abdominal Wall

The anatomy of the fully developed abdominal wall is very familiar to any surgeon repairing hernias. The vertical midline of the abdomen consists of the linea alba, which is the midline confluence of the aponeuroses of the rectus muscles and the oblique muscles. The composition of the rectus sheath changes depending on the location. Superior to the umbilicus, the anterior sheath is composed of the aponeurosis of the external oblique muscle, as well as the anterior aponeurotic lamina of the internal oblique muscle. Inferior to the arcuate line of Douglas, which is a variable distance below the umbilicus,[10] the anterior sheath consists of all aponeurotic layers (internal/external oblique, and transversus abdominis). Conversely, the posterior sheath superior to the arcuate line of Douglas consists of the posterior aponeurotic lamina of the internal oblique and the aponeurosis of the transversus abdominis. Inferior to the arcuate line, the posterior sheath consists only of the transversalis fascia. Patterns of midline decussation of the aponeuroses can vary. Normal anatomy is thought to consist of triple lines of decussation anteriorly and posteriorly (**Fig. 2**).

ETIOLOGY

A hernia is defined as a protrusion of a structure or part of structure through the tissues normally containing it. In general, a hernia is either congenital or acquired. There are multiple theories of how and why hernias develop over time, and most likely each hernia has a multifactorial etiology. Furthermore, it is currently not possible in most cases to determine which factors are most important for a given patient at a given point in time. Etiologic factors are different among patients and even different for a single patient over time. For example, a patient may develop a traumatic hernia from a direct blow to the abdominal wall at one point in time, but develop an incisional hernia at another point in time due to a postoperative wound infection and/or closure technique. Even knowing the likely etiologies for those 2 clinical scenarios leaves us in the dark about an undiagnosed collagen disorder that otherwise has no clinical manifestations (**Fig. 3**).[11]

Congenital

Congenital ventral abdominal wall hernias are hernias present at birth, and include omphalocele and gastroschisis, which are not covered in this article. Congenital hernias also include small primary umbilical or epigastric defects. Umbilical hernias are quite common in infancy, and represent the only time hernias can be cured without

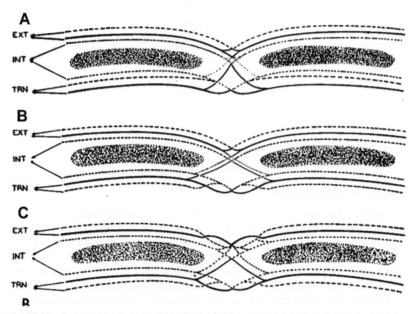

Fig. 2. (*A*) Single anterior and single posterior lines of decussation. (*B*) Single anterior and triple posterior lines of decussation. (*C*) Triple anterior and triple posterior lines of decussation. (*From* Askar OM. Surgical anatomy of the aponeurotic expansions of the anterior abdominal wall. Ann R Coll Surg Engl 1977;59:313–21.)

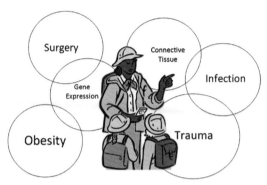

Fig. 3. Multifactorial etiology of hernia development.

an operation; most defects are small and more than 80% will close spontaneously by the age of 5.[12–16] Because of this, umbilical hernia repair is generally recommended only if the defect persists past the age of 5, or before the age of 5 if the defect is larger than 1 to 2 cm.[13,15] Contrary to this, epigastric hernias are often incarcerated and surgical repair is indicated.[14,17]

Acquired: Primary Ventral Hernia

For this article, we define acquired midline hernias as all those diagnosed during adulthood, recognizing the fact that some of these will have been present at birth, and gone unnoticed by the patient and/or medical community for years. Pregnancy, weight gain, obesity, intra-abdominal tumors, and ascites can all increase the pressure inside the abdomen, causing an increase in size of an umbilical or epigastric abdominal wall defect.[18–21] The other consequence of this increased pressure may be an increased likelihood of incarceration or strangulation of preperitoneal fat (falciform or umbilical ligaments), omentum, or bowel.

Patients will sometimes complain of feeling a hernia "come out" suddenly, especially those who participate in lifting heavy items at work, weight lifting, coughing, or any other events that cause significant straining of the abdomen. In the past, it was thought the transient extreme increase in intra-abdominal pressure caused the hernia,[15,19] but more recent studies have shown that is probably not the case. There has been research to suggest that patients with hernias have less type I collagen and more elastin in the linea alba than patients without hernias.[22,23] This type of connective tissue disorder is not otherwise clinically apparent, but likely predisposes certain individuals to developing a hernia. Of course, more obvious sources of trauma, such as blunt force from a motor vehicle collision or heavy blow to the abdomen, can cause a hernia as well.

Umbilical hernia

An umbilical hernia is a ventral hernia located at or near the umbilicus. These are sometimes referred to as a "periumbilical" hernia, because they are not always located immediately at the base of the umbilicus. Umbilical hernias, or "ruptures" as they were referred to in the past, were described in some of the earliest surgical literature, dating as far back as 1500 BC.[24] In 1915, Dr Moschcowitz of New York authored an article[25] regarding the etiology if umbilical hernias, in which he suggested the pathogenesis is related to weaknesses at the umbilicus from the passage of the umbilical cord vessels. According to Gray's anatomy, the area surrounding the cicatrix filling the umbilical defect is weaker than the cicatrix itself, thus making all ventral hernias at the umbilicus "peri-umbilical."[26]

More recently, in 2011, Fathi and colleagues[27] attempted to characterize the abdominal wall at the umbilical ring to determine what may predispose patients to developing umbilical hernias. They combined 2 previous umbilical ring classification systems into 5 types in an attempt to better define the morphologic characteristics at the umbilical ring and its relationship to the adjacent umbilical and falciform ligaments. It appears that the falciform (or round) ligament may function to protect against hernia when it crosses and covers the umbilical ring, inserting along the inferior border of the ring (Type 3 configuration) (**Fig. 4**).

Epigastric hernia

An epigastric hernia is a ventral hernia through the linea alba between the umbilicus and the xiphoid process. Controversy has surrounded the etiology of epigastric herniae, and the 2 main hypotheses are the vascular lacunae hypothesis and the tendinous fiber decussation hypothesis.[28] The first descriptions of the former were by Moschcowitz in 1914.[29] He theorized that vascular lacunae formed when small blood vessels penetrated the linea alba. These left a small space where preperitoneal fat from the falciform ligament could begin to herniate and enlarge over time. He found that a perforating blood vessel could always be found in the course of the dissection of epigastric hernias. The decussation hypothesis was popularized by Askar in 1978.[19,30] He found that epigastric herniae occur exclusively in patients who do not have triple lines of decussation, and this is what predisposes patients to develop an epigastric hernia (see **Fig. 2**). Most likely, an element of both hypotheses likely predisposes certain patients to an epigastric hernia. These factors, coupled with undiagnosed collagen disorders and significant intra-abdominal pressure, and/or operative therapy requiring a midline incision turn these theories into the reality of a clinical hernia.

Acquired: Incisional Hernia

Another source of hernia is very prevalent in today's society: iatrogenically caused hernias due to incisions. It is germane to discuss incisional hernia in this article because laparoscopic operations frequently use the umbilicus for an incision, and many open procedures involve the midline. Clinical experience shows that incisional hernias at the umbilicus are then frequently diagnosed and treated the same way a primary umbilical hernia would be. Incisional hernias began to be the subject of research beginning in the second half of the nineteenth century, the beginning of the era of modern abdominal surgery.[24] Incisional hernias can vary widely in their size and extent. The fact that scar is not as strong as the initial tissue is taught to every surgeon in the earliest stages of practice. In 2006, Hollinsky and Sandberg,[31] exposed tensile loads to resected linea alba, rectus sheath, and scar tissue. They found that scar tissue has a significantly lower loading capacity and concluded that this poses a permanent risk for herniation.

Hernias have been described from all types of abdominal incisions, but midline incisions through the linea alba have significantly higher rates of subsequent hernia defects.[32,33] Often a hernia will be noted at or near the umbilicus through a previous vertical midline incision, which may be above, below, or span the umbilicus. This is likely due to difficulties closing the fascia at the level of the umbilicus because of excessive subcutaneous fat, the umbilical stalk, the falciform, and the umbilical ligaments. It may also be due to an unrecognized existing hernia near the umbilicus (**Fig. 5**). Further complicating matters is that almost half of patients with incisional

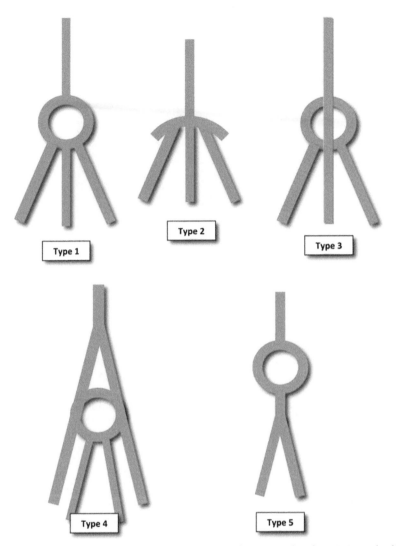

Fig. 4. Type 1: 1 Round or oval UR, RL attached to the top and MdLs, MnL to the lower border of UR. Type 2: Obliterated or slitted UR with all ligaments attached to slit. Type 3: Round or oval UR, RL covered the whole ring and terminated at the inferior border of it with MdLs and MnL. Type 4: Round or oval UR, RL bifurcated and fused to both sides of the ring; MdLs and MnL attached to the lower border of it. Type 5: Round or oval UR, RL attached to top, MnL and MdLs joined before UR and attached as a single ligament to inferior border. Abbreviations: MdL, medial umbilical ligament; MnL, median umbilical ligament; RL, round ligament (falciform); UR, umbilical ring. (*From* Fathi AH, Soltanian H, Saber AA. Surgical anatomy and morphologic variations of umbilical structures. Am Surg 2012;78(5):540–4; with permission.)

hernias will have defects not palpable on physical examination as determined by laparoscopic abdominal wall exploration.[34]

Therefore, repair of a defect only at the umbilicus when it is part of a larger incision will have a higher rate of recurrence compared with covering the entire old incision, but

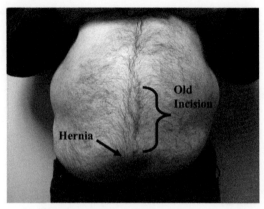

Fig. 5. Patient with previous upper midline incision terminating at the umbilicus, now with a hernia defect at the inferior most portion of the incision. This could be mistakenly treated in the same fashion as a primary umbilical hernia.

may be an option in select clinical circumstances. One example of this would be a patient with a xiphoid to pubis midline incision with a long-standing (20-year) small defect at the umbilicus who is a very high surgical risk because of advanced age, debility, and multiple comorbidities, and presents with progressively symptomatic hernia.

With the increased use of laparoscopy, an increasing number of trocar site hernias are being seen. In a recent meta-analysis by Helgstrand and colleagues,[35] it was found that 96% of these hernias occur through trocar sites 10 mm or larger, and 82% were located at or near the umbilicus. Based on the size of the laparoscopic access incision, additional defects are less likely, but still include the potential for adjacent primary defects in the periumbilical region, a fact that must be considered during the evaluation and treatment process for port site hernias in this area.

EPIDEMIOLOGY

The exact incidence of primary midline hernias (umbilical and epigastric) is unknown owing to a variety of factors, among which are the definition of a hernia (physically visible, radiologically diagnosed, presence of symptoms, or those undergoing treatment) and the ability to track data for diagnosis and procedures in both the inpatient and outpatient setting.[36–38] Whatever the definition, the incidence of primary midline hernias in the adult population is most likely variable among geographic regions, and probably has to do with many factors, such as the incidence of birth defects of the abdominal wall, and issues known to affect the acquisition and consequence of midline abdominal wall hernias, such as obesity, aortic aneurysm disease, access to surgical care, and HIV disease.[39–42]

Radiological and physical examination screening can find umbilical hernias in 23% to 50% of the adult population in some countries, and up to 90% of pregnant women. The true incidence in the United States is unknown, and even the number of repairs is difficult to ascertain. In 2003, estimates of the number of hernia repairs were 175,000 for umbilical and 80,000 for epigastric/Spigelian.[36] 2010 data compiled by a health care analytics firm revealed that of a total of 988,483 hernia repairs, 504,845 were for ventral hernias of all types.[43] Estimating from the 2003 data that umbilical and epigastric hernia repair make up roughly 22% of all ventral hernia repairs,[36] this would yield 217,466 repairs of primary midline hernias for 2010 in the United States.

According to reports from other data analytics companies, ventral hernias comprised 32% of all hernia repairs in the United States in 2011 and 2012.[44] Using Current Procedural Terminology and International Classification of Diseases, Ninth revision, coding information for 2012, there were 180,730 umbilical and 8994 epigastric hernia repairs (total = 189,724) identified in the United States.[45] Sales data for deployable prosthetics designed for small ventral hernias (Ventralex; Bard, Proceed Ventral Patch; Ethicon, and V-Patch; Atrium) reveal that 127,424 units were sold in 2011.[46]

Examining these data in aggregate and using clinical experience and logic, we recognize that incidence of umbilical and epigastric hernias will be higher for radiological and physical examination screening programs compared with incidence data from those who have had the diagnosis coded or the condition treated. Determining the incidence of the disease may be important for estimating prevalence, determining the burden to the health care system, and allowing industry to develop sensible business planning regarding research and development. Therefore, we have compiled a table with variable incidence rates (which would depend on definition and diagnostic methods) so as to make quick reference to the US population as a whole (**Table 1**). The table includes the percentage of existing primary midline hernias that are repaired based on variable estimates of the true incidence. Physical examination and ultrasound studies have shown that 23% to 50% of patients screened specifically for umbilical hernia actually had one. This study was performed at King Saud University in Riyadh, Saudi Arabia, over a 2-year period and included 302 patients.[37] A physical examination study was conducted in Nigeria by the division of pediatric Surgery at the University of Texas Southwestern Medical Center.[38] A noted that 49% of nonpregnant adults older than 18 had an "outie," defined as "any protrusion of the umbilical tip past the periumbilical skin," but only 8% had an umbilical hernia defined as "protrusion of at least 5 mm and diameter of at least 10 mm." The data from Lau and colleagues[40] reviewed diagnosis records from 14 California hospitals and identified those with the diagnosis of a ventral hernia (umbilical, incisional, ventral, epigastric, or Spigelian). There were a total of 2,807,414 patients in the regional database, of which 0.9% (25,267) had one of the specified diagnoses, and 74% (18,697; 0.7% of total) of those patients had an umbilical hernia. This suggests the prevalence of umbilical hernia in California is 0.7% of the population, and we could extrapolate this data to the US population as a whole (see **Table 1**).

Table 1	
If the true incidence in the United States is 1%, representing 2,395,164 people, and 189,724 repairs were performed, this would be 7.9% of the total umbilical and epigastric hernias available for repair*	
True Incidence of Adult Umbilical and Epigastric Hernia: Varies Depending on Method and Definition of Diagnosis (Based on 2012 Census Data)	2012 Umbilical and Epigastric Hernia Repairs, n (%)
1%, n = 2,395,164	189,724 (7.9)
10%, n = 23,951,641	189,724 (0.8)
20%, n = 47,903,282	189,724 (0.5)
30%, n = 71,854,923	189,724 (0.3)
40%, n = 95,806,565	189,724 (0.2)
50%, n = 119,758,207	189,724 (0.16)

* 189,724 number is based on data from Aileron Solutions 2012.[45]
Data from Refs.[36–38,45,47]

Since we know the approximate number of umbilical hernia repairs in the United States and the prevalence of umbilical hernia in California (0.07%), we can estimate the number of diagnosed umbilical hernias in the United States (US census 2012 population >18 years = 239,516,413)[47] to be approximately 1,676,615. Estimating 189,724 repairs in 2012, the national percentage of diagnosed umbilical hernias repaired is about 11% (189,724/1,676,615).

Interestingly, the annual number of umbilical and epigastric hernia repairs seems to be decreasing. In 2003, there were an estimated 255,000 repairs, in 2010 an estimated 217,466 repairs, and in 2012 an estimated 189,724 repairs. If accurate, the reasons for the declining number of repairs are unknown. Regarding the repair technique, and using 2012 estimated repairs and 2011 US sales data, about 67% (127,474/189,724) of umbilical/epigastric hernia repairs use a deployable prosthetic. Given that some prosthetic repairs use a flat sheet, the overall percentage of repairs with a prosthetic is probably somewhat higher than this.

We have surmised that reasons for low use and potentially decreasing number of repairs of umbilical hernia include lack of symptoms, no diagnosis, outdated knowledge of surgical options, small size, fear of surgical procedures, and economic recession.

CLASSIFICATION

In 2009, the European Hernia Society (EHS) developed a classification system for all types of ventral hernias.[48] This included primary and incisional. Epigastric and umbilical hernias are considered primary ventral hernias if they are not caused by an incision. Ventral hernias through a previous abdominal incision should be considered an "incisional hernia." Primary umbilical and epigastric hernias are classified (1) by their location (either at or near the umbilicus or in the epigastrium) and (2) by the size of the defect. The EHS suggested that a primary hernia should be considered small if it is smaller than 2 cm in diameter, medium if it is between 2 and 4 cm, or large if it is larger than 4 cm.

CLINICAL PRESENTATION

The presentation of primary ventral hernias is highly variable and patient dependent, and no different than incisional hernias. Patients will often know about a primary umbilical or epigastric hernia for years before seeking medical attention. As symptoms, such as pain, discomfort, or an increase in the size of the herniated contents, develop, patients may seek medical attention.

Primary ventral hernias can also present as an acutely incarcerated hernia. Incarceration is the state of a hernia whereby the contents cannot be reduced into the abdomen.[49] Patients will typically present with a painful bulge at the hernia site. This may be associated with variable amounts of tenderness, and occasionally changes in the skin, such as erythema, ulceration, or ischemic changes. There may be an associated bowel obstruction, but this may not be fully apparent if the symptoms have been present for a short period of time, even if small bowel is incarcerated. Regardless of whether or not the herniated contents are fat or intestine, acutely incarcerated hernias represent a scenario whereby urgent or emergent operation is warranted. Chronically incarcerated primary ventral hernias are considerably different from the acute variety, but may still present with emergent problems, such as bowel obstruction. The highly variable clinical situation dictates that the surgeon be aware of these issues, and apply the best course of action for the given scenario (**Figs. 6 and 7**).

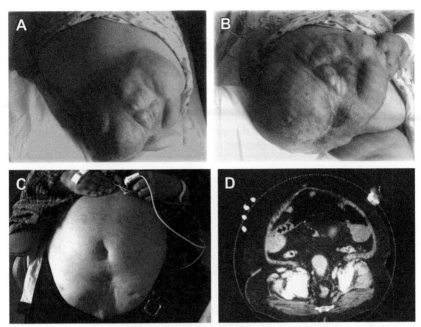

Fig. 6. Primary umbilical hernia. The patient with this chronically incarcerated primary ventral hernia allowed this to enlarge because of a lack of symptoms, and reluctantly agreed to repair only after repeated bouts of small bowel obstruction. (*A, B*) Preoperative. (*C*) Five years postoperative. (*D*) Computed tomography scan 5 years postoperative.

SURGICAL TECHNIQUE
Preoperative Planning

When a patient presents to the surgeon's office with a hernia, the visit must involve much more than a physical examination of the hernia itself. Although it is important

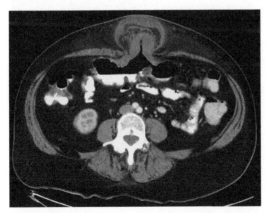

Fig. 7. An axial computed tomographic image showing a ventral hernia with incarceration of the anterior transverse colonic wall, consistent with a Richter hernia. There is surrounding edema of the herniated wall. There is also passage of contrast distally and lack of bowel dilatation. (*From* Kim R, McCoy M, Bistolarides P, et al. Richter's epigastric hernia with transverse colon strangulation. Am Surg 2012;78(5):E301–3; with permission.)

that symptoms, such as pain, enlargement, and so forth, are delineated, we believe it is *more* important to explicitly identify the patient's goals for repair, and then align those goals with the surgical team. This will allow the surgeon to select the best approach for the specific patient. A patient with a large hernia sac at the umbilicus could undergo a laparoscopic repair and adequately repair the hernia, but the patient might consider the operation a failure if the large bulge and excess skin is not resolved (**Fig. 8**), especially if the patient's goal is to have a normal abdominal wall contour. This issue will be different among all patients, regardless of age, body habitus, and activity level, and underscores the fact that the simple and explicit identification of their goals will help align expectations and plan the appropriate operation.

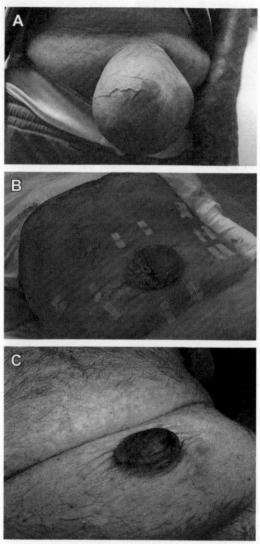

Fig. 8. Large hernia sac at umbilicus after laparoscopic repair. (*A*) Preoperative: umbilical hernia with larger hernia sac. (*B*) Appearance of sac immediately postoperatively. (*C*) Appearance of sac at 1 year postoperatively.

Generally, the surgical options include an open or laparoscopic repair, with or without mesh, and with or without defect closure. A laparoscopic-assisted approach could be used for a large hernia sac with a relatively small defect. In the future, we may be able to offer a Natural Orifice Translumenal Endoscopic Surgery (NOTES) approach.[50–55]

Selection of the approach will in part be directed by the explicitly defined patient goals, but must also take in to account the medical/surgical history, as well as the details of the hernia, particularly related to the size of the defect and the hernia sac. For example, a patient with a 2-cm periumbilical defect with an associated epigastric diastasis who wants to (or should) avoid general anesthesia will be better served with an open approach using a prosthetic designed for this approach (**Fig. 9**) compared with a laparoscopic approach (**Fig. 10**).

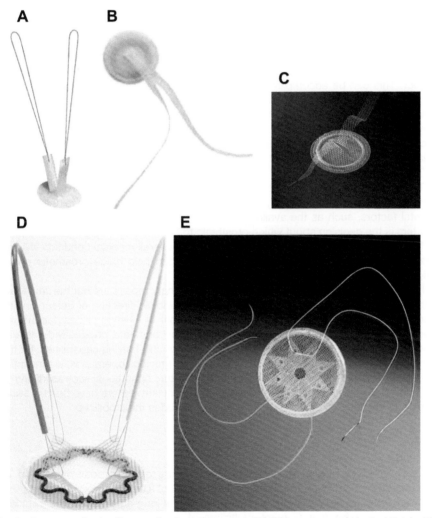

Fig. 9. Open prosthetics (for repair of small hernias). (*A*) Ethicon Proceed Ventral Patch. (*B*) Atrium Medical Corp. V-Patch. (*C*) Bard Ventralex ST Hernia Patch. (*D*) Covidien Composite Ventral Patch. (*E*) CA.B.S. Air Surgical Mesh. (*Courtesy of* [*A*] Ethicon, Cincinnati, OH, with permission; [*B*] Atrium Medical Corp, Hudson, NH, with permission; [*C*] Bard, Warwick, RI. © 2013 C.R. Bard, Inc. Used with permission; and [*D*] Covidien, Mansfield, MA, with permission.)

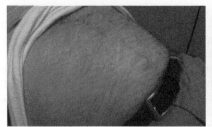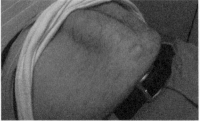

Fig. 10. Small ventral primary ventral hernia at the umbilicus with associated epigastric rectus diastasis seen only with Valsalva maneuvers. Primary repair will probably have a higher recurrence rate compared with prosthetic repair in this setting.

Mesh Repair Versus Primary Repair

From an anatomic standpoint, the goal of an umbilical or epigastric hernia repair is to stop and/or prevent intra-abdominal contents from protruding through the hernia defect. This can be accomplished by closing the defect primarily, sealing it with a prosthetic, or a combination of these two. Detailing all of the options regarding suture selection and placement, direction of defect closure, and prosthetic placement is beyond the scope of this article. Although the issues are outlined, we highlight operative details of common and increasingly important techniques. Pertinent issues related to the advantages and disadvantages of primary versus prosthetic repair are in **Table 2**.

The choice on whether or not to use a prosthetic should be based on clinical factors related to the patient's anatomy, physiology, and presentation, as well as environmental factors, such as the availability of prosthetics (**Box 1**). Further complicating matters is the decision about which prosthetic to use. Having an algorithm that takes in to account patient goals, anatomic factors, and overall medical condition will help the surgeon choose a technique, which in turn can help guide prosthetic choice (**Fig. 11**).

It is important, however, to recognize that all primary repairs are not the same, and variability exists among suture choice, suture technique, direction of defect closure, and number of layers closed. There are also a host of existing clinical factors that come in to play, such as obesity, strenuous work environments, physically demanding sporting or leisure activities, smoking status, and wound-healing capabilities. Further complicating matters are historical events, such as previous operations, wound infections, and issues that may predict a higher risk of future operations, such as inflammatory bowel disease and planned pregnancies, particularly if there have been previous cesarean sections that involve an incision that includes the umbilicus.

Surgical Procedure

Primary repair

Primary repair of umbilical and epigastric hernia refers to suture repair without the use of a prosthetic. It is important to note that these are not a uniform group of repairs. This can be accomplished with permanent, short-acting or long-acting absorbable sutures. The sutures can be monofilament, multifilament, or barbed sutures. Additionally, the defect can be closed vertically or transversely using a short or long suture technique with continuous or interrupted sutures. One additional variable of primary repair is the use of multiple suture lines, with overlapping or imbricated fascial layers. The relative advantages and disadvantages of these options are listed in **Table 3**.

Table 2
Relative advantages and disadvantages of prosthetic versus primary repair

	Advantage	Disadvantage	Comment
Prosthetic repair	Lower recurrence rate	—	—
	—	Availability of prosthetics	Short-term cost, geographic location, and administrative decisions all affect prosthetic availability. Increased cost may be offset by lower recurrence rate.
	—	Learning about prosthetic choices and new techniques	Should be part of standard practice. Variables include flat mesh vs preformed "ventral" patch; preperitoneal vs intraperitoneal placement; defect closure vs nonclosure.
	—	Potential prosthetic-related complications	Mesh contraction, mesh infection, chronic pain— all very low incidence.
Primary repair	Ubiquitous availability	—	Availability of a wide range of high-quality suture material varies among geographic locations.
	Lower procedure cost	—	May be offset by higher recurrence rates.
	No prosthetic-related complications (depends on suture type)	—	Complications related to permanent sutures are similar in terms of incidence and morbidity compared with prosthetics.
	—	Higher recurrence rate	—
	—	Multiple techniques available	Permanent vs absorbable suture; simple closure vs layered closure; transverse vs vertical closure; running vs interrupted suture; short vs long stitch technique.

Long-term cost may be the same considering lower recurrence rates with a prosthetic. A simple list, however, does not take in to account the complexity of the issue due to continuously changing variables among patients, surgeons, and facilities.

Mayo[18] originally described a repair with multiple suture lines: some interrupted permanent sutures and some running absorbable sutures. He found that the transverse direction of closure was also advantageous, as it allowed for closure of larger defects, and seemed to have less tension, and presumably better results. This is logical given that all vertical incisions will have perpendicular tension with bilateral oblique muscle contraction with Valsalva maneuvers, whereas transverse incisions are not subject to this. Additionally, the linea alba is more compliant longitudinally

---

Box 1
Factors that in most clinical scenarios would favor primary versus prosthetic repair. Departure from these factors does not constitute a breach in the standard of care, but should be accompanied by a logical thought process specifically designed achieve the goals of repair in the unique clinical situation

Favors Use of Prosthetic Repair

Larger-size defect (>2–4 cm)

Any size defect associated with the following:

Increased intra-abdominal pressure

- Strenuous work environment
- Physically demanding sports or leisure activities
- Chronic cough (severe allergies, chronic obstructive pulmonary disease, and so forth)
- Planned pregnancies

Etiology is previous operation (incisional hernia)

- Previous port site with defect closure
- Previous postpartum tubal ligation

Anticipated poor wound healing

- Chronic steroid use
- History of poor wound healing
- Poorly controlled ascites

Known collagen disorders

- Ehlers-Danlos syndrome
- Marfan disease
- Personal history of multiple hernias

Associated midline diastasis rectus

Informed patient choice, particularly if recurrence is a concern

Favors Primary Repair

Smaller size (<2–4 cm) without associated conditions mentioned above

Active skin infection, especially at the site of hernia repair

Emergent indication with strangulated omentum or bowel

Skin ulceration with leaking ascites

No appropriate prosthetic available (typically due to administrative and/or financial constraints)

Informed patient choice—any reason

Data from Earle D, Romanelli J. Prosthetic materials for hernia: what's new. Contemp Surg 2007;63(2):63–9.

---

compared with transversely, a fact that would also favor less tension on a transverse suture line.[56,57]

Although prosthetic repair in North America is common, recent European reports state that in Sweden and Denmark, primary repair is performed in 70% to 77% of cases,[58,59] thus making it worthwhile to detail this technique.

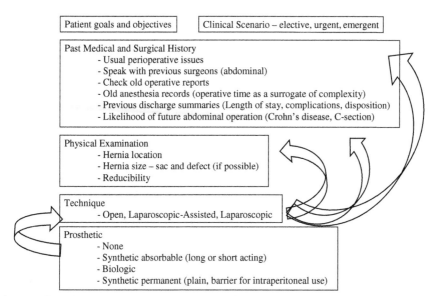

Fig. 11. Algorithm to help determine the type of hernia repair and prosthetic.

COMMON TECHNIQUES

One technique is a simple apposition of the edges. One investigator in 1959 found this technique to reduce tissue ischemia and improve suture line strength compared with methods with multiple suture lines in a rabbit model.[60] There are still variables associated with this that are related to suture technique, defect closure direction, and suture type (see **Table 3**). One early method of a multiple suture line repair was described by William J. Mayo in Rochester, Minnesota.[18] He began by vertically closing the edge of one side of the umbilical ring to the opposite side 1.0 to 1.5 inches from the edge with nonabsorbable silver wire interrupted horizontal mattress sutures. The free remaining edge of the ring was then closed with running, absorbable (gut) suture (**Fig. 12**).

Dr Mayo subsequently found that closing the defect transversely allowed closure of larger defects, as the tension was generally less with the transverse closure. His recurrence rates were reported to be 2 of 75, and a modern case series revealed 0% to 5.4% recurrence with this technique at 24 to 70 months of follow-up.[59,61] Others have reported higher recurrence rates with this method.[19,62,63] Interestingly, some of these higher recurrence rates are for different clinical scenarios, such as incisional and emergency umbilical hernia repairs,[64,65] which may have an impact on perceptions regarding repair of elective primary ventral hernias.

Open Prosthetic Repair

Using a prosthetic for open repair of a primary ventral hernia (umbilical or epigastric) is not as simple as it sounds. Options for prosthetic choice include a variety of raw materials and designs, and can be placed in a variety of locations with or without defect closure. Options for open prosthetic repair are listed in **Table 4**.

In the fairly recent past, small primary ventral hernias using a prosthetic were difficult to perform with a small incision, prompting many surgeons to adopt a laparoscopic approach, a technique we detail later. New prosthetic designs, however, have made prosthetic deployment easier and quicker than using a flat sheet.[66–70]

Table 3
Variables in primary repair of umbilical and epigastric hernia

| Technique | Primary Repair Considerations | | |
	Advantages	Disadvantages	Comments
Suture selection			
Permanent	No loss of suture strength	Increased risk of long-term suture sinus formation	Risk of infection and sinus formation slightly increased with braided vs monofilament sutures
Long-acting absorbable	Higher tensile strength through wound-healing period	• Only available in monofilament suture • More inelastic memory often perceived as poorer handling characteristics	• Barbed monofilament sutures are also available • Has the best chance for long term wound strength and avoiding suture sinus formation
Short-acting absorbable	Available in both braided and monofilament	• Lower tensile strength through wound-healing period • Braided suture has slightly increased risk of infection	May appeal to a larger group of surgeons' preference for braided suture

Suture technique

Short stitch technique (5–8 mm bites of tissue in terms of depth and travel, avoids muscle)	• Distributes tension over larger area
	• Higher suture line strength compared with long-stitch technique
	• Tissue pull-through results in small defect
	• Shown to reduce hernia rates by almost 25%*
	• Shown to reduce surgical site infection rate by 50%*
		• Requires a minor practice modification
		• Slightly increases operative time
			• Important to avoid muscle in the closure line
			  ○ Data for reducing hernia and infection rates based on primary laparotomy closure*
			  ○ May not be useful for defects smaller than 1 cm as a running suture, but concepts still apply

Long stitch technique ("standard" technique of 1-cm bites of tissue on terms of depth and travel)	• Reduced area of tension distribution • Weaker suture line strength compared with short-stitch technique	Theoretically will have a higher recurrence rate, generate more tissue ischemia, and have a higher infection rate	Data extrapolated from primary laparotomy closure still applies regarding tissue ischemia, but outcomes in hernia repair are unknown
Single layer closure	Technically easy	No redundancy	Commonly practiced for years with reasonable outcomes for small defects
Multiple layer closure	Distributes tension over 2 areas creating redundancy	More difficult	• Should be transverse orientation • Care must be taken to avoid deep bites for final layer to avoid visceral injury

* The data referring to the primary laparotomy closure is ref.[71]

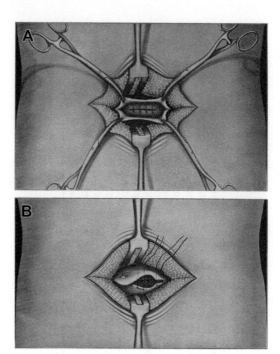

Fig. 12. Original graphics from Mayo's 1901 description of "An Operation for the Radical Cure of Umbilical Hernia." (*A*) Depiction of the closure of the peritoneum. (*B*) Depiction of the closure of the aponeurosis. (*From* Mayo WJ. VI. An operation for the radical cure of umbilical hernia. Ann Surg 1901;34(2):276–80.)

These "ventral patches" are designed to allow a prosthetic larger than the defect to be deployed under the fascia, then anchored to the fascia with or without defect closure with attached suture straps. The prosthetics are designed for intraperitoneal use by using barrier-coated or partially absorbable prosthetics (see **Fig. 9**). **Table 5** is a list of currently available prosthetics designed specifically for use in small ventral hernias.

We highlight only one technique of repair using a newly designed ventral patch. A skin incision is made over the defect, the size and direction depending on the size of the defect, previous scars, and degree of obesity. The herniated contents are resected and/or reduced, as appropriate. A space large enough for the prosthetic is then dissected between the abdominal wall and the umbilical and/or falciform ligaments. If using a monopolar energy device for hemostasis, take appropriate precautions to avoid thermal injury of the underlying viscera. We believe it is not important to avoid breaching the peritoneal cavity when using a prosthetic designed for intraperitoneal use. The purpose of the preperitoneal dissection is primarily to allow the prosthetic to lie flat, in intimate contact with the abdominal wall fascia. Occasionally, the defect is enlarged slightly in a transverse orientation to allow for a proper dissection. The prosthetic is then folded, and placed in the preperitoneal space. The fixation straps are pulled up through the fascial defect, cut the appropriate length, and the defect is then closed transversely with a short running suture, incorporating the shortened fixation tabs in to the closure. We use a long-acting, absorbable, barbed suture with the short-stitch technique for defect closure.[71] If the umbilical skin was elevated by the hernia and/or dissection, it is tacked down to the subcutaneous and/or abdominal wall fascia with

Table 4
Options and considerations for open prosthetic repair of primary midline ventral hernias

Prosthetic Types	Options	Design	Comments
Permanent	• Polypropylene • Polyester • PTFE • Composite	• Barrier • Deployment design for subfascial placement • Fixation tabs	Prosthetic deployment designs allow for easier subfascial placement compared to equivalent sized flat sheets.
Absorbable	• Synthetic • Biologic	• Short acting • Long acting	• Should use in an augmentation, rather than bridging fashion, ie, close the defect over or under the prosthetic. • May be more useful for contaminated cases.
Prosthetic placement	• Intraperitoneal • Extraperitoneal (subfascial) • Inlay (edge to edge): not recommended • Onlay: anterior aspect of fascia	—	Subfascial, extraperitoneal location may be intraperitoneal or extraperitoneal, but the prosthetic should lay flat against the abdominal wall, and superficial to umbilical and falciform ligaments. Onlay technique requires small skin flaps.
Defect closure	• None • Transverse • Vertical	• Single vs multiple suture lines • Short-stitch vs long-stitch technique • Running vs interrupted • Permanent vs absorbable sutures • Absorbable short vs long acting	• Running suture technique may not be feasible for very small defects. • Defect may be closed with onlay or subfascial mesh placement.

Prosthetics may be used with or without defect closure.
Abbreviation: PTFE, polytetrafluoroethylene.

Table 5
Listing of currently marketed prosthetics specifically designed for open, retro-fascial placement during repair of umbilical and epigastric hernias

Prosthetic Trade Name	Manufacturer	Materials	Shape and Sizes	Features
Ventralex ST Hernia Patch	CR Bard - Davol; Warwick, RI	PP and PGA fibers, PDO ring, absorbable barrier (HA, CMC, PEG)	• Round • 4.3 cm • 6.4 cm • 8.0 cm	• Partially absorbable, barrier coated • 102 g/m² and 37 g/m² layers of PP creating a "pocket" for fixation tacks • Stiff at implantation • Pair of fixation straps • Absorbable component short acting (30 d)
Proceed Ventral Patch	Ethicon; Cincinnati, OH	PP, PGA, PDO rings, sutures and film, absorbable barrier (oxygenated regenerated cellulose)	• Round • 4.3 cm • 6.4 cm	• Multiple layers of polymers laminated together • 45 g/m² PP after absorption • Stiff at implantation • Pair of fixation straps anchored at center • Absorbable component short acting (30 d)
C-Qur V-Patch	Atrium Medical; Hudson, NH	PP, fully coated with omega 3 fatty acids (absorbable)	• Round • 4.3 cm • 6.4 cm • 8.0 cm	• 2 layers of 85 g/m² creating a "pocket" • Fixation straps • Absorbable O3FA ring for deployment
Parietex Composite Ventral Patch	Covidien; Mansfield, MA	PET, PGLA ring, absorbable barrier (porcine collagen and glycerol)	• Round • 4.6 cm • 6.6 cm • 8.6 cm	• Partially absorbable (ring only) • 4 fixation tabs located near center • Removable positioning handles • 80 g/m² PET after absorption • Absorbable barrier
Biomesh CA.B.S. Air	Cousin Biotech; Saddle Brook, NJ	• PP • PP/PTFE	• Round • 6.8 cm (PP) • 5, 7, and 9 cm (PP/PTFE)	• Balloon deployment • Comes with 2 or 4 preplaced sutures • PP version: 2 layers of mesh • PP/PTFE version: 2 layers of PP, 1 layer ePTFE • Each PP layer <40 g/m²

Abbreviations: CMC, carboxymethyl cellulose; HA, hyaluronic acid; O3FA, omega-3 fatty acid; PDO, polydioxanone; PEG, polyethylene glycol; PET, polyethylene terephthalate; PGA, polyglycolic acid; PGLA, polyglycolic-co-L-lactic) acid; PP, polypropylene; PTFE, polytetrafluoroethylene.

at least 2 short-acting, interrupted absorbable sutures. We use more than one suture to avoid disruption in the unlikely event of a subcutaneous hematoma or seroma.

Laparoscopic Repair

Laparoscopic repair of small, readily identifiable primary midline ventral hernias in thin patients is generally not necessary, and often more invasive than the open mesh repair described previously. There are circumstances, however, when a laparoscopic approach is warranted. These include incisional hernias, incarcerated hernias (acute or chronic), suspicion for multiple defects, suspicion for a defect larger than 4 cm, and obesity. Incisional hernias that are present at the umbilicus, but are part of a longer midline incision that traverses or ends at the umbilicus are frequently associated with multiple defects discovered during laparoscopic exploration,[34] but not detected clinically. Acutely or chronically incarcerated hernias can be difficult to repair laparoscopically, but a laparoscopic approach may be beneficial to assess viability of the gastrointestinal tract compared with a small incision immediately over the hernia defect. Occasionally, there is suspicion for multiple or large defects based on history and/or physical examination, including obesity and chronically incarcerated hernias, which can also increase the uncertainty regarding defect size and number. In these scenarios, a diagnostic laparoscopy can help determine whether or not the defect is large or small. For larger and/or multiple defects, a larger prosthetic may be required, and the surgeon can proceed with a laparoscopic, or laparoscopic-assisted, technique. If the defect turns out to be single and small, the surgeon could then proceed with a less painful open repair with a deployable prosthetic designed for this purpose.

We will make a few points about the technical aspects of diagnostic laparoscopy and laparoscopic repair of small midline ventral hernias. It is important to dissect the falciform and/or umbilical ligaments away from the abdominal wall to identify other defects, and allow the prosthetic to intimately adhere to the abdominal wall, rather than the peritoneum and fat in these embryologic remnants. Identification of all defects will allow use of the most appropriately sized prosthetic. We also believe it is important to use a prosthetic that extends to the lateral border of the rectus muscles to avoid fixation injury to the epigastric vessels or muscle, and to give the prosthetic a better mechanical advantage, particularly if there is a diastasis of the rectus muscles (**Fig. 13**). It is our practice to use both suture and tack fixation, and place a prosthetic large enough to extend to the lateral borders of the rectus muscles to avoid fixation injury to the epigastric vessels. Prosthetic size, as well as fixation type and amount, should be appropriate for the defect and patient, keeping in mind that recurrence rates will be higher for smaller mesh:defect size ratio, larger defects, and recurrent hernias.[72]

Pain Management

Commonly, local anesthetic administered at the hernia location by the surgeon is sufficient for intraoperative and early postoperative pain relief. Longer-term postoperative pain relief is accomplished by orally administered nonsteroidal anti-inflammatory, acetaminophen, and/or narcotic-based medications. Recently there has been research in regional anesthetic blocks for umbilical hernia repair. The rectus sheath block, first described in 1899, is the subject of many scientific articles, mostly in the pediatric surgery literature.[73] Many studies have shown a benefit to using a rectus sheath block in pediatric patients undergoing umbilical hernia repair in the form of decreased postoperative pain scores and use of narcotic pain medication.[74,75] The rectus sheath block involves injecting local anesthetic into the potential space between the rectus muscle and the posterior rectus sheath bilaterally. It has classically been described as a procedure performed blindly, but more recently there have been

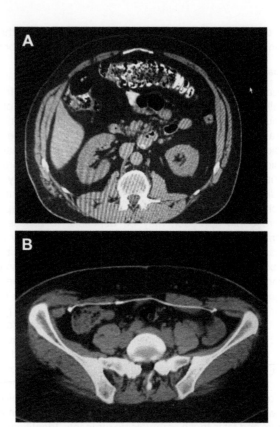

Fig. 13. Case (*A*) Although the mesh is flat, and covering the defect, it is at higher risk for failure because it does not extend lateral to the rectus muscles. Case (*B*) Six-year follow-up after LVHR with mesh extending beyond lateral borders of rectus muscles. Much lower risk of recurrence.

descriptions of performing the block in an open fashion during the umbilical hernia repair,[74] or using an ultrasound probe to visualize the muscles, fascia, and peritoneal cavity.[73] The goal is to infiltrate local anesthetic into the area where the sensory nerves of the abdominal wall travel.

Another regional abdominal wall anesthetic technique is the transversus abdominis plane (TAP) block. It was first described as a blind technique, using anatomic landmarks, by Rafi in 2001.[76] The technique is now commonly performed using ultrasound guidance.[77–80] The anesthetic is injected into the space between the internal oblique muscle and the transversus abdominis muscle, and is usually performed bilaterally so as to achieve midline anesthesia (**Table 6**).[78]

Our practice is to use local anesthetic infiltration into the wound for all small and medium umbilical and epigastric hernias in adults, when approaching the repair in an open fashion. If a laparoscopic procedure is performed, or when using an open technique for a larger hernia, we (surgical team) perform an ultrasound-guided bilateral TAP block at the conclusion of the procedure.

Immediate Postoperative Care and Recovery

After performing a small to medium-sized open umbilical or epigastric hernia repair, the postoperative care is rather routine. The wound should be dressed as the

Table 6		
Anesthetic options for umbilical and epigastric hernia repair		
	Anesthesia	
Local	Skin, subcutaneous tissue, and fascia at hernia location	• Administered by surgeon • Duration usually less than 6 h
Regional block	Rectus sheath, TAP	• Administered by surgeon or anesthesia • Lasts up to 24 h • TAP usually performed with ultrasound guidance
IV medication	NSAIDs, narcotics, acetaminophen	• Administered by nurse in hospital setting
PO medication	NSAIDs, narcotics, acetaminophen	• Self-administered at home
Topical	NSAIDS, narcotics	• Administered at home

Abbreviations: IV, intravenous; NSAIDs, nonsteroidal anti-inflammatory drugs; PO, oral; TAP, transversus abdominus plane.

operating surgeon sees fit. We ask the patients to refrain from getting the wound wet for 24 to 48 hours, or at least until there is no drainage. We also recommend returning to normal activities as tolerated by pain, and do not dictate specific restrictions. Because return to work has many factors that weigh in to the decision, we engage the patient in that decision-making process.

Complications

Even though umbilical and epigastric hernia repairs are often considered "minor" procedures, our experience at a referral center has demonstrated that they can be fraught with complications. Most problems are wound related, including seromas, hematomas, superficial or deep surgical site infections, and mesh infections.[58,81–86] Patients also may experience chronic pain at the site of the repair.[87] Many of these complications do not require specialized treatment, but are often associated with multiple visits to the surgeon's office, medical therapy, hospital admission, or additional operative procedures. Long-term complications related to suture sinuses are probably no different from laparotomy closure, making long-acting absorbable suture material an attractive choice. Long-term complications specifically related to the prosthetic are very uncommon, even when used for emergent repair of incarcerated and strangulated hernias.[87–89]

Another major source of morbidity is hernia recurrence. Hernia rates of up to 54% have been quoted in the past literature for a simple sutured repair.[64,90–92] More recent studies have found recurrence rates to be from as low as 0% to 3% with a mesh repair,[91,93–96] to up to 14% for a sutured repair.[90,97] Cost and availability influence prosthetic use; however, the cost of another hernia repair because of recurrence should also be considered[98] when looking at economic issues. Additionally, issues from a patient perspective, such as inconvenience and morbidity of a second operation, are also important.

SPECIAL CONSIDERATIONS
Acutely Incarcerated Hernia

Acutely incarcerated umbilical and epigastric hernias range from life-threatening conditions requiring emergent operation, to simple reduction of the hernia with outpatient follow-up. It is important to keep in mind that the typical patient goal of treatment of an acutely incarcerated hernia is pain relief, and there is also a desire to fix the problem so it does not return. This scenario requires the surgeon to balance the risk of prosthetic use in a potentially contaminated operative field versus risk of a recurrent hernia. Because of the higher recurrence rates when repaired without mesh, recent research has shown that prosthetics can actually be placed in the setting of an incarcerated hernia. In 2007, Abdel-Baki and colleagues[99] randomized 42 patients with acutely incarcerated paraumbilical hernia into 2 groups: one with onlay polypropylene mesh repair, and one with tissue repair only. Over an average of 16 months, 19% of the tissue repair group had a hernia recurrence, whereas no patients in the mesh repair group recurred. There were no significant differences in rates of wound infections, seromas, or any other complications. A retrospective study from The Netherlands[100] found that suture repair had more than twice (24%) the rate of wound infection compared with mesh repair (11%) for acutely incarcerated umbilical hernias. Furthermore, only 1 of 99 patients with mesh repair had to have their mesh removed. Univariate and multivariate analysis revealed, however, that the type of repair (mesh vs suture) did not have an impact on wound infection, rather bowel resection was associated with an odds ratio of 3.5 for development of a wound infection. In spite of this, the overall wound infection rate for all cases was only 12.3%. It appears that mesh implantation can be safe, even in an acutely incarcerated hernia, and should always be considered to decrease recurrence rates. Further research and analysis regarding type of prosthetic and prosthetic placement technique are warranted to improve outcomes even further.

Pregnancy

The challenge of the hernia diagnosed during pregnancy lies in deciding when to operate. Generally, a watchful waiting approach is encouraged for asymptomatic patients until the postpartum period. Buch and colleagues[101] found that there were no complications with 12 patients who underwent postpartum inguinal or umbilical hernia repairs anywhere from 4 to 52 weeks after delivery. All of the hernias were diagnosed during pregnancy and none of the patients had incarceration of their hernia before it was repaired. Four patients had subsequent uncomplicated pregnancies.

A more difficult problem is the pregnant patient presenting with an acutely incarcerated hernia. There is very little literature published regarding this circumstance, but general surgical principles still apply.[102] It is important to remember that the health of the mother is of paramount importance to the survival of both mother and fetus. Careful consideration should be paid to the age of the pregnancy, anesthesiology issues, pain intensity, duration of incarceration, and ability to reduce the hernia. The contents of the hernia are also an important factor in the decision making. In later stages of pregnancy, the uterus will protect the umbilical area from incarceration of the intestine, but it is still possible to have incarcerated omentum that can be quite painful.[103] As always, a clear discussion should be had with the patient and family regarding the issues involved in the decision making and the risks and benefits of observation versus operative repair should be detailed.

Diastasis Recti

The surgeon should always assess every patient with a primary midline ventral hernia for the presence of diastasis recti, a fact that we have seen commonly overlooked during examination of a relatively "simple" problem (see **Fig. 10**). The patient should be examined while standing and while lying down, with and without Valsalva maneuvers. As the diagnosis of diastasis alone is not a surgical problem, when it accompanies the presence of a hernia, the problem becomes more complex. By definition, having a separation between the 2 rectus muscles in the midline naturally causes a thinning of the linea alba.[104–106]

It is logical that suturing together a thinned out linea alba will have a higher recurrence rate than suture repair with a normal linea alba. Therefore, we believe that a patient with an umbilical or epigastric hernia that resides within or at the terminus of a rectus diastasis should generally undergo a prosthetic repair versus a primary suture repair.

Cirrhosis and Ascites

Umbilical hernia repair in the cirrhotic patient with ascites has been the topic of much debate and literature. Classical surgical teaching of a "wait and see" approach is no longer recommended, as the consequences of skin necrosis and ascites leak are disastrous (**Fig. 14**). Most studies since 2000 advocate for early, elective repair of umbilical hernias in patients with cirrhosis and ascites[107–112]; the patient needs to be optimized for the surgery and ascites controlled. Many different techniques have been used for surgical repair, and it is unclear at this time if any method is superior. A study by Ammar in 2008[113] showed that cirrhotic patients who had a mesh repair had a trend of more wound infections compared with those repaired without mesh, but a significantly decreased recurrence rate. More recently, Cho and colleagues[114] found that the Model for End-Stage Liver Disease (MELD) score was very important to predict preoperative mortality for elective hernia repair in patients with portal hypertension. Patients with a MELD score higher than 15 had a mortality rate of 11.1% compared with a rate of 1.3% in those patients with a MELD score lower than 15.

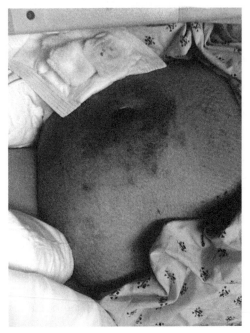

Fig. 14. Patient with umbilical hernia that was not repaired due to presence of cirrhosis and ascites. Patient developed rupture of umbilical hernia sac with leaking ascites, as shown.

SUMMARY

Umbilical and epigastric hernias are primary midline defects that are present in up to 50% of the population when screened for with physical examination and radiological studies. In the United States, only about 1% of the population carries this specific diagnosis, and only about 11% of these end up being repaired, which would be approximately 263,000 per year. Actual data regarding repairs, however, reveal as low as 189,000 repairs in 2012, but accurate data collection is very difficult because of the lack of a robust national medical record.

The repair of these hernias are aimed at symptom relief and/or prevention, and the patient's goals and expectations should be explicitly identified and aligned with the health care team. Although the overall success rates of prosthetic versus suture repair are high, use of a prosthetic repair consistently offers lower recurrence rates compared with suture repair in both elective and emergent situations, with a very low prosthetic-related complication rate. Precise technical issues related to both types of repair are complex, and highly variable. Some of this variability is related to an endless number of unpredictable clinical scenarios related to the patient, the surgeon, and the institution, such as urgency of repair, associated diastasis recti, pregnancy, ascites, surgeon preference, and product availability.

Although reducing variability can be good when considering poor outcomes, it can also adversely affect outcomes by stifling innovation. With so many assumptions in the diagnosis and treatment of umbilical and epigastric hernias, use of a continuous quality improvement program may help to improve poor outliers, and maintain innovation in techniques and policies that improve outcomes even further.

REFERENCES

1. Ghomrawi HM, Mancuso CA, Westrich GH, et al. Discordance in TKA expectations between patients and surgeons. Clin Orthop Relat Res 2013;471(1): 175–80.
2. Jones KR, Burney RE, Peterson M, et al. Return to work after inguinal hernia repair. Surgery 2001;129(2):128–35.
3. Lledo R, Rodriguez-Ros T, Targarona EM, et al. Perceived quality of care of inguinal hernia repair: assessment before and after the procedure. Int Surg 2000;85(1):82–7.
4. Ibrahim MS, Khan MA, Nizam I, et al. Peri-operative interventions producing better functional outcomes and enhanced recovery following total hip and knee arthroplasty: an evidence-based review. BMC Med 2013;11:37.
5. Burney RE, Jones KR, Coon JW, et al. Core outcomes measures for inguinal hernia repair. J Am Coll Surg 1997;185(6):509–15.
6. Jones KR, Burney RE, Christy B. Patient expectations for surgery: are they being met? Jt Comm J Qual Improv 2000;26(6):349–60.
7. Danquah G, Mittal V, Solh M, et al. Effect of Internet use on patient's surgical outcomes. Int Surg 2007;92(6):339–43.
8. Brewer S, Williams T. Finally, a sense of closure? Animal models of human ventral body wall defects. Bioessays 2004;26(12):1307–21.
9. Sadler TW. Langman's medical embryology. 9th edition. Baltimore (MD): Lippincott Williams & Wilkins; 2004.
10. Loukas M, Myers C, Shah R, et al. Arcuate line of the rectus sheath: clinical approach. Anat Sci Int 2008;83(3):140–4.
11. Wagh PV, Read RC. Collagen deficiency in rectus sheath of patients with inguinal herniation. Exp Biol Med 1971;137(2):382.

12. Katz DA. Evaluation and management of inguinal and umbilical hernias. Pediatr Ann 2001;30(12):729–35.
13. Zendejas B, Kuchena A, Onkendi EO, et al. Fifty-three-year experience with pediatric umbilical hernia repairs. J Pediatr Surg 2011;46(11):2151–6.
14. Graf JL, Caty MG, Martin DJ, et al. Pediatric hernias. Semin Ultrasound CT MR 2002;23(2):197–200.
15. Jackson OJ, Moglen LH. Umbilical hernia—a retrospective study. Calif Med 1970;113(4):8–11.
16. Hall DE, Roberts KB, Charney E. Umbilical hernia—what happens after age 5 years. J Pediatr 1981;98(3):415–7.
17. Muschaweck U. Umbilical and epigastric hernia repair. Surg Clin North Am 2003;83(5):1207–21.
18. Mayo WJ. VI. An operation for the radical cure of umbilical hernia. Ann Surg 1901;34(2):276–80.
19. Askar OM. New concept of etiology and surgical repair of para-umbilical and epigastric hernias. Ann R Coll Surg Engl 1978;60(1):42–8.
20. Shlomovitz E, Quan D, Etemad-Rezai R, et al. Association of recanalization of the left umbilical vein with umbilical hernia in patients with liver disease. Liver Transpl 2005;11(10):1298–9.
21. McAlister V. Management of umbilical hernia in patients with advanced liver disease. Liver Transpl 2003;9(6):623–5.
22. Fachinelli A, Trindade MR. Qualitative and quantitative evaluation of total and types I and III collagens in patients with ventral hernias. Langenbecks Arch Surg 2007;392(4):459–64.
23. Fachinelli A, Trindade MR, Fachinelli FA. Elastic fibers in the anterior abdominal wall. Hernia 2011;15(4):409–15.
24. Sanders DL, Kingsnorth AN. From ancient to contemporary times: a concise history of incisional hernia repair. Hernia 2012;16(1):1–7.
25. Moschcowitz AV. The pathogenesis of umbilical hernia. Ann Surg 1915;61:570–88.
26. Gray H. Gray's Anatomy. Revised American Edition from the 15th English Edition ed.
27. Fathi AH, Soltanian H, Saber AA. Surgical anatomy and morphologic variations of umbilical structures. Am Surg 2012;78(5):540–4.
28. Lang B, Lau H, Lee F. Epigastric hernia and its etiology. Hernia 2002;6(3):148–50.
29. Moschcowitz AV. Department of Technique. The pathogenesis and treatment of herniae of the linea alba. Surg Gynecol Obstet 1914;18:504–7.
30. Askar OM. Aponeurotic hernias—recent observations upon paraumbilical and epigastric hernias. Surg Clin North Am 1984;64(2):315–33.
31. Hollinsky C, Sandberg S. Measurement of the tensile strength of the ventral abdominal wall in comparison with scar tissue. Clin Biomech 2007;22(1):88–92.
32. Bickenbach KA, Karanicolas PJ, Ammori JB, et al. Up and down or side to side? A systematic review and meta-analysis examining the impact of incision on outcomes after abdominal surgery. Am J Surg 2013. Available at: http://dx.doi.org/10.1016/j.amjsurg.2012.11.008.
33. Samia H, Lawrence J, Nobel T, et al. Extraction site location and incisional hernias after laparoscopic colorectal surgery: should we be avoiding the midline? Am J Surg 2013;205(3):264–7.
34. Saber AA, Rao AJ, Itawi EA, et al. Occult ventral hernia defects: a common finding during laparoscopic ventral hernia repair. Am J Surg 2008;195(4):471–3.

35. Helgstrand F, Rosenberg J, Bisgaard T. Trocar site hernia after laparoscopic surgery: a qualitative systematic review. Hernia 2011;15(2):113–21.
36. Rutkow IM. Demographic and socioeconomic aspects of hernia repair in the United States in 2003. Surg Clin North Am 2003;83(5):1045–51.
37. Bedewi MA, El-Sharkawy MS, Al Boukai AA, et al. Prevalence of adult paraumbilical hernia. Assessment by high-resolution sonography: a hospital-based study. Hernia 2012;16(1):59–62.
38. Meier DE, OlaOlorun DA, Omodele RA, et al. Incidence of umbilical hernia in African children: redefinition of "normal" and reevaluation of indications for repair. World J Surg 2001;25(5):645–8.
39. Sundstrom A, Mortimer O, Akerlund B, et al. Increased risk of abdominal wall hernia associated with combination anti-retroviral therapy in HIV-infected patients—results from a Swedish cohort-study. Pharmacoepidemiol Drug Saf 2010;19(5):465–73.
40. Lau B, Kim H, Haigh PI, et al. Obesity increases the odds of acquiring and incarcerating noninguinal abdominal wall hernias. Am Surg 2012;78(10):1118–21.
41. Papadimitriou D, Pitoulias G, Papaziogas B, et al. Incidence of abdominal wall hernias in patients undergoing aortic surgery for aneurysm or occlusive disease. Vasa 2002;31(2):111–4.
42. Erdas E, Dazzi C, Secchi F, et al. Incidence and risk factors for trocar site hernia following laparoscopic cholecystectomy: a long-term follow-up study. Hernia 2012;16(4):431–7.
43. Innovations in healthcare analytics. SDI; 2010.
44. Millennium Research Group Inc; 2012. Available at: www.mrg.net.
45. Aileron Solutions; 2012.
46. IMS Health Solutions; 2011.
47. US Census Bureau. State and County QuickFacts. 2013. Available at: http://quickfacts.census.gov/qfd/states/00000.html.
48. Muysoms FE, Miserez M, Berrevoet F, et al. Classification of primary and incisional abdominal wall hernias. Hernia 2009;13(4):407–14.
49. Kulah B, Kulacoglu IH, Oruc MT, et al. Presentation and outcome of incarcerated external hernias in adults. Am J Surg 2001;181(2):101–4.
50. Wood S, Panait L, Bell R, et al. Pure transvaginal umbilical hernia repair. Surg Endosc 2013.
51. Jacobsen GR, Thompson K, Spivack A, et al. Initial experience with transvaginal incisional hernia repair. Hernia 2010;14(1):89–91.
52. Buck L, Michalek J, Van Sickle K, et al. Can gastric irrigation prevent infection during NOTES mesh placement? J Gastrointest Surg 2008;12(11):2010–4.
53. Earle DB, Desilets DJ, Romanelli JR. NOTESA (R) transgastric abdominal wall hernia repair in a porcine model. Hernia 2010;14(5):517–22.
54. Earle DB, Romanelli JR, McLawhorn T, et al. Prosthetic mesh contamination during NOTESA (R) transgastric hernia repair: a randomized controlled trial with swine explants. Hernia 2012;16(6):689–95.
55. Sherwinter DA, Gupta A, Eckstein JG. Natural orifice translumenal endoscopic surgery inguinal hernia repair: a survival canine model. J Laparoendosc Adv Surg Tech A 2011;21(3):209–12.
56. Grassel D, Prescher A, Fitzek S, et al. Anisotropy of human linea alba: a biomechanical study. J Surg Res 2005;124(1):118–25.
57. Foerstemann T, Trzewik J, Holste J, et al. Forces and deformations of the abdominal wall—a mechanical and geometrical approach to the linea alba. J Biomech 2011;44(4):600–6.

58. Bisgaard T, Kehlet H, Bay-Nielsen M, et al. A nationwide study on readmission, morbidity, and mortality after umbilical and epigastric hernia repair. Hernia 2011; 15(5):541–6.
59. Dalenbäck J, Andersson C, Ribokas D, et al. Long-term follow-up after elective adult umbilical hernia repair: low recurrence rates also after non-mesh repairs. Hernia 2012.
60. Farris JM, Smith GK, Beattie AS. Umbilical hernia—an inquiry into the principle of imbrication and a note on the preservation of the umbilical dimple. Am J Surg 1959;98(2):236–42.
61. Lau H, Patil NG. Umbilical hernia in adults—laparoscopic vs open repair. Surg Endosc 2003;17(12):2016–20.
62. Kelly HA. An operation for umbilical hernia. Ann Surg 1910;51:694–6.
63. DuBose FG. A new operation for umbilical hernia. Surg Gynecol Obstet 1915;771.
64. Paul A, Korenkov M, Peters S, et al. Unacceptable results of the Mayo procedure for repair of abdominal incisional hernias. Eur J Surg 1998;164(5):361–7.
65. Garcia M, Rico P, Seoane I. Hernia umbilical del adulto. Resultados a largo plazo en pacientes operados de urgencia. World J Surg 1994;(21):62–5.
66. Berrevoet F, D'Hont F, Rogiers X, et al. Open intraperitoneal versus retromuscular mesh repair for umbilical hernias less than 3cm diameter. Am J Surg 2011; 201(1):85–90.
67. Martin DF, Williams RF, Mulrooney T, et al. Ventralex mesh in umbilical/epigastric hernia repairs: clinical outcomes and complications. Hernia 2008;12(4):379–83.
68. Tollens T, Den Hondt M, Devroe K, et al. Retrospective analysis of umbilical, epigastric, and small incisional hernia repair using the Ventralex (TM) hernia patch. Hernia 2011;15(5):531–40.
69. Steinemann D, Limani P, Ochsenbein N, et al. Suture repair of umbilical hernia during caesarean section: a case-control study. Hernia 2013.
70. Ambe P, Meyer A, Koehler L. Repair of small and medium size ventral hernias with a proceed ventral patch: a single center retrospective analysis. Surg Today 2013;43(4):381–5.
71. Millbourn D, Cengiz Y, Israelsson LA. Effect of stitch length on wound complications after closure of midline incisions a randomized controlled trial. Arch Surg 2009;144(11):1056–9.
72. SAGES guidelines for laparoscopic ventral hernia repair, in press.
73. de Jose Maria B, Gotzens V, Mabrok M. Ultrasound-guided umbilical nerve block in children: a brief description of a new approach. Paediatr Anaesth 2007;17(1):44–50.
74. Clarke FK, Cassey JG. Paraumbilical block for umbilical herniorraphy. ANZ J Surg 2007;77(8):659–61.
75. Gurnaney HG, Maxwell LG, Kraemer FW, et al. Prospective randomized observer-blinded study comparing the analgesic efficacy of ultrasound-guided rectus sheath block and local anaesthetic infiltration for umbilical hernia repair. Br J Anaesth 2011;107(5):790–5.
76. Rafi AN. Abdominal field block: a new approach via the lumbar triangle. Anaesthesia 2001;56(10):1024–6.
77. Hebbard P, Fujiwara Y, Shibata Y, et al. Ultrasound-guided transversus abdominis plane (TAP) block. Anaesth Intensive Care 2007;35(4):616–7.
78. Young MJ, Gorlin AW, Modest VE, et al. Clinical implications of the transversus abdominis plane block in adults. Anesthesiol Res Pract 2012;2012:731645.
79. Abdallah FW, Chan VW, Brull R. Transversus abdominis plane block—a systematic review. Reg Anesth Pain Med 2012;37(2):193–209.

80. Borglum J, Maschmann C, Belhage B, et al. Ultrasound-guided bilateral dual transversus abdominis plane block: a new four-point approach. Acta Anaesthesiol Scand 2011;55(6):658–63.

81. Yavuz N, Ipek T, As A, et al. Laparoscopic repair of ventral and incisional hernias: our experience in 150 patients. J Laparoendosc Adv Surg Tech A 2005; 15(6):601–5.

82. Farrow B, Awad S, Berger DH, et al. More than 150 consecutive open umbilical hernia repairs in a major Veterans Administration Medical Center. Am J Surg 2008;196(5):647–51.

83. Courtney CA, Lee AC, Wilson C, et al. Ventral hernia repair: a study of current practice. Hernia 2003;7(1):44–6.

84. Love H, Kumar A. Complications of incisional hernia repair: delaminated mesh with incarcerated hernia. ANZ J Surg 2004;74(8):705–6.

85. Tagaya N, Mikami H, Aoki H, et al. Long-term complications of laparoscopic ventral and incisional hernia repair. Surg Laparosc Endosc Percutan Tech 2004;14(1):5–8.

86. Tsimoyiannis EC, Tsimogiannis KE, Pappas-Gogos G, et al. Seroma and recurrence in laparoscopic ventral hernioplasty. JSLS 2008;12(1):51–7.

87. Erritzoe-Jervild L. Long-term complaints after elective repair for small umbilical or epigastric hernias. Hernia.

88. Kulacoglu H, Yazicioglu D, Ozyaylali I. Prosthetic repair of umbilical hernias in adults with local anesthesia in a day-case setting: a comprehensive report from a specialized hernia center. Hernia 2012;16(2):163–70.

89. Bessa SS, Abdel-Razek AH. Results of prosthetic mesh repair in the emergency management of the acutely incarcerated and/or strangulated ventral hernias: a seven years study. Hernia 2013;17(1):59–65.

90. Halm JA, Heisterkamp J, Veen HF, et al. Long-term follow-up after umbilical hernia repair: are there risk factors for recurrence after simple and mesh repair. Hernia 2005;9(4):334–7.

91. Edelman DS, Bellows CF. Umbilical herniorrhaphy reinforced with biologic mesh. Am Surg 2010;76(11):1205–9.

92. Luijendijk RW, Lemmen MH, Hop WC, et al. Incisional hernia recurrence following 'vest-over-pants' or vertical Mayo repair of primary hernias of the midline. World J Surg 1997;21(1):62–6.

93. Asolati M, Huerta S, Sarosi G, et al. Predictors of recurrence in veteran patients with umbilical hernia: single center experience. Am J Surg 2006;192(5):627–30.

94. Stabilini C, Stella M, Frascio M, et al. Mesh versus direct suture for the repair of umbilical and epigastric hernias. Ten-year experience. Ann Ital Chir 2009;80(3): 183–7.

95. Sanjay P, Reid TD, Davies EL, et al. Retrospective comparison of mesh and sutured repair for adult umbilical hernias. Hernia 2005;9(3):248–51.

96. Eryilmaz R, Sahin M, Tekelioglu MH. Which repair in umbilical hernia of adults: primary or mesh? Int Surg 2006;91(5):258–61.

97. Venclauskas L, Silanskaite J, Kiudelis M. Umbilical hernia: factors indicative of recurrence. Medicina (Kaunas) 2008;44(11):855–9.

98. Aslani N, Brown CJ. Does mesh offer an advantage over tissue in the open repair of umbilical hernias? A systematic review and meta-analysis. Hernia 2010;14(5):455–62.

99. Abdel-Baki NA, Bessa SS, Abdel-Razek AH. Comparison of prosthetic mesh repair and tissue repair in the emergency management of incarcerated paraumbilical hernia: a prospective randomized study. Hernia 2007;11(2):163–7.

100. Nieuwenhuizen J, van Ramshorst GH, ten Brinke JG, et al. The use of mesh in acute hernia: frequency and outcome in 99 cases. Hernia 2011;15(3):297–300.
101. Buch KE, Tabrizian P, Divino CM. Management of hernias in pregnancy. J Am Coll Surg 2008;207(4):539–42.
102. Pearl J, Price R, Richardson W, et al. Guidelines for diagnosis, treatment, and use of laparoscopy for surgical problems during pregnancy. Surg Endosc 2011;25(11):3479–92.
103. Perry Z, Netz U, Yitzhak A, et al. Pros and cons in the approach to an incarcerated umbilical hernia in the pregnant woman. Am Surg 2011;77(3):E43–4.
104. Hickey F, Finch JG, Khanna A. A systematic review on the outcomes of correction of diastasis of the recti. Hernia 2011;15(6):607–14.
105. Rath AM, Attali P, Dumas JL, et al. The abdominal linea alba: an anatomo-radiologic and biomechanical study. Surg Radiol Anat 1996;18(4):281–8.
106. Beer GM, Schuster A, Seifert B, et al. The normal width of the linea alba in nulliparous women. Clin Anat 2009;22(6):706–11.
107. Fagan SP, Awad SS, Berger DH. Management of complicated umbilical hernias in patients with end-stage liver disease and refractory ascites. Surgery 2004; 135(6):679–82.
108. Carbonell AM, Wolfe LG, DeMaria EJ. Poor outcomes in cirrhosis-associated hernia repair: a nationwide cohort study of 32,033 patients. Hernia 2005;9(4): 353–7.
109. Gray SH, Vick CC, Graham LA, et al. Umbilical herniorrhapy in cirrhosis: improved outcomes with elective repair. J Gastrointest Surg 2008;12(4):675–81.
110. McKay A, Dixon E, Bathe O, et al. Umbilical hernia repair in the presence of cirrhosis and ascites: results of a survey and review of the literature. Hernia 2009;13(5):461–8.
111. Eker HH, van Ramshorst GH, de Goede B, et al. A prospective study on elective umbilical hernia repair in patients with liver cirrhosis and ascites. Surgery 2011; 150(3):542–6.
112. Choi SB, Hong KD, Lee JS, et al. Management of umbilical hernia complicated with liver cirrhosis: an advocate of early and elective herniorrhaphy. Dig Liver Dis 2011;43(12):991–5.
113. Ammar SA. Management of complicated umbilical hernias in cirrhotic patients using permanent mesh: randomized clinical trial. Hernia 2010;14(1):35–8.
114. Cho SW, Bhayani N, Newell P, et al. Umbilical hernia repair in patients with signs of portal hypertension surgical outcome and predictors of mortality. Arch Surg 2012;147(9):864–9.

Laparoscopic Ventral Hernia Repair

Andrea Mariah Alexander, MD, Daniel J. Scott, MD*

KEYWORDS

- Incisional hernia • Ventral hernia • Laparoscopic hernia repair • Laparoscopy
- Recurrent hernia

KEY POINTS

- Laparoscopic ventral hernia repair provides low recurrence rates, shorter hospital stays, and decreased wound complications.
- Appropriate patient selection and meticulous technique are essential to achieve successful outcomes.
- Adhesiolysis should be performed using sharp dissection to avoid thermal injury.
- Wide mesh overlap and secure fixation of the mesh are important.

INTRODUCTION

The laparoscopic approach was first introduced by LeBlanc and Booth in the early 1990s.[1] Since its introduction, it has continued to evolve and has become an important option in the hernia surgeon's armamentarium. However, only 27.4% of ventral hernia repairs are performed laparoscopically, likely because of the relatively advanced nature of this procedure and because all hernias may not be suitable for a laparoscopic approach.[2] Using current techniques, numerous studies have documented the safety and efficacy of this approach. Some data suggest that the laparoscopic approach results in a shorter hospital stay and lower recurrence rates compared with open approaches. However, pain may still be significant after laparoscopic repairs and there are not significant advantages from this standpoint. Nonetheless, it is well accepted that the primary advantage of the laparoscopic approach is that wound infections are less frequent compared with open approaches.

Disclosures: Ethicon: licensing agreement, research grants, Covidien: research grants, Storz: research/equipment grants, Accelerated Technologies: consultant, NeatStitch: consultant (D.J. Scott).
Department of Surgery, Southwestern Center for Minimally Invasive Surgery, University of Texas Southwestern Medical Center, 5323 Harry Hines Boulevard, Dallas, TX 75390-9092, USA
* Corresponding author.
E-mail address: daniel.scott@utsouthwestern.edu

The laparoscopic repair is based on the principles applied in the open underlay approach, which has been touted as the gold standard by the American Hernia Society.[3] This approach places the mesh in a retrorectus, preperitoneal, or intraperitoneal location, which serves to reinforce a substantial portion of the abdominal wall. By placing the mesh posteriorly, the underlay technique applies Pascal's law, which states that pressure exerted on an enclosed fluid is transmitted undiminished throughout the fluid and acts equally in all directions. Accordingly, as the intra-abdominal pressure increase, equal amounts of force are dispersed across the mesh. This situation is different from the onlay technique, whereby intra-abdominal pressure exerts lifting forces against the mesh. Thus, the underlay technique seems mechanically advantageous. In the laparoscopic repair, the mesh is placed intraperitoneally with wide overlap, allowing even distributions of forces along the surface of the mesh. This procedure results in a solid repair.

There is controversy surrounding the importance of restoring the midline apposition of the abdominal wall muscles during ventral hernia repair. The laparoscopic approach bridges the defect using sound mechanical principles, as outlined earlier. However, proponents of open repairs, such as a components separation with underlay buttressing, suggest that a better functional outcome may be achieved. However, few to no data are available to clearly support one method over the other in terms of functional outcome. In our experience, the laparoscopic approach results in favorable outcomes from this standpoint. Because the laparoscopic approach avoids creation of large skin flaps or soft tissue dissections, the advantage of fewer wound complications makes this approach attractive.

Although the laparoscopic approach is the technique of choice for many surgeons, care must be taken to ensure that patients are well selected and that meticulous technique is followed.

INDICATIONS AND PATIENT SELECTION

All patients with a ventral hernia may be considered for a repair via a laparoscopic or open approach, unless medically unfit for such an operation. For the laparoscopic approach, several absolute and relative contraindications exist (**Box 1**).

The laparoscopic approach is not indicated for most emergent situations, especially if hemodynamic instability or compromise of intestinal blood supply is present.

Box 1
Contraindications to LVHR

Absolute
- Medically unsuitable for a major operation
- Strangulated hernia with gangrenous bowel
- Uncontrolled coagulopathy
- Hostile abdomen

Relative
- Multiple previous mesh hernia repairs
- Incarcerated hernia
- Loss of domain
- Infected or contaminated fields

Similarly, laparoscopic approaches are not well suited to coagulopathic patients. An open approach may be required for patients with a hostile abdomen. For instance, enterocutaneous fistula, previous open abdomen, history of severe abdominal injuries, or previous extensive operations may be associated with diffuse adhesions and make safe laparoscopic access difficult or impossible. However, most patients who are candidates for a laparoscopic ventral hernia repair (LVHR) have had previous operations. The decision to proceed should be based on the surgeon's experience and the expectation that safe access may be obtained. Adhesions may be dense in patients with previous mesh repairs, although a laparoscopic approach may be feasible in some cases.

Incarcerated hernias may be difficult to reduce laparoscopically and may require an open approach; however, under general anesthesia, it may be possible to reduce the hernia using a combination of manual external pressure and careful laparoscopic adhesiolysis. Loss of domain is also a relative contraindication. If adhesiolysis is successful, once the viscera are reduced, there may be exceptionally little working space; in this situation, it is often impossible to proceed laparoscopically with mesh placement and fixation. For infected or contaminated fields, the standard laparoscopic repair may not be feasible, because a synthetic mesh is usually implanted. Most surgeons would opt for an open approach, using an alternative technique or implantation of a nonpermanent reinforcement material. Although not yet widely performed, there have been recent reports of successfully implanting biological mesh laparoscopically in such circumstances.[4] Some patients may wish to have excessive skin or disfiguring scars excised at the time of surgery. In these instances, an open approach may be more suitable.

PREOPERATIVE PLANNING

Several patient factors should be addressed preoperatively such that patient outcomes may be optimized. In particular, smoking and obesity are known risk factors for recurrence. Some surgeons require smoking cessation before proceeding with an open or a laparoscopic repair; however, because wound infections are less frequent for laparoscopic repairs, this approach may be advantageous in patients who are unable to stop smoking. The laparoscopic approach has been touted by some experts as the superior approach for obese individuals for similar reasons. However, obesity still poses an increase in both wound complications and recurrences rates, even using the laparoscopic approach.[5,6] It is therefore desirable for patients to lose weight preoperatively if possible. For morbidly obese individuals, it may be prudent to approach ventral hernias in a staged approach. A weight loss operation may be first performed, often with temporary hernia closure using primary repair or absorbable mesh.[7] A definitive hernia repair, using a laparoscopic or open approach, may be performed 6 to 18 months after the weight loss operation, when the patient has lost substantial weight and has fewer comorbidities.

Once the decision has been made to proceed laparoscopically, patient education is paramount to provide realistic expectations. All complications should be discussed, with emphasis on postoperative pain, possible seroma formation, risk of enterotomy, and management options, and the risk of conversion to open. These complications are discussed in more detail later.

Routine imaging may not be necessary in most cases, but can be performed at the discretion of the surgeon. For complex hernias, including recurrent hernias or those along the abdominal borders, knowing the proximity to viscera or bony landmarks may be useful in planning the approach for mesh fixation.

SURGICAL TECHNIQUE
Preparation

A mechanical bowel preparation may be performed at the discretion of the surgeon, especially if colonic adhesions are expected; however, most surgeons do not routinely prepare their patients for this operation. Sequential compression devices are placed for deep vein thrombosis prophylaxis. In addition, obese and high-risk patients with complex hernias requiring longer operative times may benefit from a preoperative dose of subcutaneous heparin. A prophylactic antibiotic to cover skin flora is given within 1 hour of the incision. Some surgeons use an iodophor adhesive barrier to decrease contact of the mesh with the skin, but many do not believe that this is necessary.

Depending on the location and complexity of the hernia, as well as the anticipated duration of the procedure, a Foley catheter may be placed. It is important to have bladder decompression when repairing lower abdominal hernias. For suprapubic hernias, having a Foley catheter is important, because the catheter allows instillation of fluid such that the bladder anatomy may be identified and dissected free from surrounding structures.

Positioning

Patients are usually placed in the supine position. Arms are tucked for all midabdominal and lower abdominal hernias to facilitate adequate external working space. For upper abdominal hernias, the arms may be placed on arm boards. For flank hernias, a bump on the ipsilateral side may improve visualization. Patients should be adequately padded and secured to the operating table such that tilting from side to side or in a Trendelenburg/reverse Trendelenburg fashion can be accomplished; such gravity retraction of visceral contents is often helpful.

Access

Access can be obtained by either an open or closed technique. Most surgeons prefer creation of a pneumoperitoneum with a Veress needle followed by entrance into the abdomen with an optical trocar. This approach can facilitate rapid initial entry without creating large cut-down incisions. However, placement of a Veress needle in a reoperative abdomen may be difficult and requires familiarity with this technique. Alternatively, an open method with a direct cut-down may be used. Both access methods are suitable and the choice should be left to the discretion of the surgeon.

The position of the first trocar should be guided by previous abdominal surgeries and the location of the hernia, in an attempt to anticipate and maximally avoid intraabdominal adhesions. The location should be at least several centimeters from all previous scars and as far from the hernia as possible, but still providing suitable instrument reach. Often, for midabdominal and lower abdominal hernias, the first trocar is optimally placed in the left (or right) upper quadrant subcostally in the miclavicular line. At such a location, the peritoneum is suspended from the costal margin, facilitating Veress needle insertion; In addition, adhesions are sparse, especially in the left subcostal area. For upper abdominal hernias, it may be necessary to access the abdomen in the lower quadrants. Regardless of the location or technique used, great care must be exercised to minimize the risk of complications such as vascular or visceral injuries. Specific to ventral hernia repair, if a visceral injury occurs, the placement of a permanent mesh prosthetic may not be possible, as discussed later.

Port Layout

For port layout (**Fig. 1**), it is important to assess the extent of the defect and anticipate the planned coverage area of the mesh to avoid interference between the ports and the mesh during mesh fixation. Once the initial trocar has been placed, the abdomen is explored to visualize the distribution of adhesions, presence of all hernia defects,

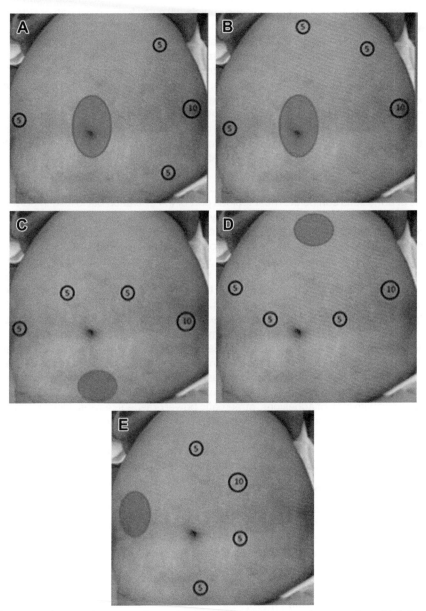

Fig. 1. Port layout. Shown are the author's preferences for port placement for midabdominal (*A, B*), suprapubic (*C*), subxiphoid (*D*), and flank (*E*) hernias (hernia location indicated by larger oval). The 10- mm trocar is used for mesh placement and therefore the location of this port is interchangeable with any of the 5 ports.

and to assess the abdomen for any unexpected incidental findings. This procedure is often best performed with a 30° or 45° laparoscope to adequately view the anterior abdominal wall. The complexity of the hernia dictates how many ports are needed, although a total of 3 or 4 ports is usually sufficient. Ideally, ports need to be placed as lateral as possible when repairing midline defects. This strategy allows better access to the anterior abdominal wall, assisting in lysis of adhesions and mesh fixation. However, ports must also be placed sufficiently away from bony or other external landmarks such that adequate range of motion is afforded. For suprapubic, subxiphoid, or more lateral defects, the port positions vary accordingly, but similar principles are followed. A 10-mm to 12-mm trocar is usually used for insertion of the mesh. Otherwise, 5-mm ports are adequate for other purposes, including the use of working instruments and camera insertion, if a 5-mm optic is used. Ports are often inserted sequentially, because lysis of adhesions permits sufficient visualization. Additional ports can be added if needed for dense adhesions. Although many hernias can be repaired using only 3 trocars, it is our preference for hernias located in the central portion of the abdomen (see **Fig. 1**A, B) to routinely use a fourth trocar located directly opposite the primary working ports to facilitate mesh fixation on the opposite side.

Lysis of Adhesions

Lysis of adhesions can be the most tedious part of the operation but is also important, because significant adverse outcomes may result if complications occur and are not recognized; this is especially true if a missed enterotomy occurs. Ideally, all dissection should be performed sharply using laparoscopic scissors. Electrocautery or other energy sources such as ultrasonic shears or bipolar coagulation devices should be avoided unless the surgeon has confirmed that bowel is not in the field of dissection. Thermal injuries may not be evident at the time of adhesiolysis, because coagulation devices may temporarily seal the edges of bowel with a delayed presentation of the enterotomy. In addition, if energy sources are used, the surgeon should remain extremely cautious, because the tip of some devices remains heated for a period. If a device is subsequently used for blunt dissection, contact between the instrument and the viscera may result in a thermal injury, even if the device is not activated. Accordingly, it may be advantageous to use nonthermal methods for hemostasis if bleeding is encountered; sutures or clips may be used for this purpose.

To assist with lysis of adhesions, atraumatic bowel graspers may be used to provide gentle traction to the bowel. Excessive traction can lead to deserosalization or bowel injury; hence, appropriate handling of the bowel is important. If there are dense adhesions between the abdominal wall or previous mesh and bowel, the mesh or part of the fascia can be excised and left attached to the bowel (**Fig. 2**).

Reduction of Hernia Contents

Atraumatic graspers should be used to gradually reduce the hernia contents. While applying gentle traction, adhesive bands can be released by sharply dividing them. Manual pressure applied externally may help in reduction. The hernia sac is normally left in situ and not excised. However, it may be necessary to excise a portion of the sac if bowel is closely adherent. If the hernia cannot be reduced, conversion to an open repair is necessary.

Management of Inadvertent Enterotomy

Bowel injury may occur during adhesiolysis. If a true enterotomy is not made and only a serosal injury has occurred, then the bowel can be oversewn laparoscopically, depending on the skill set of the surgeon. In this case, the lumen is not entered and

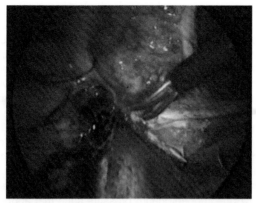

Fig. 2. Laparoscopic adhesiolysis. In this case, the bowel was densely adhered to the abdominal wall. Rather than risking an enterotomy, part of the fascia was left attached to the bowel.

there is no contamination; it is usually acceptable to proceed with mesh placement. If a full-thickness injury occurs, subsequent management depends on several factors, including the defect size, amount of spillage, and surgeon experience. In this situation, there should be a low threshold for converting to an open operation if such an approach is needed to ensure adequate repair of the injury. If an open approach is used, then the hernia may be repaired either primarily or by implanting a biological mesh.[8] However, several laparoscopic options have also been described. It may be possible to repair the injury laparoscopically, complete the adhesiolysis, and delay the hernia repair. For this protocol, the patient is admitted to the hospital, kept on antibiotics, and returned to the operating room in 2 to 6 days for laparoscopic mesh placement.[9,10] In select cases with minimal or no spillage, several reports documented successful outcomes after proceeding with synthetic mesh placement after laparoscopic repair of the enterotomy during the same operation.[11,12]

Providing Clearance for Mesh

To ensure adequate overlap of mesh, additional clearance may be necessary. A minimum of 3 cm of mesh overlap is considered acceptable. Because most meshes are associated with significant postoperative shrinkage, many experts recommend at least 5 cm of mesh overlap. Adequate overlap may also be important to avoid hernia recurrence if the mesh shifts or moves for any reason. Accordingly, it is optimal to clear the peritoneal surface widely in terms of freeing up adhesions well away from the defect. Normal anatomic fat or other attachments may also require dissection such that the mesh may be positioned directly against the peritoneal surface, thereby enhancing fixation and ingrowth. For hernias near the upper midline, the falciform ligament should be dissected off the abdominal wall; this can usually be achieved with judicious use of electrocautery or other energy sources. For hernias in the lower abdomen, excessive fat on the abdominal wall above the bladder may need to be carefully reflected in a caudal direction to fully expose the muscular wall. Additional exposure and clearance strategies for suprapubic, flank, and subxiphoid hernias are discussed later.

Defect Size Measurement

The size of the defect should be accurately measured such that a suitable piece of mesh may be selected and adequate overlap may be afforded. This procedure can be difficult, because measurements on the external abdominal wall are larger than those taken on the peritoneal surface. This phenomenon exists because of the curved shape of the abdomen and the distance between the inner and outer surfaces. For instance, in obese patients with thick abdominal walls, the internal and external hernia defect size measurements may vary substantially. Accordingly, care must be taken to determine the internal defect size, because mesh is placed at this level. One method is to introduce a ruler into the peritoneal cavity and directly measure the defect (**Fig. 3**). To obtain the most accurate measurements, the pneumoperitoneum is reduced to 5 to 8 mm Hg so that the abdominal wall is minimally stretched. A plastic ruler is usually cut in half lengthwise such that the ruler fits through either a 5 mm or 10 mm trocar. Graspers are used to stretch the ruler taut and measurements in the transverse and longitudinal axes are obtained. Alternatively, spinal needles may be placed percutaneously at the periphery of the defect; the distance between the needles is measured externally with a low pneumoperitoneum pressure such that abdominal wall stretch is minimized. Although the first method requires a moderate degree of skill to manipulate the ruler intracorporeally, it avoids the use of needles and potential inaccuracies associated with external measurements. However, the spinal needle method may be simpler and is preferred by some experts. Regardless of the method, it is critical to identify all hernia defects and to include all defects within the measured distances; this allows the mesh to be sized appropriately to cover all of these areas. For this purpose, it is helpful to mark externally the extent of all defects.

After defect measurement, it is also helpful to create a diagram on the abdominal wall surface to aid mesh placement (**Fig. 4**). Once the defects have been marked, lines are drawn to designate the transverse and longitudinal axes of the repair (centered on the defect area). Next, a line is drawn about 5 cm from the edge of the hernia defect on all sides; this line represents the area that is covered by the mesh. Although it is not necessarily expected that the transfascial sutures all lie on this line, it is expected that all sutures lie in a symmetric fashion in relation to the transverse and longitudinal axes. For most repairs, a symmetric piece of mesh is used and symmetric overlap of the defect is important. If the mesh is off center to any significant extent, then the overlap on 1 side may not be adequate, whereas excessive overlap is afforded on the other side.

In addition, some experts recommend mesh overlap of the entire original incision, even if a hernia is detected in only a portion of an incision; for instance, some surgeons suggest covering an entire lower midline incision even if only a periumbilical defect is identified.[13] Proponents of this approach cite that such incisions are inherently at risk for subsequent hernia formation and that a preemptive repair avoids future hernias.

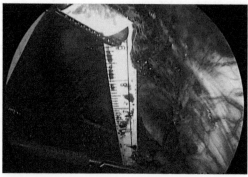

Fig. 3. Defect size measurement. A ruler may be placed intraperitoneally to directly measure the fascial defect. Before measurement, the pneumoperitoneum is reduced to 5 to 8 mm Hg.

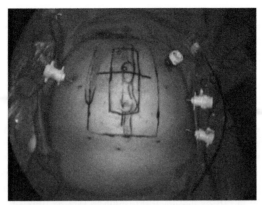

Fig. 4. Abdominal wall diagram. The diagram drawn on the external abdominal wall guides placement of transfascial sutures to ensure symmetric coverage of the defect.

However, providing such additional overlap may require substantially more dissection and may not always be practical if a larger mesh prosthetic is required.

Mesh Selection and Preparation

A mesh prosthetic that is suitable for intraperitoneal placement is required for this repair. Typically a permanent mesh that has an antiadhesion barrier is used. Ideally, these materials promote tissue ingrowth on the abdominal wall side and minimize adhesions to the visceral side. Although only expanded polytetrafluoroethylene (ePTFE) was available when LVHR was first gaining popularity, a variety of suitable meshes are available (**Table 1**). A detailed review of permanent meshes is covered

Table 1
Common prosthetics used for LVHR

Mesh Type (Manufacturer)	Tissue Ingrowth Component	Antiadhesion Barrier Component
Composix E/X (Davol, A Bard Company, Warwick, RI)	PP	ePTFE
Composix L/P (Davol, A Bard Company, Warwick, RI)	PP (lower density)	ePTFE
DUALMESH (W. L. Gore & Associates, Inc, Newark, DE)	ePTFE (~22 μm)	ePTFE (<3 μm)
C-Qur (Atrium Medical Corporation, Hudson, NH)	PP	Omega 3 fatty acid
Proceed (Ethicon, Cincinnati, OH)	PP, encapsulated by PDS	Oxidized regenerated cellulose
Sepramesh IP (Davol, A Bard Company, Warwick, RI)	PP coknitted with PGA	Hydrogel barrier
Pariatex (Covidien, Mansfield, MA)	PET (polyester)	Collagen, PEG, glycerol
Physiomesh (Ethicon, Cincinnati, OH)	PP encapsulated by PDS	Polyglecaprone-25 (monocryl) layer on both sides of PP

Abbreviations: PDS, polydioxanone; PEG, polyethylene glycol; PET, polyethylene terephthalate; PGA, polyglycolic acid; PP, polypropylene.

in a separate article elsewhere in this issue. However, handling characteristics vary between meshes, and each particular material may have unique advantages and disadvantages. For instance, the antiadhesion barrier on some meshes may be fragile and become dislodged during insertion or manipulation. Some meshes may have sufficiently large interstices to afford visualization of the underlying anatomy, whereas other meshes are completely opaque. Regardless of the specific characteristics, the surgeon should be familiar with the type of mesh being used, such that an optimal repair may be achieved.

The correct size of mesh is chosen based on the size of the hernia defects, as detailed earlier. It may be necessary to place 2 separate pieces of mesh if the defects are not close; in this case, essentially, 2 different repairs are performed in the same patient. However, if multiple defects or a very large defect are present, it is ideal to select a single piece of mesh large enough to cover all areas of concern. If a sufficiently large piece of mesh is not available, then multiple pieces may be sutured together. However, recurrences may occur if the junction between pieces tears apart.

The mesh should be marked to ensure correct orientation once it is placed intraperitoneally (**Fig. 5**). This strategy is important for routine repairs and becomes especially helpful if the defect is asymmetrical or if the mesh is cut in an asymmetrical fashion to accommodate anatomic considerations. At a minimum, it is recommended that the transverse and longitudinal axes are marked with permanent ink on the mesh. Marks may be placed at the corners and along the periphery of the mesh to designate the planned locations for transfascial suture fixation. Marks may also be used to identify the side designed to be in contact with the viscera.

Four axial sutures are then placed for use in initial suspension of the mesh once it has been placed intra-abdominally. Additional sutures may be placed in the mesh before intra-abdominal placement; however, these may be difficult to manage and are not necessarily recommended for routine repairs. The sutures are placed less than a centimeter from the edge and 3 to 4 knots are thrown. The tails are left at least 12 to 15 cm long. Permanent sutures are most widely used; for instance, many surgeons choose 0-sized polyester sutures. Alternatively, there have been reports of using absorbable sutures to decrease the risk of chronic pain, but this is not widely accepted.

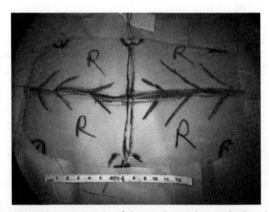

Fig. 5. Mesh preparation. The rough side of the mesh may be marked with an R to designate which side faces the abdominal wall. The vertical axis is marked with arrows. Additional sites for transfascial suture placement have been marked at the corners.

Mesh Insertion

The mesh is then rolled to place it within the abdomen. The antiadhesive barrier (smooth side) is kept protected on the inner aspect such that abrasive forces to this material are minimized. Most surgeons use a 10-mm or 12-mm port for mesh insertion, although some meshes may be placed through a 5-mm port. Direct insertion using a grasper may be feasible. Alternatively, a grasper can be inserted through a 5-mm port and guided out of a 10-mm port, such that the mesh may be pulled into the abdomen; this technique is often easier than trying to push the mesh through the port. Lubrication of the mesh using a water-soluble lubricant and increasing the pneumoperitoneum pressure back to 15 mm Hg may be helpful. Once the mesh is intra-abdominal, it may then be unrolled and oriented appropriately, with the antiadhesive barrier positioned toward the bowel.

Mesh Fixation

The most widely accepted method of mesh fixation is transfascial sutures. Those who advocate transfascial sutures believe that it is necessary to prevent mesh migration, and this practice is widely accepted. There have been reports of fixating mesh with tacks alone to decrease postoperative pain; however, most experts believe that sutures are critical to prevent recurrence.

   The goal of mesh fixation is to suspend the mesh with equal overlap over all hernia defects and in a taut fashion, with no wrinkles or folds. This strategy aims to maximize mesh coverage of the defect and to obviate the chance of mesh protruding into the defect. Accordingly, the pneumoperitoneum pressure is set at 5 to 8 mm Hg to minimize stretch on the abdominal wall. The mesh is then suspended and held taut using graspers to identify the retrieval locations for the first 2 axial sutures; typically the longitudinal axis is suspended first, because this tends to be the longer of the 2 axes. These locations are referenced to the previously drawn diagram on the skin surface to ensure that all defects are equally covered. Stab incisions are made in the skin and the sutures previously placed in the mesh are brought externally through the abdominal wall with a transfascial suture retrieval device (**Fig. 6**). These sutures may be held externally with a hemostat, but grasping the suture at any part that will remain in the patient should be avoided to prevent fracturing and weakening of the suture. The sutures of each pair are retrieved individually and should encompass a 1-cm-wide bite

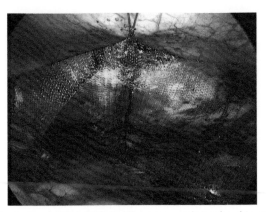

Fig. 6. Transfascial suture retrieval. Stab incisions are made in the skin and the sutures are brought externally with a transfascial suture device.

of fascia such that a horizontal mattress configuration is achieved; larger bites should be avoided, because they may be associated with an increased risk of pain, either by creating an increased area of compression on the muscular tissue or via entrapment of nerves innervating the cutaneous tissue. To avoid the latter situation, it may also be helpful to orient retrieval of the sutures in a transverse fashion, such that fixation is accomplished in a manner parallel to the path of cutaneous nerves. Once the first set of axial sutures has been determined to be suitable, they are tied down, with care being taken to push the knots down through the subcutaneous tissue; the knots should lie directly against the anterior fascia and air knots should be avoided. The second set of axial sutures may be retrieved and secured in a similar fashion. Care is again taken to identify suitable locations for retrieval of this second set, ensuring equal overlap of all defects.

Tacks are then placed circumferentially around the mesh at approximately 1-cm intervals and within 2 to 5 mm of the edge to prevent the bowel from becoming incarcerated between the mesh and abdominal wall (**Fig. 7**). Many surgeons use additional tacks to provide further mesh fixation to the peritoneal surface. A second row of tacks may be placed at approximately 2-cm intervals and 2 cm from the edge (see **Fig. 7**) for this purpose. Such additional fixation may aid in stabilizing the mesh during subsequent passage of additional transfascial sutures. Some surgeons suggest that additional tack fixation may also help eliminate dead space and decrease the size or incidence of postoperative seroma formation. To assist in tack placement, external pressure is applied to the abdominal wall; ideally, the abdominal wall is manipulated such that the peritoneal surface becomes relatively parallel to the end of the tacking device. Such an orientation avoids skiving and fosters secure tack placement. Tacks are placed in 1 quadrant of the mesh at a time. Subsequently, the opposing quadrant of mesh is stretched and fixated in a similar fashion. Care is taken to prevent stretching the mesh overzealously in 1 direction over another, because doing so can favor overlap of 1 area over another.

Permanent or absorbable tacks may be used, at the discretion of the operating surgeon. One of the most widely used permanent tacks consists of titanium helical fasteners, which are 3.8 mm long and are deployed using a 5-mm disposable instrument. This construct provides 2.8 mm of tissue penetration using most currently available meshes, which have a thickness of about 1 mm. This degree of penetration equates to the construct anchoring fully into the peritoneal layer but minimally into

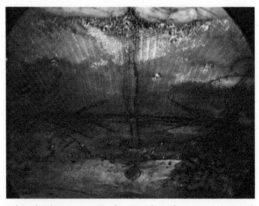

Fig. 7. Circumferential tack placement. Tacks are placed at 1-cm intervals at the perimeter of the mesh. A second row may also be placed.

the myofascial layers.[3] For this reason, many surgeons do not believe that tack fixation should be relied on for long-term prevention of mesh migration. The advantages of absorbable tacks, at least theoretically, include possibly fewer adhesions and less pain. For instance, titanium is an adhesiogenic material and often at least flimsy adhesions to these tacks are visualized during reoperations. In addition, although penetration is minimal, the potential for nerve damage exists in some locations. However, some surgeons believe that currently available absorbable tacks do not offer sufficiently robust fixation because of their technical design, and such devices are often more expensive.

As mentioned earlier, most surgeons suggest that placement of additional transfascial sutures is important to providing the repair with long-term durability. Additional sutures are usually placed every 5 cm around the perimeter of the mesh (**Fig. 8**). The number of sutures may be modified according to the degree of concern over hernia recurrence and the specific type of hernia. For instance, placement of numerous sutures may be useful if wide overlap is not feasible, or in patients who are smokers or obese. Similarly, additional suture fixation may help prevent mesh bulging or dislodgement in the setting of large solitary defects; this is in contrast to Swiss cheese defects, which present a diminished tendency for the mesh to protrude into the defect postoperatively.

Once the mesh has been fixated, the adequacy of the repair may be evaluated intraoperatively. The axial markings on the mesh should lie essentially at the center of the defects. If a concern exists as to inadequate overlap, an additional piece of mesh may be implanted and fixated to strengthen the repair. However, it is preferable to plan and execute the initial repair in a successful fashion to avoid this situation.

Closure

After completion of mesh fixation, the abdominal cavity is evaluated for signs of bleeding or other complications. The 10-mm trocar site is closed either laparoscopically or in an open fashion, although this may not be necessary if a dilating (noncutting) trocar is used. It is important to use a hemostat or other instrument to elevate the skin of each of the stab incisions made for transfascial suture placement. This strategy prevents skin dimpling. The pneumoperitoneum is released. The port

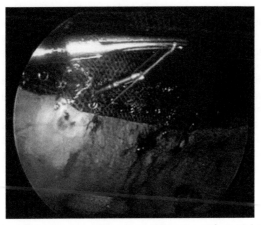

Fig. 8. Additional transfascial suture placement. After circumferential tacking, additional transfascial sutures are placed every 3 to 5 cm.

incision sites are then closed with interrupted or running subcuticular sutures. A liquid skin adhesive or adhesive strips are then placed over the port sites and the stab incisions.

HERNIAS IN DIFFICULT LOCATIONS

Laparoscopic repair of defects located at the periphery of the abdomen may present unique challenges with regard to exposure and mesh fixation, but may be feasible depending on the level of surgeon experience and specific patient factors. General strategies for repair of such defects are discussed in detail in a separate article elsewhere in this issue. A few concepts that are most relevant to laparoscopic repairs are described in the following sections.

Subxiphoid

The proximity of subxiphoid hernias to the diaphragm and ribs challenge fixation of the mesh. As with most upper abdominal hernias, the falciform ligament must be dissected for adequate exposure. Transfascial suture fixation is not advised above the costal margin for fear of pneumothorax or intercostal nerve entrapment. The caudal and lateral aspects of the mesh are fixated in a traditional fashion, with transfascial sutures placed through the muscular and fascial layers of the abdomen. The cephalad portion of the mesh may be partially fixated by placing several transfascial sutures to the rim of fascia (or periosteum) that is usually present adjacent to the xiphoid and central costal margins. A wide overlap of mesh is then created cephalad to the defect internally, such that the superior border of mesh reaches 8 to 10 cm above the costal margin, overlapping the diaphragm. This portion of the mesh may be fixated to the diaphragm by careful laparoscopic placement of sutures; alternatively, the use of fibrin sealants has been reported.[14–16]

Lumbar/Flank

Flank hernias are frequently associated with urologic or other retroperitoneal procedures. They occur between the costal margin and iliac crest, often close to adjacent viscera and bony landmarks, including the ribs, pelvis, and spine. Lateral positioning of the patient is usually required to provide access to the paraspinous muscles.

Depending on the location of the defect, a peritoneal flap along with medial mobilization of the colon may be necessary. The plane between the retroperitoneal organs and paraspinal musculature is developed. Points of fixation should be planned according to the defect. For lower defects, the mesh may be fixed to the Cooper ligament or to the iliac crest periosteum. Tacks and transfascial sutures are placed superior to the iliopubic tract, avoiding the triangle of pain.

For more superior defects near the costal margin, fixation can be applied to a rim of fascia just below the costal margin, with mesh overlapping cephalad, as in the subxiphoid repair. Bone anchoring has also been described. Transfascial sutures are placed along the paraspinous muscle in the standard fashion.[17] Most experts suggest using wide overlap of mesh beyond the points of fixation in the areas where the hernia abuts bony landmarks. Overlapping portions of mesh in areas that cannot be directly fixated can often be held in place by closure of the peritoneal flap initially used to gain exposure.

Suprapubic

Suprapubic hernias are seen after previous pelvic surgery and are often associated with extensive scar tissue involving the bladder, colon, or rectum; not all cases may be amenable to laparoscopic approaches. For patients deemed suitable candidates, caution must be exercised during the dissection to avoid injuring the bladder, iliac vessels, or other nearby structures. To assist in identifying the bladder, it may be helpful to instill approximately 200 cc of saline into the bladder through a Foley catheter. The proximal and lateral borders of the bladder can then be identified. Peritoneal flaps are created to mobilize the bladder off the anterior abdominal wall in a manner similar to a transabdominal preperitoneal laparoscopic inguinal hernia repair. Once initial mobilization is completed, the bladder is decompressed to provide working space.

The Cooper ligament and the pubic bone are then exposed and serve as points of mesh fixation. It is considered essential to provide 3 to 5 cm of mesh overlap posterior to the pubic bone.[18,19] Transfascial sutures are placed to anchor the mesh to the periosteum or fascia directly adjacent to the pubis, and tacks are most often used for fixation to Cooper ligaments bilaterally. Alternatively, bone anchors may be used. Once the cephalad and lateral portions of the mesh are fixated using transfascial sutures placed through the abdominal wall in a traditional fashion, the peritoneal flap is closed and serves to hold the posterior overlapping piece of mesh in the appropriate location.

RECURRENT HERNIAS

Before repair of a recurrent ventral hernia with previous mesh placement, it is beneficial to review all available operative notes and consider computed tomography (CT) imaging to help guide the approach. The old mesh can be left in place or excised, depending on several factors. If the mesh is not palpable and well incorporated, it can be left in situ. If the mesh is partially unincorporated or has a curled-up edge, a portion of the mesh may be excised. If the mesh is bulky, it may be useful to excise a portion of the mesh to facilitate a flat layout of the new mesh repair, in hopes of achieving suitable tissue ingrowth (**Fig. 9**). For mesh that is palpable externally and bothersome to the patient, it may be possible to excise this portion of the mesh laparoscopically; however, an open repair many be needed. If a piece of mesh is densely adherent to the bowel, a small piece of mesh may be excised and left attached to the bowel to prevent deserosalization or an enterotomy.

POSTOPERATIVE CARE

The size and complexity of the hernia dictates the postoperative care. For small defects, it may be possible to discharge the patient home on the same day. However,

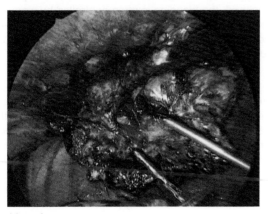

Fig. 9. Excision of old mesh.

for most hernias and for larger hernias and those requiring extensive lysis of adhesions, patients may require several days of hospitalization. Pain can initially be intense from the transfascial sutures, requiring intravenous (IV) narcotics for the first 24 hours. Oral medications and IV antiinflammatories may also be used. Other adjuncts include muscle relaxants such as cyclobenzaprine or diazepam to relieve muscle spasms related to suture sites.

Diet may be advanced as tolerated in most cases, depending on the surgeon's preference and the extent of adhesiolysis; a clear liquid diet may be started immediately after surgery for most cases. Routine postoperative care includes early ambulation, subcutaneous low-molecular-weight heparin, sequential compression devices, and incentive spirometry. An abdominal binder is placed postoperatively, and the patient is advised to wear it for 3 to 14 days, which may decrease the size and duration of seromas.[20] Patients are discharged when tolerating a regular diet, and pain is controlled on oral medications. Pain medications may need to be continued for up to several weeks postoperatively, because improvement is often a slow but steady process. Patients are encouraged to resume normal activity after surgery, but advised not to lift heavy objects (>9.07 kg [20 lbs]) or engage in strenuous activities for 4 to 6 weeks.

COMPLICATIONS
Bleeding

Intraoperative bleeding most often is seen with insertion of the trocars, adhesiolysis, or mesh fixation and is usually controlled with simple measures. Trocar bleeding usually resolves with tamponade from the trocar itself. However, if it continues after removal, a suture placement or electrocautery may be necessary.

During adhesiolysis, in an attempt to avoid thermal injury to the surrounding viscera, bleeding may occur from the cut omentum or adhesive bands. A suction irrigator may be necessary to identify bleeding locations, especially if substantial raw omental surfaces are present. If no bowel is close, points of bleeding can be controlled carefully using a thermal energy device such as electrocautery or ultrasonic shears. However, it may be necessary to apply clips or use suture ligation if the source of bleeding is close to visceral structures. Similarly, if the bleeding source is on the bowel or mesentery, suture ligation may be the most prudent means of achieving hemostasis.

During mesh fixation, an attempt should be made to identify the epigastric vessels to avoid injury during passage of transfascial fixation sutures or placement of tacks. If these vessels are injured, the bleeding is often controlled by simply tying the suture. They may also be ligated by placing additional simple or figure-of-eight transfascial sutures. Before completion of the procedure, the abdomen should be inspected to ensure that adequate hemostasis has been achieved.

Intestinal Injury

The management of a recognized injury was discussed earlier. The reported incidence of an incidental enterotomy is between 1% and 3%, which is higher than that reported for open ventral hernia repairs.[8] It is therefore paramount that surgeons are vigilant in preventing, recognizing, and treating this potentially lethal complication. An unrecognized enterotomy has been reported to occur in 0.33% of repairs.[9] Leblanc reported that the mortality of an uncomplicated ventral hernia was reported as 0.05%; this increased to 1.7% with a recognized enterotomy and to 7.7% with an unrecognized injury. Presentation may include increasing pain, abdominal distention, or signs of sepsis such as tachycardia, fever, hypotension, or decreased urine output. Diagnostic studies may be indicated, depending on the clinical scenario, but the surgeon should not hesitate to take the patient directly to the operating room if a bowel injury is suspected. At exploration, if contamination is found, a laparotomy may be necessary to repair the injury, wash out the abdomen, and remove the mesh; a primary abdominal closure or an alternative method, such as absorbable or biological mesh placement, may be performed.

Seromas

Because the hernia sac is left in place and drains are not traditionally used during a laparoscopic hernia repair, most patients develop a seroma postoperatively. In the early postoperative period, fluid fills the space between the mesh and the skin and slowly becomes resorbed as scar tissue forms and obliterates this cavity. As a preventative measure, most surgeons place an abdominal binder to compress the hernia sac area starting immediately postoperatively and continuing for at least 2 weeks. This strategy may decrease the size and duration of seromas, but most patients still have one. Most seromas are asymptomatic and resolve spontaneously. A study by Susmallian and colleagues[21] followed 20 consecutive patients with routine ultrasound examinations over a 90-day period. Although seromas formed in 100% of patients, only 35% were detectable on physical examination. This study documented that the peak in seroma volume was at 7 days and that 80% of the seromas resolved by 90 days. Other studies have reported an incidence of 0.7% to 12% for persistent or symptomatic seromas.[5,9,22] The higher percentage reported in some studies is likely because many surgeons do not consider a seroma as a complication unless an intervention such as aspiration is required. Most experts recommend the avoidance of aspiration, because even using sterile conditions poses a risk of contamination of an otherwise sterile fluid collection in contact with the mesh prosthetic. Instead, patients are reassured that most collections resolve, and a CT scan may be obtained if there is any concern over a recurrence. Aspiration may be considered in patients with significant symptoms of pain or pressure or with persistent seromas after 3 months of observation, but in practice this is rarely needed.

Persistent Pain

Even although a large incision is not used, LVHR may be associated with significant abdominal pain, which is usually muscular in nature and related to mesh fixation using transfascial sutures and tacks. As mentioned earlier, patients may require analgesics or muscle relaxants for the first few weeks postoperatively. Significant pain persisting beyond the first 6 to 12 weeks is rare, with several studies indicating an incidence of 1% to 2%.[23–25] The pain is usually located at 1 of the suture sites, may be relatively intense, and is exacerbated with physical activity. In this case, conservative treatment is indicated and is likely be successful. If further treatment is needed, injection therapy may be useful using local anesthetics.[5,26] Cobb and colleagues[5] recommended injecting the site with 25 to 30 mL of 0.25% bupivacaine with 1:200,000 epinephrine and 1% lidocaine using a 22-gauge needle. Although rarely required, exploratory laparoscopy with removal of tacks or transfascial sutures has been described with success. Other potential causes of persistent pain include a seroma or hernia recurrence; CT scan imaging may be indicated if the diagnosis is not clinically evident.

Wound and Mesh Infections

Most wound complications after LVHR are seromas, and infections are rare. In a meta-analysis (N = 4582 LVHRs) published by Pierce and colleagues,[25] the overall wound complications were reported as 3.8% to 5.3%, which did not include seromas. These investigators reported an incidence of wound infections in only 1.3% to 2.3% of patients, and mesh infections in only 0.9% to 1.3% of patients. This incidence includes data from the study by Heniford and colleagues[22] (N = 819 LVHRs), which reported an overall infection rate of 1.8%, including both wound and mesh infections.

Because trocar sites are usually located remotely in relation to the mesh, infections at these locations may be treated with packing and antibiotics, with minimal risks of involvement of the mesh. For the mesh to become infected is a rare event. CT imaging may show gas and fluid collections, with extensive inflammatory changes. Such circumstances usually require open abdominal exploration, with identification of any concomitant intra-abdominal complications, washout and drainage, and mesh removal. In select cases, some investigators have described management of limited mesh infections with percutaneous or open drainage and prolonged antibiotics with salvage of the mesh.[27–29] However, most infected meshes require excision.

Recurrence

Recurrence rates associated with LVHR have been acceptably low. Several studies have shown better results for laparoscopic repairs compared with open repairs. In the meta-analysis by Pierce and colleagues,[25] the recurrence rates for paired laparoscopic (N = 619) versus open (N = 758) cases was 3.1% and 12.1%, respectively. In a meta-analysis by Forbes and colleagues[30] comparing 8 randomized controlled trials evaluating laparoscopic versus open repair, the recurrence rates were similar at 3.4% and 3.6%, respectively.

Several factors have been shown to increase the risk of recurrence. As would be expected, recurrent hernias, larger defects, and morbid obesity are associated with an increased risk of recurrence.[22] In a retrospective review of 270 LVHRs, Cobb and colleagues[5] reported an overall recurrence rate of 4.7%. Patients with a body mass index (BMI), calculated as weight in kilograms divided by the square of height in meters, of less than 40 (N = 225) had a recurrence rate of 3.5% to 4.5%, compared with 9.4% in patients with a BMI greater than 40 (N = 52). Patients with previous hernia repairs (N = 257) had a recurrence rate of 7.3% compared with 2.2% for initial repairs (N = 138). Technical factors known to correlate with decreased recurrence include adequate exposure of the defect with the mesh in contact with the fascia, appropriate overlap, and adequate fixation.

Most experts advocate the use of transfascial sutures as a critical step in preventing recurrence. Some investigators have reported low recurrence rates using tacks only.[12,31–33] They advocate this technique to decrease the risk of persistent pain that has been associated with transfascial suture fixation. However, other expert surgeons have reported high recurrences early in their career with the use of only tacks.[22,24] Therefore, most experts advise transfascial fixation.

SUMMARY

LVHR has established itself as a well-accepted option in the treatment of hernias. Clear benefits have been established regarding the superiority of LVHR in terms of fewer wound infections compared with open repairs. Meticulous technique and appropriate patient selection are critical to obtain the reported results.

REFERENCES

1. LeBlanc KA, Booth WV. Laparoscopic repair of incisional abdominal hernias using expanded polytetrafluoroethylene: preliminary findings. Surg Laparosc Endosc 1993;3:39–41.

2. Colavita PD, Tsirline VB, Belyansky I, et al. Prospective, long-term comparison of quality of life in laparoscopic versus open ventral hernia repair. Ann Surg 2012; 256:714–23.
3. Jin J, Rosen MJ. Laparoscopic verses open ventral hernia repair. Surg Clin North Am 2008;88:1083–100.
4. Franklin ME, Trevino JM, Portillo G, et al. The use of porcine small intestinal submucosa as a prosthetic material for laparoscopic hernia repair in infected and potentially contaminated fields: long-term follow-up. Surg Endosc 2008;22: 1941–6.
5. Cobb WS, Kercher KW, Matthews BD, et al. Laparoscopic ventral hernia repair: a single center experience. Hernia 2006;10:236–42.
6. Tsereteli Z, Pryor BA, Heniford BT, et al. Laparoscopic ventral hernia repair in morbidly obese patients. Hernia 2008;12:233–8.
7. Newcomb WL, Polhil JL, Chen AY, et al. Staged hernia repair preceded by gastric bypass for the treatment of morbidly obese patients with complex ventral hernias. Hernia 2008;12:465–9.
8. LeBlanc KA, Elieson MJ, Corder JM III. Enterotomy and mortality rates of laparoscopic incisional and ventral hernia repair: a review of the literature. JSLS 2007; 11:408–14.
9. LeBlanc KA. Laparoscopic incisional and ventral hernia repair; complications–how to avoid and handle. Hernia 2004;8:323–31.
10. Berger D, Bientzle M, Müller A. Postoperative complications after laparoscopic incisional hernia repair. Surg Endosc 2002;16:1720–3.
11. Heniford TB, Park A, Ramshaw BJ, et al. Laparoscopic ventral and incisional hernia repair in 407 patients. J Am Coll Surg 2000;190:645–50.
12. Carbajo MA, Martp del Olmo JC, Blanco JI, et al. Laparoscopic approach to incisional hernia. Surg Endosc 2003;17:118–22.
13. Wassenaar EB, Schoenmaeckers EJ, Raymakers JT, et al. Recurrences after laparoscopic repair of ventral and incisional hernia: lessons learned from 505 repairs. Surg Endosc 2009;23(4):825–32.
14. Ferrari GC, Miranda A, Sansonna F, et al. Laparoscopic repair of incisional hernias located on the abdominal borders. Surg Laparosc Endosc Percutan Tech 2009;19:348–52.
15. Eisenberg D, Popescu WM, Duffy AJ, et al. Laparoscopic treatment of subxiphoid incisional hernias in cardiac transplant patients. JSLS 2008;12:262–6.
16. Losanoff JE, Basson MD, Laker S, et al. Subxiphoid incisional hernias after median sternotomy. Hernia 2007;11:473–9.
17. Edwards C, Geiger T, Bartow K, et al. Laparoscopic transperitoneal repair of flank hernias: a retrospective review of 27 patients. Surg Endosc 2009;23:2692–6.
18. Carbonell AM, Kercher KW, Matthews BD, et al. The laparoscopic repair of suprapubic ventral hernias. Surg Endosc 2005;19:174–7.
19. Palanivelu C, Rangarajan M, Parthasarathi R, et al. Laparoscopic repair of suprapubic incisional hernias: suturing and intraperitoneal composite mesh onlay. Hernia 2008;12:251–6.
20. Chowbey RK, Sharma A, Khullar R, et al. Laparoscopic ventral hernia repair. J Laparoendosc Adv Surg Tech A 2000;10:79–84.
21. Susmallian S, Gewurtz G, Ezri T, et al. Seroma after laparoscopic repair of hernia with PTFE patch: is it really a complication? Hernia 2001;5:139–41.
22. Heniford BT, Park A, Ramshaw BJ, et al. Laparoscopic repair of ventral hernias: nine years' experience with 850 consecutive hernias. Ann Surg 2003;238: 391–9.

23. Bageacu S, Blanc P, Breton C, et al. Laparoscopic repair of incisional hernias. Surg Endosc 2002;16:345–8.
24. LeBlanc KA, Whitaker JM, Bellanger DE, et al. Laparoscopic incisional and ventral hernioplasty: lessons learned from 200 patients. Hernia 2003;7:118–24.
25. Pierce RA, Spitler JA, Frisella MM, et al. Pooled data analysis of laparoscopic vs. open ventral hernia repair: 14 years of patient data accrual. Surg Endosc 2007; 21:378–86.
26. Carbonell AM, Harold KL, Mahmutovic A, et al. Local injection for the treatment of suture site pain after laparoscopic ventral hernia repair. Am Surg 2003;69: 688–92.
27. Paton BL, Novitsky YW, Zerey M, et al. Management of infections of polytetrafluoroethylene-based mesh. Surg Infect (Larchmt) 2007;8(3):337–41.
28. Trunzo JA, Ponsky JL, Jin J, et al. A novel approach for salvaging infected prosthetic mesh after ventral hernia repair. Hernia 2009;13:545–9.
29. Collage RD, Rosengart MR. Abdominal wall infections with in situ mesh. Surg Infect (Larchmt) 2010;11(3):311–8.
30. Forbes SS, Eskicioglu C, McLeod RS, et al. Meta-analysis of randomized controlled trials comparing open and laparoscopic ventral and incisional hernia repair with mesh. Br J Surg 2009;96:851–8.
31. Sanchez LJ, Bencini L, Moretti R. Recurrences after laparoscopic ventral hernia repair: results and critical review. Hernia 2004;8:138–42.
32. Baccari P, Nifosi J, Ghirardelli L, et al. Laparoscopic incisional and ventral hernia repair without sutures: a single-center experience with 200 cases. J Laparoendosc Adv Surg Tech A 2009;19(2):175–9.
33. Olmi S, Scaini A, Cesana GC, et al. Laparoscopic versus open incisional hernia repair. Surg Endosc 2007;21:555–9.

Open Ventral Hernia Repair with Component Separation

Eric M. Pauli, MD[a], Michael J. Rosen, MD[b],*

KEYWORDS

- Ventral hernia • Incisional hernia • Abdominal wall reconstruction
- Retromuscular hernia repair • Transversus abdominis release (TAR)
- Rives-Stoppa technique

KEY POINTS

- Incisional hernias are the most common complication after laparotomy and the most common indication for reoperation after laparotomy.
- Recent advancements in mesh technology and technical refinements in the methods of herniorraphy have dramatically changed the way open hernia surgery is conducted.
- Abdominal wall reconstructive procedures, which typically include separation of the abdominal wall layers and release of one or more myofascial planes, require a clear understanding of the anatomy of the abdominal wall.
- The authors' favored approach to open ventral hernia repair is a posterior component separation (retrorectus dissection with release of the transversus abdominis aponeurosis and muscle) with sublay of appropriately selected mesh between layers of vascularized tissues and subsequent reconstruction of the linea alba.
- Retromuscular hernia repairs have been shown in multiple studies to have a low recurrence rate (3%–6%) at long-term follow-up and have been accepted as the gold standard technique for open ventral hernia repair by the American Hernia Society.

INTRODUCTION

Despite improved outcomes in many other areas of surgery, abdominal wall hernia formation still complicates 11% to 50% of all laparotomies.[1–6] It remains the most common complication following laparotomy and is the most common indication for reoperation by a 3:1 margin over bowel obstruction.[7] With more than 2 million laparotomies performed in the United States annually, general surgeons are faced with

Disclosures: Eric Pauli is a speaker for Bard and Synthes. Michael Rosen is a speaker for Covidien, Bard, and Lifecell. He receives research support from Lifecell, Davol, W.L. Gore, and Cook.
^a Department of Surgery, Penn State Hershey Medical Center, 500 University Drive, H149, Hershey, PA 17036, USA; ^b Department of Surgery, Case Comprehensive Hernia Center, University Hospitals Case Medical Center, 11100 Euclid Avenue, Cleveland, OH 44106, USA
* Corresponding author.
E-mail address: michael.rosen@uhhospitals.org

epidemic numbers of patients requiring ventral herniorraphy.[8] A reliable method with a low recurrence rate is still clearly necessary for the estimated 200,000 patients undergoing ventral hernia repairs annually.[9]

Traditional methods of hernia repair have unacceptably high recurrence rates.[10,11] Primary open suture repair of ventral hernias with simple fascial reapproximation results in recurrence rates in excess of 50% in long-term follow-up.[6,12–19] Fifty-five years ago, the mesh herniorraphy was introduced.[20] The principle of a tension-free mesh reinforced herniorraphy has undergone technical refinements since this time and is still considered to be the gold standard repair.[11,21] Despite the widespread implementation of this "gold standard," the addition of mesh to open repairs still results in long-term recurrence rates as high as 32%.[17–19] Moreover, the ideal method of mesh implantation is the subject of ongoing debate.

With the advent of laparoscopic ventral hernia repair in 1993, minimally invasive techniques became the preferential method for many surgeons.[22] Intuitively, these repairs had the advantage: they provided wide mesh overlap of the hernia defect without significant soft tissue dissection. Short-term data suggested decreased morbidity and a lower recurrence rate.[23] Sadly, these data were not borne out in the long term, where recurrence rates in well-selected populations still reach 14% to 17%.[24–27] As a consequence, one of the most pressing controversies of ventral hernia repair is whether to approach the problem in an open or laparoscopic fashion.[11]

Parallel with the evolution of laparoscopic ventral hernia repair, novel methods of abdominal component separation were being developed. In 1990, Ramirez and colleagues[28] originally described techniques of medial fascial advancement to aid in definitive reconstruction. In their components separation, Ramirez and colleagues[28] first released the posterior rectus sheath. In 30% of their patients, this was insufficient to permit midline closure, and they therefore created large skin flaps to expose and release the external oblique muscle. Recurrence rates after such component separation hernia repairs range from 10% to 22%, with mean follow-up periods of 9.5 months to 4.5 years.[29–31] Modifications of these myofascial advancement flaps have been developed to reduce the morbidity incurred by creating these skin flaps (and by default reduce the recurrence rate). Such methods include periumbilical perforator sparing (PUPS) methods, endoscopic release of the external oblique muscle, and, more recently, posterior component separation methods that avoid any skin undermining.[32–38]

Posterior component separation methods are based on the Rives-Stoppa-Wantz retrorectus repair, which used the 6-cm-wide to 8-cm-wide potential space between the posterior rectus sheath and the rectus muscle to permit mesh positioning in a sublay fashion.[39–42] Given its superior track record, this approach was deemed to be the gold standard method for open ventral hernia repair by the American Hernia Society in 2004.[11,38] Although durable, the Rives-Stoppa-Wantz technique does not permit dissection beyond the lateral border of the posterior rectus sheath, making it insufficient to permit adequate mesh overlap and tension-free repair of larger abdominal wall defects.[38,42] Methods to extend this potential space have been described and include preperitoneal dissection, intramuscular plane formation, and release of the transversus abdominis muscle.[35,37,38,43] Using these methods, surgeons have been able to achieve recurrence rates as low as 3% to 6%.[35,36,38,43]

In this article, we describe our current operative technique for open ventral hernia repair using component separation. Although we describe methods of anterior component separation, in our current practice, we primarily use posterior component separation with transversus abdominis release to permit dissection beyond the retrorectus space. This method adheres to the literature supported principles of a tension-free midline fascial closure with wide mesh overlap of mesh positioned in a sublay position. Our experience with this method supports a low recurrence rate and reduced wound morbidity.

PREOPERATIVE PLANNING

Physical Examination
- Defect size, location of prior incisions or stomas, draining sinuses, exposed mesh, skin issues (eg, thinning, ulceration, cellulitis) should all be ascertained from physical examination.

Operative History
- Review of old operative reports is mandatory to identify what types of repairs have been previously attempted, what type of mesh was used (if any), and into which plane it was placed.

Abdominal Wall Imaging
- Computed tomography (CT) of the abdomen and pelvis remains the gold standard preoperative imaging modality for ventral hernia repair. Typically no contrast is required.
- CT scans demonstrate the size and location of the hernia sac(s), identify synthetic mesh as well as signs of mesh infection (fluid collections, inflammatory stranding, sinus tracts), and provide information about the remaining abdominal musculature.
- CT angiography can identify the periumbilical perforating vessels and may help in deciding between classical or PUPS anterior component separation.

Managing Medical Comorbidities
- Comorbidities associated with higher rates of recurrence and complication should be medically optimized; diabetic blood sugar control, cardiac risk factors, obesity, malnutrition, pulmonary function, methicillin-resistant *Staphylococcus aureus* (MRSA) colonization.
- Smoking cessation is an absolute requirement. Supplemental oxygen use also precludes surgery.
- Obese patients, especially those with a body mass index higher than 45, should undergo a medical bariatric evaluation to facilitate weight loss, improve exercise tolerance, reduce protein malnutrition, and possibly steer the patient to surgical weight loss surgery before herniorraphy is attempted.

Preoperative Counseling
- A frank discussion with the patient about the likelihood of one or more complications is part of the informed consent process. Hernia recurrence, mesh infection (and its potential consequences), abdominal compartment syndrome, and requirement for postoperative ventilation are all reviewed.
- We specifically address "unacceptable outcomes" with patients as part of our determination of what mesh (synthetic or biologic) to use. Some patients will accept the risk of synthetic mesh infection or draining sinus for a lower hernia recurrence rate; others will not.

CLINICAL ANATOMY

A thorough understanding of the anatomy of the abdominal wall is mandatory when performing ventral herniorraphy with component separation. This includes not only an understanding of the neurovascular supply to muscle, fat, and skin, but also knowledge of force vectors each of the muscular layers generates. Such knowledge results in the best clinical outcomes by providing a well-vascularized, innervated, and correctly oriented abdominal wall reconstruction.

Normally, 2 vertically oriented rectus abdominis muscles originate at the pubic symphysis and insert on the costal cartilage of ribs 5 to 7. These muscles should lie on either side of the intact, midline linea alba. On each side of the rectus, 3 flat semihorizontally oriented muscles are found layered on one another: the external oblique muscle, the internal oblique muscle, and the transversus abdominis muscle (from superficial to deep). Disruption of the linea alba permits unopposed lateral pull on the recti by the lateral musculature and contributes to increase in size of incisional midline hernias.

At the lateral boarder of the rectus muscle, the aponeurosis of the lateral abdominal muscles alternately separate or fuse to contribute to the rectus sheath. Here, the external oblique aponeurosis and rectus sheath fuse to form the linea semilunaris. Above the arcuate line, the internal oblique aponeurosis splits to contribute to both the anterior and posterior rectus sheaths (**Fig. 1**). Below the arcuate line, the aponeurosis does not split but rather fuses with the external oblique fascia to form the anterior rectus sheath alone (see **Fig. 1**). The transversus abdominis muscle's medial aponeurosis merges with the posterior lamina of the internal oblique to form the posterior sheath. For retrorectus repair, it is important to note that the transversus abdominis does not contribute to the linea semilunaris. Its muscle belly extends medial to the linea semilunaris, behind the rectus muscle, in the upper one-third of the abdomen (**Fig. 2**).

Each rectus muscle receives blood supply from the inferior and superior epigastric arteries as well as intercostal arterial branches that enter the muscle belly laterally. These intercostal branches are also the main blood supply to the lateral musculature. They travel with the thoracoabdominal nerves (branches of T7–T12) in the "neurovascular plane" located between the internal oblique and transversus abdominis muscles. In addition to supplying the lateral abdominal musculature and skin, these branches innervate the rectus muscle posteriorly and slightly medial to the linea semilunaris. Both anterior and posterior component separations are able to preserve these intercostal neurovascular bundles due to their location deep to the internal oblique.

For anterior component separation, where lipocutaneous flaps are created, knowledge of the skin vascularity is also critical. For a classic component separation (external oblique release), transection of the deep epigastric perforating vessels leaves the central abdominal wall without its major blood supply. PUPS component separation preserves these vessels to reduce the risk of ischemia-related wound complications.

CHOICE OF MESH

- For patients with clean wounds, we prefer a large (30.5 × 30.5-cm) lightweight, macroporous, polypropylene mesh. There is emerging evidence that use of this mesh is also acceptable in patients with multiple comorbidities (diabetes, obesity, prior mesh infection) or in clean-contaminated circumstances (fistula takedown, enterotomy closure, small bowel resection, stoma formation or relocation).
- Use of synthetic mesh with an antiadhesive coating can be considered if the viscera will be exposed to the mesh, but this is rarely necessary with either technique to be described.

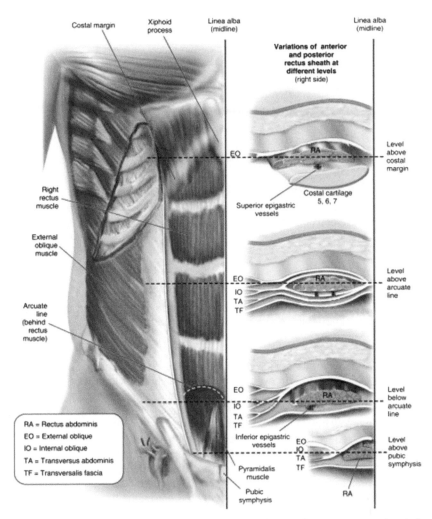

Fig. 1. Normal anatomic positions of the abdominal wall musculature. Cross-sectional views (*left*) show the division and fusion of the lateral muscle fascial sheaths at the linea semilunaris both above and below the arcuate line. (*From* Rosen M, editor. Atlas of abdominal wall reconstruction. New York: Saunders; 2011; with permission.)

- Biologic mesh is appropriately considered for patients with a higher risk of developing a postoperative surgical site infection (SSI). This includes potentially contaminated or contaminated fields, patients with medical comorbidities (diabetes, obesity, immunosuppression, steroid use) or history of MRSA infection.

SURGICAL TECHNIQUE: POSTERIOR COMPONENT SEPARATION

Positioning and Marking
- The patient is positioned in a supine position with arms abducted.
- A Foley catheter and an orogastric tube are placed.
- The abdomen is clipped of hair and is widely sterilized with a 2% chlorhexidine gluconate and 70% isopropyl alcohol solution.

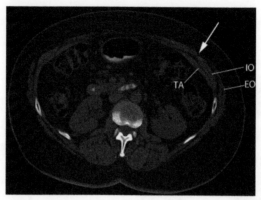

Fig. 2. CT scan of the upper abdomen. Note that the transversus abdominis (TA) muscle does not insert into the lateral boarder of the rectus muscle but rather passes medial to the linea semilunaris (*arrow*) and posterior to the rectus itself. EO, external oblique; IO, internal oblique.

- All old incisions (including old laparoscopic port sites and drain locations) are marked. Excess skin and old scar to be excised are similarly marked.
- An iodophor-impregnated adhesive drape is used.

Incision
- A full midline laparotomy incision is made, with an elliptical skin component to remove old scar, thin skin over the hernia, or ulcerated wounds.
- In the morbidly obese, several other considerations are made:
  - The incision is stopped at the level of the pubis; we do not extend the incision onto or below the pannus where skin care issues may compromise the incision
  - The umbilicus is typically removed during the repair
  - Unless there is a compelling indication, we do not perform a panniculectomy concomitantly with the hernia repair because of the higher risk of SSI.
- Safe access to the abdominal cavity is critical to avoid bowel injury and is best achieved by traversing fascia in an area remote from the hernia (above or below the old incision).

Adhesiolysis and Foreign Body Excision
- Visceral adhesions to the anterior abdominal wall and pelvis are fully lysed. This is critical to allow full medial mobility of the posterior abdominal wall components.
- Care must be taken to avoid excess injury to the posterior layers of the abdominal wall (peritoneum and transversalis fascia) during this portion of the procedure.
- Interloop adhesions are typically ignored unless the patient has a history of adhesive related small bowel obstruction.
- Any encountered foreign bodies (tacks, suture material, old mesh) are fully removed.
- A sterile towel is packed over the viscera to protect them during the component separation.

Retrorectus Dissection
- Using electrocautery, an incision is made in the posterior rectus sheath within 0.5 cm of its medial boarder. This incision is extended superiorly and inferiorly, spanning the entire length of the rectus muscle (**Fig. 3**A).

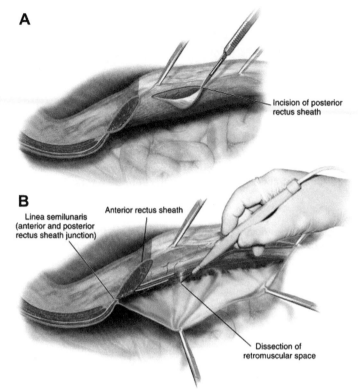

Fig. 3. (*A*) Retrorectus dissection begins by incision of the posterior rectus sheath just medial to the linea alba. (*B*) Electrocautery dissection extends the plane to the linea semilunaris, taking care to preserve the epigastric vessels on the posterior aspect of the rectus muscle. (*From* Rosen M, editor. Atlas of abdominal wall reconstruction. New York: Saunders; 2011; with permission.)

- Working medial to lateral, the plane is continued using blunt and electrocautery dissection. Care must be taken to avoid injury to the epigastric vessels, which should remain with the muscle, not the posterior sheath, during the dissection (see **Fig. 3**B).
- The lateral limit of this dissection is the linea semilunaris at the lateral boarder of the rectus muscle, where the anterior and posterior rectus sheaths fuse (see **Fig. 3**B).
- Identification and preservation of the intercostal neurovascular structures as they enter the posterior aspect of the rectus muscle is crucial.
- Superiorly, this plane is extended into the retroxyphoid/retrosternal space (**Fig. 4**A). Inferiorly, the plane extends into the space of Retzius (see **Fig. 4**B). Blunt dissection in this avascular plane permits exposure to the midline symphysis pubis and Cooper's ligaments bilaterally. Care must be exercised here to avoid injury to the inferior epigastric vessels at their origin on the iliac vessels.

Transversus Abdominis Release
- In many circumstances, dissection in the retrorectus space just to the linea semilunaris is insufficient to permit adequate abdominal wall reconstruction because of the following considerations:
  - Non-midline ventral hernias may occur lateral to this landmark
  - There may be insufficient retrorectus space to permit adequate prosthetic reinforcement of the hernia

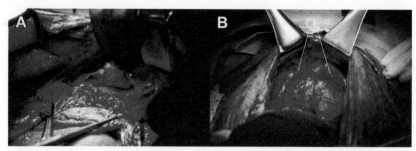

Fig. 4. Extension of the retrorectus plane into the (*A*) retroxyphoid/retrosternal space and (*B*) the space of Retzius. Note the exposure of Coppers ligaments (CL) bilaterally. (*From* Rosen M, editor. Atlas of abdominal wall reconstruction. New York: Saunders; 2011; with permission.)

- ○ There may be insufficient medial advance of both the posterior rectus sheath (to exclude the mesh from the peritoneal cavity) and of rectus muscles (to permit reconstruction of the linea alba anterior to the mesh)
- Methods to extend the retrorectus dissection lateral to the linea semilunaris include intramuscular dissection (by dividing the internal oblique muscle), dissection within the preperitoneal plane, or transversus abdominis release (TAR), which we favor.
- Approximately 0.5 cm medial to the linea semilunaris, electrocautery is used to incise the posterior sheath, exposing the transversus muscle (**Fig. 5**A). This is most easily accomplished in the upper half of the abdomen, where the muscle belly is well defined.
- Using a tonsil (Schnidt) or right-angled clamp to assist dissection, electrocautery is used to hemostatically transect the transversus abdominis muscle (see **Fig. 5**B). Care must be taken to avoid injury to the transversalis fascia/peritoneal layer that lays deep to this.
- Once divided, the muscle can be retracted anteriorly and the avascular retromuscular plane developed bluntly. Superiorly, this plane extends beyond the costal margin to the diaphragm, inferiorly to the myopectineal orifice, and laterally to the psoas muscle.
- The TAR is then completed on the contralateral side.

Reconstruction of Posterior Layer
- The posterior rectus sheath is reapproximated in the midline using running 2-0 polyglycolic acid (vicryl) suture (**Fig. 6**).
- Any holes created in the posterior layer during dissection must be closed; this prevents bowel from contacting the unprotected mesh and prevents bowel from slipping in-between the posterior layer and the mesh, which can result in a bowel obstruction from internal herniation.
- Fenestrations in the posterior layer are common in areas where the abdominal wall has been traversed (laparoscopic port sites, drain sites, old incisions) and below the arcuate line (where there is no transversus abdominis muscle within the posterior layer).
- Small holes that cannot be repaired primarily with suture can be closed with native tissue (omentum, colon epiploicae, hernia sac). Larger holes are best closed by patching the defect with absorbable mesh (vicryl) secured with a running absorbable suture.

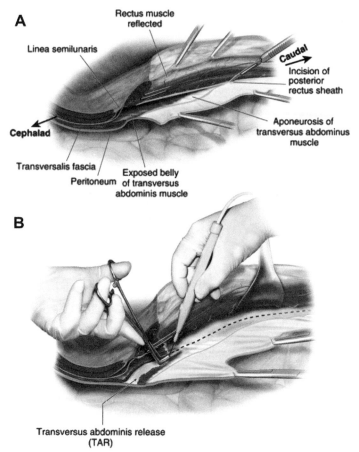

A
Rectus muscle reflected

Linea semilunaris

Caudal

Incision of posterior rectus sheath

Cephalad

Aponeurosis of transversus abdominus muscle

Transversalis fascia

Peritoneum

Exposed belly of transversus abdominis muscle

B

Transversus abdominis release (TAR)

Fig. 5. (*A*) Incision of the posterior rectus sheath exposes the transversus abdominis muscle. (*B*) Transversus abdominis release exposes the transversalis fascia/preperioneal plane, which can be extended to the psoas muscle. (*From* Rosen M, editor. Atlas of abdominal wall reconstruction. New York: Saunders; 2011; with permission.)

- The newly created visceral sac and abdominal wall are irrigated with 3 L of antibiotic lavage solution.

Mesh Placement
- The mesh is turned into a diamond configuration and is anchored inferiorly using a single transfascial stitch just above the pubic ramus or bilateral sutures placed into Cooper's ligaments. We typically use slow-absorbing 0 monofilament absorbable suture (polyglyconate or polydioxanone) to secure the mesh.
- For inferior midline defects, the mesh can be positioned deep in the space of Retzius and the anchoring stitch(es) backed off the edge to permit adequate overlap (at least 4 cm). For concurrent inguinal or femoral hernias, the mesh can be positioned to cover the myopectineal orifice(s).
- For superior midline defects, the mesh is positioned well beyond the costal margin (at least 4 cm to allow adequate overlap of the defect) and is anchored with transfascial sutures placed around the xyphoid process.

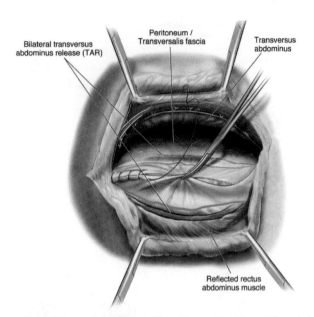

Fig. 6. Reconstruction of the posterior layer. (*From* Rosen M, editor. Atlas of abdominal wall reconstruction. New York: Saunders; 2011; with permission.)

- Working on one side and then the other, full-thickness transfascial sutures are placed to secure the mesh in 3 cardinal points (**Fig. 7**). We prefer using a Reverdin needle (**Fig. 8**) to facilitate transfascial suture placement.
- Kocher clamps are placed on the medial edge of the rectus muscle on the ipsilateral side and the abdominal wall is pulled toward the midline as the transfascial sutures are placed. This permits the mesh to be tensioned "physiologically," which has several advantages in the repair:
  - The mesh absorbs much of the force needed to move the rectus muscles toward the midline. This not only permits primary fascial closure over the mesh, but also reduces the tension on the midline closure.

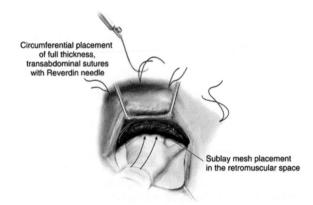

Fig. 7. Mesh is secured in the retromuscular space using the Reverdin needle to place transfascial sutures in cardinal locations. (*From* Rosen M, editor. Atlas of abdominal wall reconstruction. New York: Saunders; 2011; with permission.)

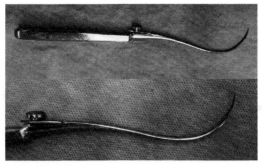

Fig. 8. Reverdin needle: curvilinear suture passer with an eye 1 cm from the distal end.

    ○ The mesh will not buckle or wrinkle when the linea alba is re-created, reducing the space for seroma to accumulate.

Reconstruction of the Anterior Layers
- With the mesh circumferentially secured, the linea alba is re-created by suturing the anterior rectus sheaths to each other in the midline using multiple figure-of-eight stitches of slow-absorbing 0 monofilament absorbable suture (**Fig. 9**).
- Before these stitches are tied, closed suction drains (typically 2) are positioned anterior to the mesh and in the dependent (inferior and lateral) portions of the repair.
- Because of the substantial rectus medialization afforded by TAR and by physiologically tensioning the mesh, it is uncommon to not complete the anterior fascial closure over the mesh.
- The subcutaneous tissues can be closed In layers with absorbable suture. The skin is stapled. Subcutaneous drains are placed only in circumstances in which there is a large dead space not effectively closed with sutures.

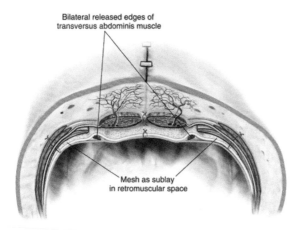

Bilateral released edges of
transversus abdominis muscle

Mesh as sublay
in retromuscular space

Fig. 9. Cross-sectional view of the completed reconstruction. Mesh is secured in a sublay position with transfascial sutures. The linea alba is recreated anterior the mesh in the midline. (*From* Rosen M, editor. Atlas of abdominal wall reconstruction. New York: Saunders; 2011; with permission.)

SURGICAL TECHNIQUE: ANTERIOR COMPONENT SEPARATION

- Incision, adhesiolysis, and foreign body (mesh) excision proceed identical to posterior component separation methods outlined previously.

Formation of Subcutaneous Flaps

- Once the fascia medial to the rectus has been identified, lipocutaneous flaps are created by dissecting the subcutaneous tissues off the anterior rectus sheath. These flaps extend superiorly to the costal margin, inferiorly to inguinal ligament, and laterally to just beyond the linea semilunaris (lateral boarder of rectus muscles) where the external oblique fascial release will occur.
- PUPS Variation
  - ○ Two subcutaneous tunnels are created just above the anterior rectus sheath with electrocautery.
    - ■ The epigastric tunnel extends from the xyphoid to 4 cm above umbilicus and runs laterally along the costal margin to just beyond the linea semilunaris.
    - ■ The suprapubic tunnel extends from the pubic tubercle to 6 cm below the umbilicus and runs laterally along the inguinal ligament to just beyond the linea semilunaris.
  - ○ The tunnels are then connected to each other lateral to the linea semilunaris. This method preserves the umbilicus and periumbilical branches of the inferior epigastric vessels (**Fig. 10**).
  - ○ Use of a fiber-optic lighted retractor greatly facilitates this dissection.

External Oblique Release

- With electrocautery, the external oblique aponeurosis and muscle fibers are divided 1 to 2 cm lateral to the linea semilunaris from just above the costal margin to just above the inguinal ligament (**Fig. 11**).

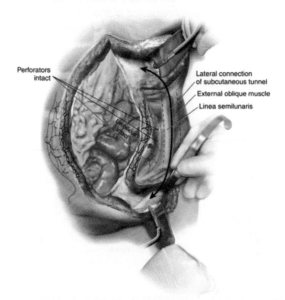

Fig. 10. PUPS technique. Superior and inferior flaps are connected with a lateral subcutaneous tunnel. (*From* Rosen M, editor. Atlas of abdominal wall reconstruction. New York: Saunders; 2011; with permission.)

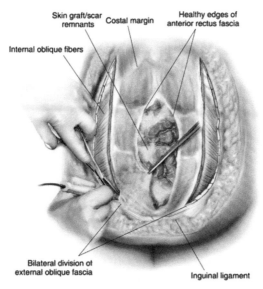

Fig. 11. Division of the external oblique fascia and muscle fibers lateral to the linea semilunaris. (*From* Rosen M, editor. Atlas of abdominal wall reconstruction. New York: Saunders; 2011; with permission.)

- This maneuver is similar whether the classic or PUPS technique is being implemented. With PUPS, the lighted retractor again facilitates visualization.
- An assessment is then made as to whether the linea alba can be re-created at the midline without undue tension.
  - If no tension is found, mesh placement and fascial closure can begin.
  - If the midline fascia will not reapproximate, retrorectus dissection (as described for posterior component separation) can be performed to permit greater medialization of the rectus muscle.

Mesh Placement
- Mesh can be placed as an underlay (within the peritoneal cavity), sublay (within the retrorectus space), or as an onlay, depending on the types of release performed, whether midline fascia can be approximated, and surgeon preference.
  - Underlay mesh is secured via transabdominal sutures passed through the lateral cut edge of the external oblique fascia. If synthetic mesh is used here, it must have an antiadhesive barrier.
  - Sublay mesh is placed within the retrorectus space after the posterior layer has been closed. Transabdominal sutures are passed through the medial cut edge of the external oblique at the level of the linea semilunaris.
  - Onlay mesh is placed over the closed midline repair, and is secured to the lateral cut edges of the external oblique bilaterally (**Fig. 12**).
- Regardless of implant location or type (biologic or synthetic), mesh should be secured with slowly absorbing monofilament suture and placed under physiologic tension.
- Drains are generally placed above the mesh regardless of its implant location.

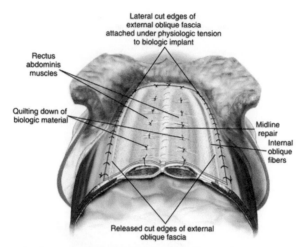

Lateral cut edges of
external oblique fascia
attached under physiologic tension
to biologic implant

Rectus
abdominis
muscles

Quilting down of
biologic material

Midline
repair
Internal
oblique
fibers

Released cut edges of external
oblique fascia

Fig. 12. Onlay mesh placement following external oblique release. The mesh is secured to the lateral cut edges of the external oblique fascia. (*From* Rosen M, editor. Atlas of abdominal wall reconstruction. New York: Saunders; 2011; with permission.)

Reconstruction of the Anterior Layers
- Because of the large skin flaps created with anterior component separation, several maneuvers have been proposed to reduce the risk of wound occurrences:
  - Subscarpa fat may be removed if ischemic.
  - Redundant skin may be removed from the midline.
  - Skin flaps may be sutured to the abdominal wall to reduce dead space.
  - Multiple closed suction drains (2–4) are placed to evacuate fluid from the dead space. These subcutaneous drains are left in place for several weeks.
    - For PUPS, drains are specifically positioned in the right, left, and central subcutaneous compartments.
- The subcutaneous tissues can be closed in layers with absorbable suture. The skin is stapled.

POSTOPERATIVE CARE

Airway Management
- In cases with prolonged operative times, patients with underlying pulmonary disease, or cases ending late in the evening, the patient is kept intubated overnight.
- If the plateau airway pressure increases more than 6 cm H_2O following approximation of the linea alba, the patient is also kept intubated for 24 hours.[44]
- The addition of 24 to 48 hours of chemical paralysis is a useful adjunct for more significant rises in plateau pressure (9 cm H_2O or greater).[44]

Pain Management
- Epidural catheters are recommended in all patients and are maintained for 3 to 4 days postoperatively.
- For patients in whom an epidural cannot be placed (or is contraindicated) or who have delayed bowel function at the time of epidural removal, an intravenous patient-controlled analgesia device is used.
- Patients are transitioned to oral narcotic analgesia when they tolerate a diet.

Diet
- We are conservative with dietary advancement to avoid retching and emesis, which can jeopardize the repair.
- Patients are kept nil per os until flatus is passed, at which time clear liquids are begun.
- When bowel function has returned, patients are advanced to an appropriate diet (eg, regular, diabetic).
- Nasogastric tube decompression is used only in patients with extensive adhesiolysis or in whom small bowel resection has been performed.

Drains (anterior component separation)
- Subfascial drains are typically removed before hospital discharge (within 7 days).
- Subcutaneous drains are left until output is less than 30 mL per day for 2 consecutive days. This can result in drains that are in place for several weeks postoperatively.

Drains (posterior component separation)
- When synthetic mesh is used, drains are removed when then the output is less than 30 mL per day or on the day of discharge (whichever is first). This typically occurs on day 4 to 7.
- When biologic mesh is used, we leave drains in place for 2 weeks irrespective of the output volume.

Abdominal Binder
- We routinely use an abdominal binder in the immediate postoperative period.
- Following discharge, the patient may wear the binder as desired.
- If there is concern for the viability of lipocutaneous skin flaps, most will not place a binder.

General Postoperative Issues
- Mechanical and pharmacologic venous thromboembolism prophylaxis is instituted in all patients beginning in the operating room.
- Following Surgical Care Improvement Project (SCIP) guidelines, prophylactic antibiotics are given within 1 hour of skin incision and are discontinued within 24 hours.
- For patients with active mesh or soft tissue infections, antibiotics are given until resolution of the infection.

POSTOPERATIVE COMPLICATIONS
Wound Complications
- SSIs are a major source of morbidity following open ventral hernia repair.[45] In the highest-risk populations, the SSI rate has been reported to be as high as 27% to 41%.[46–49]
- Wound complications are more common and more severe in anterior component separation than posterior component separation techniques.[43]
- Cellulitis is managed with appropriate antibiotics.
- Infected collections (including seromas and hematomas) are drained percutaneously or operatively.
- Asymptomatic fluid collections are generally followed conservatively.
- Necrosis of skin or subcutaneous tissues is addressed with early operative debridement.
- Prophylactic use of negative-pressure vacuum therapy on a closed surgical incision does not reduce the 30-day SSI rate following abdominal wall reconstruction.[50]

Pulmonary Complications
- Diaphragm function and pulmonary toilet are both negatively affected by abdominal wall reconstruction, leaving patients vulnerable to pulmonary complications.
- On evaluation of the 2007 National Inpatient Sample, ventral hernia patients discharged with a diagnosis of respiratory failure and mechanical ventilation had a 4-fold greater length of stay and an 18-fold greater death rate.[44]
- As many as 20% of patients will experience a postoperative respiratory complication following component separation hernia repair.[44]
- Aggressive pulmonary toilet, including incentive spirometer use, chest physiotherapy, adequate analgesia, and upright posture, are all critical to minimizing these complications.

Gastrointestinal Complications
- Paralytic ileus is common following ventral hernia repair, although the exact rate is not reported.
- Prolonged ileus, or symptoms suggestive of an early small bowel obstruction, should prompt further investigation. A CT scan of the abdomen and pelvis will demonstrate an internal hernia (bowel is seen protruding through a rent in the posterior layer). Prompt surgical reexploration in this case is mandatory.

Intra-Abdominal Hypertension
- Except in the smallest ventral hernia repairs, some degree of intra-abdominal hypertension (IAH) is likely created in the course of reapproximating the linea alba.
- We do not routinely follow bladder pressure measurements, but are aggressive in our management of the secondary consequences of IAH, including the following:
  ○ Liberal use of paralytic agents if needed to permit adequate ventilation
  ○ Aggressive fluid resuscitation to permit adequate urine output
  ○ Maintaining endotracheal intubation for 24 to 48 hours postoperatively (as outlined previously)

Death
- Mortality following open ventral hernia repair is uncommon (0%–1%).
- Cardiac, pulmonary, and thromboembolic events are the leading sources of postoperative mortality.

OUTCOMES

Polarizing opinions are common among hernia specialists, and are driven by the lack of well-designed comparative trials evaluating outcomes of open ventral hernia repairs with the techniques described previously. Most of the available literature is retrospective in nature. Techniques vary greatly among investigators, as do definitions of postoperative events and duration of follow-up. The addition of innumerable types and sizes of mesh into this equation makes it difficult to draw firm conclusions. There is still a clear need to address these issues in well-designed, prospective randomized trials.

Anterior Component Separation

The separation of components technique described by Ramirez and colleagues[28] has undergone many technical refinements since its original description. This method permits mobilization and medial advancement of the abdominal wall musculature, permitting reconstruction of the midline and obliteration of the hernia defect. Anterior component separation has gained wide acceptance today. **Table 1** summarizes the

Table 1
Outcomes of anterior component separation hernia repair

Author, Year	n	Method	Wound Complication, %	Mortality, %	Mean Follow-up, mo	Recurrence Rate, %
Ramirez et al,[28] 1990	11	ACS	—	—	4–42	0
Jernigan et al,[51] 2003	73	Modified ACS	—	0	24	5.5
de Vries Reileigh,[52] 2003	43	ACS	32.6	2.3	15.6	32
Girotto et al,[53] 2003	96	ACS with onlay mesh	26	—	26	22
Gonzalez et al,[9] 2005	42	ACS with onlay mesh	63	0	16	3
Hultman et al,[54] 2005	13	ACS ± mesh	—	—	11.5	15.4
Jin et al,[55] 2007	22	ACS with onlay or underlay AHDM	—	0	21.4	9.7
Espinosa-de-los-Monteros et al,[56] 2007	39	ACS with onlay AHDM	26	—	15	5
Diaz et al,[57] 2009	31	ACS with onlay AHDM	41.9	—	10.5	6.5

Abbreviations: ACS, anterior component separation; AHDM, acellular human dermal matrix.
Data from Refs.[9,28,51–57]

salient results from a number of trials involving anterior component separation. The major drawback to anterior component separation remains the need to create extensive skin flaps, which predisposes the patient to a variety of surgical site events. Wound complication rates as high as 26% to 63% have been found.[9,53,56] Other investigators cite difficulty managing subxyphoid, suprapubic, and non-midline defects with this technique because of the absence of a reliable space for prosthetic reinforcement with wide overlap.[38]

PUPS Method

PUPS component separation has the advantage of preservation of the lipocutaneous blood supply while permitting external oblique release. **Table 2** summarizes the largest reports involving PUPS component separation. These studies have been generally retrospective comparisons of classic anterior separation methods with the PUPS technique. Although recurrence rates were not different between the groups, these studies have highlighted statistically significant differences in rate and severity of surgical site occurrences (skin necrosis, wound infection, abscess). Clarke[59] noted a 25% rate of skin necrosis when using classical methods and 0% with PUPS technique. Similarly, Dumanian and colleagues[32] at Northwestern University outlined their results from a series of 41 patients who had a 2% rate of wound complications compared with a 20% rate when using classic anterior component separation methods.[58] Data suggest that with longer-term follow-up, the recurrence rate after PUPS rises to as high as 13.8%.[59]

Posterior Component Separation

Although PUPS techniques address the wound-related morbidity of anterior component separation, it does not address issues with non-midline defects, suprapubic or subxyphoid hernias, or the need for a large space to permit wide mesh overlap of the hernia defect. Posterior component separation addresses all of these concerns. **Table 3** summarizes the available data on posterior component separation methods. Overall, these studies consistently demonstrate a long-term recurrence rate well below 10%, far superior to the other techniques described.[35–38,61–63] Although the wound complication rate appears to be no different from anterior component separation rates, it should be emphasized that the severity of the complications noted was far

Table 2
Outcomes of PUPS hernia repair

Year	n	Method	Wound Complication, %	Mortality, %	Mean Follow-up, mo	Recurrence Rate, %
Sukkar et al,[58] 2001	51	PUPS	13.7	—	24	3.9
Saulis et al,[32] 2002	41	PUPS	4.9	—	—	7.3
Clarke,[59] 2010	56	Modified PUPS	3.1	1.5	38	13.8
Butler & Campbell,[60] 2011	38	PUPS	26.3	0	12.4	3

Abbreviation: PUPS, periumbilical perforator sparing.
    Data from Refs.[32,58–60]

Table 3
Outcomes of posterior component separation hernia repair

Year	n	Method	Wound Complication, %	Mortality, %	Mean Follow-up, mo	Recurrence Rate, %
Paajanen & Hermunen,[61] 2004	84	Retrorectus dissection only	6	0	18	5
Israelsson et al,[62] 2006	228	"Sublay Mesh"	—	—	12–24	7.3
Novitsky et al,[35] 2006	128	Preperitoneal	12.5	0	28.1	3.1
Iqbal et al,[36] 2007	254	Retrorectus dissection only	13	0	70	5
Carbonell et al,[37] 2008	20	Posterior component, intramuscular	15	5	12	5
Wheeler et al,[15] 2009	90	Retrorectus dissection only	31	0	53	7
Krpata et al,[43] 2012	55	Posterior Component with TAR	25.5	0	6.8	3.6
Mehrabi et al,[63] 2010	174	Retrorectus dissection only	3.4	0	91	1.1
Novitsky et al,[38] 2012	42	Posterior Component with TAR	23.8	0	26.1	4.7

Abbreviation: TAR, transversus abdominis release.
Data from Refs.[15,35–38,43,61–63]

less. Few patients required operative debridement, and many of these data were prospectively collected to assess for a wide variety of wound related issues.

SUMMARY

Open ventral hernia repair with component separation represents a group of complex surgical techniques developed to address the ever-growing population of patients requiring abdominal wall reconstruction. The methods described share similar key elements: (1) fascial release permits myofascial advancement and reconstruction of the linea alba, and (2) the creation of vast spaces within the abdominal wall ensure wide overlap of mesh to maximize surface ingrowth. The key difference between anterior and posterior component separation techniques is the location of this potential space. Anterior separation methods create large lipocutaneous flaps and are usually accompanied by onlay of mesh. Posterior separation methods create no such flaps and permit a sublay of mesh. Differences in wound complications and recurrence rates are likely directly related to these 2 facts.

Posterior component separation with TAR detailed previously has several advantages over anterior component separation and other methods of posterior separation. First, it permits extensive lateral dissection in the avascular potential space beneath the transversus abdominis muscle. This creates an ideal space for mesh implantation, while at the same time preserving the entire neurovascular supply to the anterior abdominal wall. The release of the transversus abdominal muscle itself permits sufficient medicalization of the rectus muscles, so as to permit complete reconstruction of the abdominal wall layers posterior and anterior to the mesh. This places the mesh in a well-vascularized pocket, remote from the skin surface. Moreover, the retromuscular position of the mesh permits wide overlap of "difficult" defects (subxyphoid, subcostal, suprapubic). Based on these advantages, as well as its quoted 3% to 5% recurrence rate, posterior component separation with transversus abdominis release has become our preferred method of choice for the management of patients requiring open ventral hernia repair.

REFERENCES

1. Cengiz Y, Israelsson LA. Incisional hernias in midline incisions: an eight-year follow up. Hernia 1998;2:175–7.
2. Mudge M, Hughes LE. Incisional hernia: a 10 year prospective study of incidence and attitudes. Br J Surg 1985;72:70–1.
3. Santora TA, Rosylin JJ. Incisional hernia. Surg Clin North Am 1993;73:557–70.
4. Pollock AV, Evans M. Early prediction of late incisional hernia. Br J Surg 1989;76:953–4.
5. Anthony T, Bergen PC, Kim LT, et al. Factors affecting recurrences following incisional herniorrhaphy. World J Surg 2000;24:95–100.
6. Cassar K, Munro A. Surgical treatment of incisional hernia. Br J Surg 2002;89:534–45.
7. Duepree HJ, Senagore AJ, Delaney CP, et al. Does means of access affect the incidence of small bowel obstruction and ventral hernia after bowel resection? Laparoscopy versus laparotomy. J Am Coll Surg 2003;197(2):177–81.
8. Wechter ME, Pearlman MD, Hartmann KE. Reclosure of the disrupted laparotomy wound; a systemic review. Obstet Gynecol 2005;106:376–83.
9. Gonzalez R, Rehnke RD, Ramaswamy A, et al. Component separation technique and laparoscopic approach; a review of two evolving strategies for ventral hernia repair. Am Surg 2005;71:598–605.

10. Cobb WS, Kercher KW, Heniford BT. Laparoscopic repair of incisional hernias. Surg Clin North Am 2005;85(1):91–103.
11. Jin J, Rosen MJ. Laparoscopic versus open ventral hernia repair. Surg Clin North Am 2008;88:1083–100.
12. Paul A, Korenkov M, Peters S, et al. Unacceptable results of the Mayo procedure for repair of abdominal incisional hernias. Eur J Surg 1998;164:361–7.
13. Flum DR, Horvath K, Koepsell T. Have outcomes of incisional hernia repair improved with time? A population-based analysis. Ann Surg 2003;237:129–35.
14. Korenkov M, Sauerland S, Arndt M, et al. Randomized clinical trial of suture repair, polypropylene mesh or autodermal hernioplasty for incisional hernia. Br J Surg 2002;89:50–6.
15. Wheeler AA, Matz ST, Bachman SL, et al. Retrorectus polyester mesh repair for midline ventral hernias. Hernia 2009;13:597–603.
16. Burger JW, Luijendijk RW, Hop WC, et al. Long-term follow-up of a randomized controlled trial of suture versus mesh repair of incisional hernia. Ann Surg 2004; 240:578–83.
17. Luijendijk RW, Hop WC, van den Tol MP, et al. A comparison of suture repair with mesh repair for incisional hernia. N Engl J Med 2000;343(6):392–8.
18. Koller R, Miholic J, Jakl RJ. Repair of incisional hernias with expanded polytetrafluoroethylene. Eur J Surg 1997;163:261–6.
19. de Vries Reilingh TS, van Goor H, Charbon JA, et al. Repair of giant midline abdominal wall hernias: "components separation technique" versus prosthetic repair: interim analysis of a randomized controlled trial. World J Surg 2007;31: 756–63.
20. Usher FC, Ochsner J, Tuttle LL Jr. Use of marlex mesh in the repair of incisional hernias. Am Surg 1958;24(12):967–74.
21. Klinge U, Conze J, Krones C, et al. Incisional hernia: open techniques. World J Surg 2005;29:1066–72.
22. LeBlanc KA, Booth WV. Laparoscopic repair of incisional abdominal hernia using expanded polytetrafluoroethylene: preliminary findings. Surg Laparosc Endosc 1993;3:39–41.
23. Heniford BT, Ramshaw BJ. Laparoscopic ventral hernia repair a report of 100 consecutive cases. Surg Endosc 2000;14(5):419–23.
24. Rosen MJ, Brody F, Ponsky JL, et al. Recurrence rate after laparoscopic ventral hernia repair. Surg Endosc 2003;17(1):123–8.
25. Greenstein AJ, Nguyen SQ, Buch KE, et al. Recurrence after laparoscopic ventral hernia repair: a prospective pilot study of suture versus tack fixation. Am Surg 2008;74(3):227–31.
26. Ballem N, Parikh R, Berber E, et al. Laparoscopic versus open ventral hernia repairs: 5 year recurrence rates. Surg Endosc 2008;22(9):1935–40.
27. Singhal V, Szeto P, VanderMeer TJ, et al. Ventral hernia repair: outcomes change with long-term follow-up. JSLS 2012;16:373–9.
28. Ramirez OM, Ruas E, Dellon AL. "Components separation" method for closure of abdominal-wall defects: an anatomic and clinical study. Plast Reconstr Surg 1990;86:519–26.
29. Lowe JB 3rd, Lowe JB, Baty JD, et al. Risks associated with "components separation" for closure of complex abdominal wall defects. Plast Reconstr Surg 2003;111:1276–83.
30. Hultman CS, Tong WM, Kittinger BJ, et al. Management of recurrent hernia after components separation: 10-year experience with abdominal wall reconstruction at an academic medical center. Ann Plast Surg 2011;66:504–7.

31. Ko JH, Wang EC, Salvay DM, et al. Abdominal wall reconstruction: lessons learned from 200 "components separation" procedures. Arch Surg 2009;144: 1047–55.

32. Saulis AS, Dumanian GA. Periumbilical rectus abdominis perforator preservation significantly reduces superficial wound complications in "separation of parts" hernia repairs. Plast Reconstr Surg 2002;109:2275–80.

33. Harth KC, Rosen MJ. Endoscopic versus open component separation in complex abdominal wall reconstruction. Am J Surg 2010;199:342–6.

34. Lowe JB, Garza JR, Bowman JL, et al. Endoscopically assisted "components separation" for closure of abdominal wall defects. Plast Reconstr Surg 2000; 105:720–9.

35. Novitsky YW, Porter JR, Rucho ZC, et al. Open preperitoneal retrofascial mesh repair for multiply recurrent ventral incisional hernias. J Am Coll Surg 2006;203: 283–9.

36. Iqbal CW, Pham TH, Joseph A, et al. Long-term outcome of 254 complex incisional hernia repairs using the modified rives-Stoppa technique. World J Surg 2007;31:2398–404.

37. Carbonell AM, Cobb WS, Chen SM. Posterior components separation during retromuscular hernia repair. Hernia 2008;12:359–62.

38. Novitsky YW, Elliott HL, Orenstein SB, et al. Transversus abdominis muscle release: a novel approach to posterior component separation during complex abdominal wall reconstruction. Am J Surg 2012;204:709–16.

39. Rives J, Pire JC, Flament JB, et al. Treatment of large eventrations. New therapeutic indications apropos of 322 cases. Chirurgie 1985;111:215–25.

40. Stoppa RE. The treatment of complicated groin and incisional hernias. World J Surg 1989;13:545–54.

41. Wantz GE. Giant prosthetic reinforcement of the visceral sac. The Stoppa groin hernia repair. Surg Clin North Am 1998;78:1075–87.

42. Stoppa R, Petit J, Abourachid H, et al. Original procedure of groin hernia repair: interposition without fixation of Dacron tulle prosthesis by subperitoneal median approach. Chirurgie 1973;99:119–23.

43. Krpata DM, Blatnik JA, Novitsky YW, et al. Posterior and open anterior components separations: a comparative analysis. Am J Surg 2012;203:318–22.

44. Blatnik JA, Krpata DM, Pesa NL, et al. Predicting severe postoperative respiratory complications following abdominal wall reconstruction. Plast Reconstr Surg 2012;130(4):836–41.

45. Finan KR, Vick CC, Kiefe CI, et al. Predictors of wound infection in ventral hernia repair. Am J Surg 2005;190(5):676–81.

46. Dunne JR, Malone DL, Tracy JK, et al. Abdominal wall hernias: risk factors for infection and resource utilization. J Surg Res 2003;111(1):78–84.

47. Kaafarani HM, Kaufman D, Reda D, et al. Predictors of surgical site infection in laparoscopic and open ventral incisional herniorrhaphy. J Surg Res 2010; 163(2):229–34.

48. Houck JP, Rypins EB, Sarfeh IJ, et al. Repair of incisional hernia. Surg Gynecol Obstet 1989;169(5):397–9.

49. Blatnik JA, Krpata DM, Novitsky YW, et al. Does a history of wound infection predict postoperative surgical site infection after ventral hernia repair? Am J Surg 2012;203(3):370–4.

50. Pauli EM, Krpata DM, Novitsky YW, et al. Negative pressure therapy for high-risk abdominal wall reconstruction incisions. Surg Infect (Larchmt) 2013. [Epub ahead of print].

51. Jernigan TW, Fabian TC, Croce MA. Staged management of giant abdominal wall defects: acute and long term results. Ann Surg 2003;238(3):349–55.
52. de Vries Reileigh TS. Components separation technique for the repair of large abdominal wall hernias. J Am Coll Surg 2003;196(1):32–7.
53. Girotto JA, Chiaramonte M, Menon NG, et al. Recalcitrant abdominal wall hernias: long-term superiority of autologous tissue repair. Plast Reconstr Surg 2003;112:106–14.
54. Hultman CS, Pratt B, Cairns BA. Multi-disciplinary approach to abdominal wall reconstruction after decompressive laparotomy for abdominal compartment syndrome. Ann Plast Surg 2005;54(3):269–75.
55. Jin J, Rosen MJ, Blatnik J, et al. Use of acellular dermal matrix for complicated ventral hernia repair: does technique affect outcomes? J Am Coll Surg 2007; 205:654–60.
56. Espinosa-de-los-Monteros A, de la Torre JI, Marrero I, et al. Utilization of human cadaveric acellular dermis for abdominal hernia reconstruction. Ann Plast Surg 2007;58:264–7.
57. Diaz JJ Jr, Conquest AM, Ferzoco SJ, et al. Multi-institutional experience using human acellular dermal matrix for ventral hernia repair in a compromised surgical field. Arch Surg 2009;144:209–15.
58. Sukkar SM, Dumanian GA, Szczerba SM. Challenging abdominal wall defects. Am J Surg 2001;181(2):115–21.
59. Clarke JM. Incisional hernia repair by fascial component separation: results in 128 cases and evolution of technique. Am J Surg 2010;200:2–8.
60. Butler CE, Campbell KT. Minimally invasive component separation with inlay bioprosthetic mesh (MICSIB) for complex abdominal wall reconstruction. Plast Reconstr Surg 2011;128(3):698–709.
61. Paajanen H, Hermunen H. Long-term pain and recurrence after repair of ventral incisional hernias by open mesh: clinical and MRI study. Langenbecks Arch Surg 2004;389(5):366–70.
62. Israelsson LA, Smedberg S, Montgomery A, et al. Incisional hernia repair in Sweden 2002. Hernia 2006;10(3):258–61.
63. Mehrabi M, Jangjoo A, Tavoosi H, et al. Long-term outcome of Rives-Stoppa technique in complex ventral incisional hernia repair. World J Surg 2010;34: 1696–701.

Atypical Hernias
Suprapubic, Subxiphoid, and Flank

William W. Hope, MD*, W. Borden Hooks III, MD

KEYWORDS

- Flank • Suprapubic • Subxiphoid • Hernia • Ventral • Incisional • Laparoscopy

KEY POINTS

- The atypical hernias most commonly encountered include subxiphoid, suprapubic, and flank hernias and can be difficult to repair because of their proximity to bony structures.
- Both laparoscopic and open techniques can be used to fix these hernias, using the principles of hernia repair, including wide mesh overlap with appropriate fixation.
- Thorough knowledge of the anatomy of the abdominal wall is essential for successful repair of these difficult hernias.

INTRODUCTION

Hernias located near bony prominences or off midline can be difficult to repair because of the challenge of obtaining a tension-free repair with wide overlap of mesh prosthetic and adequate fixation. The most common locations for these atypical hernias are in the subxiphoid, suprapubic, and flank, and the location is often related to previous incisions. The 2 techniques most often used for repair are the open and laparoscopic approach. Although there are several different techniques described for these hernias, several principles are important to review.

- Goals of the repair should be individualized and discussed with the patient preoperatively, which can help the surgeon decide between the open and laparoscopic approach.
- Although not mandatory, computed tomography (CT) scanning can help with surgical planning and decisions regarding surgical technique.
- Because of lower recurrence rates,[1,2] mesh use should be considered in all cases, unless the hernia is small or there is a contraindication. Wide overlap of

Disclosures: No funding was received for this work.
Dr Hope's disclosures: Research support Ethicon, honorarium eMedicine. Dr Hooks has nothing to disclosure.
Department of Surgery, New Hanover Regional Medical Center, South East Area Health Education Center, University of North Carolina-Chapel Hill, 2131 South 17th Street, PO Box 9025, Wilmington, NC 28401, USA
* Corresponding author.
E-mail address: William.Hope@seahec.net

Surg Clin N Am 93 (2013) 1135–1162
http://dx.doi.org/10.1016/j.suc.2013.06.002
0039-6109/13/$ – see front matter © 2013 Elsevier Inc. All rights reserved.

surgical.theclinics.com

mesh with appropriate fixation is essential for success in these difficult hernias, and the use of bridging techniques with mesh is discouraged.

- In general, synthetic mesh is used, because there are few data regarding the use of biological meshes in atypical hernias, and the data available lack long-term follow-up.[3] When synthetic mesh is not applicable, biological or bioabsorbable mesh can be used. Mesh choice should be based on clinical factors and the surgeon's preference.[4]
- Adjunctive maneuvers for fascial closure, such as component separation, often cannot be used in atypical hernias because of the location of the fascial defects.

PREOPERATIVE PLANNING

Patients should be prepared as with any patient undergoing a ventral hernia repair, with a few special caveats.

- Patients undergoing flank hernia repair require elevation of the ipsilateral side of the hernia for adequate exposure of the hernia and adequate mesh fixation. This can be achieved by placing a bump or with the use of a bean bag.
- In patients undergoing laparoscopic repair of subxiphoid and suprapubic hernias, tucking and padding both arms help the surgeon and assistant move freely on the side of the patient.
- The use of a 3-way Foley catheter is helpful during laparoscopic suprapubic hernia repair, because many patients require laparoscopic takedown of the bladder.

Patients undergoing repair of atypical hernias should have preoperative antibiotics, deep vein thrombosis prophylaxis, and β-blockers depending on the clinical situation.

SURGICAL TECHNIQUE

The surgical techniques most likely to produce a successful repair facilitate a wide overlap with mesh of the hernia defect with adequate fixation. Whether this is performed using the laparoscopic or open approach should be determined by various patient factors and the goals of the repair.

Suprapubic Hernia

Open approach
Many techniques are used for the treatment of ventral hernias. The 2 most common techniques are an underlay (the mesh is placed posterior to the hernia defect intraabdominal, preperitoneal, or retrorectus) and an overlay (the hernia defect is closed, and the mesh is placed above the defect). The bridging-type repair, in which the mesh is sewn to the fascia, results in a high recurrence rate and should be used only in special clinical circumstances (**Fig. 1**).[5]

Our preferred technique for open repair of a suprapubic hernia is the underlay technique, with the mesh in the retromuscular position. The preperitoneal space is dissected to the pubic bone, allowing mesh placement and fixation to the pubis. Thorough knowledge of the relative anatomy and myofascial components of the abdominal wall are essential for a successful operation.

Preoperative planning
- Abdominal CT is useful to assess the size and location of the hernia, occult incarceration of bowel or bladder, previous mesh material, and the integrity of abdominal wall musculature.

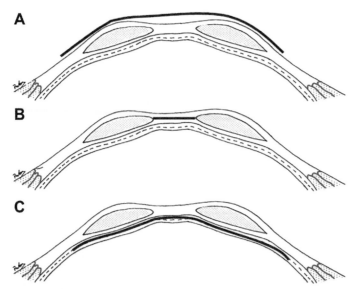

Fig. 1. Techniques of mesh placement. (*A*) Onlay technique. (*B*) Inlay or bridge technique. (*C*) Retrorectus or underlay technique. (*From* Shell DH 4th, de la Torre J, Andrades P, et al. Open repair ventral Incisional hernias. Surg Clin North Am 2008;88:69; with permission.)

- Screening colonoscopy is needed in some clinical situations before abdominal wall reconstruction.
- Nutritional evaluation and smoking cessation are important, because these are risk factors for wound issues after this surgery.[6]

Positioning

- The patient is positioned supine with arms to the side, a Foley catheter is placed, and antibiotics and deep vein thrombosis prophylaxis are given based on surgeon preference and the clinical situation.
- Most suprapubic hernias are incisional hernias from lower midline or Pfannenstiel-type incisions (**Fig. 2**).

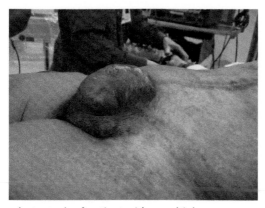

Fig. 2. Preoperative photograph of patient with a multiple recurrent suprapubic incisional hernia.

Abdominal access

- A lower midline incision is often used and can be extended superior to the umbilicus depending on the size of the hernia. If there is a large scar from previous surgery, this can be excised.
- As in all open hernia surgery, careful abdominal entry is required to avoid iatrogenic injury, because intestinal contents and, in the case of suprapubic hernias, the bladder, can be in the hernia sac.

Lysis of adhesions

- After the abdomen is safely entered, adhesiolysis is performed sharply with scissors to clear the right and left side of the abdomen and the superior and inferior borders of the incision.
- All abdominal adhesions should be cleared, if possible, depending on the clinical situation.

Retromuscular dissection

- Obtaining preperitoneal or retrorectus access is an essential skill for hernia surgeons. Creating these planes allows the surgeon to place the mesh in the retromuscular position without contact with the abdominal viscera and is a well-accepted method for hernia repair.[7,8] Another theoretic advantage of the retromuscular position of mesh, compared with an onlay position, is that in the case of a superficial wound infection, the mesh is still covered by muscle and fascia and potentially avoids mesh infections.
- The retrorectus plane is often easier to obtain in patients with previous surgery. The posterior rectus sheath is incised approximately 0.5 cm from its edge. This incision is usually made at the level of the umbilicus or in the midportion of the wound if the incision is a lower midline. The rectus muscle and the glistening white posterior rectus sheath should be visible (**Fig. 3**).
- The incision of the posterior rectus sheath is extended superiorly and inferiorly and laterally to the linea semilunaris. Dissection is usually performed bluntly with finger dissection or a peanut. Care must be taken to identify and preserve the intercostal nerves and vessels to maintain a functional abdominal wall.
- The retrorectus plane is taken all the way to the pubis above the bladder. The superior extent of dissection depends on the size of the hernia but should be

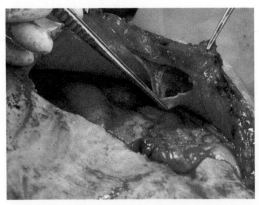

Fig. 3. Starting the dissection to enter the retrorectus space. The posterior rectus sheath is incised at the midportion of the abdominal incision and incised superiorly and inferiorly.

dissected at least 4 to 5 cm above the edge of the facial defect to allow for appropriate mesh overlap.

- Preperitoneal dissection is also an option, although it is often more technically difficult. If the thin layer of peritoneum can be dissected, it should be dissected laterally as far as needed for sufficient mesh overlap, to the pubic bone inferiorly, and 4 to 5 cm above the fascial defect superiorly.
- One benefit of the preperitoneal space compared with the retrorectus space is the ability to place larger pieces of mesh, because the lateral dissection plane is not confined by the lateral border or the rectus sheath, and dissection all the way toward the retroperitoneum and kidney can be performed.
- One drawback of preperitoneal placement is not cutting the posterior rectus sheath, which does not produce the component release that may be needed to help close the midline fascia above the mesh.
- One potential solution to these problems may be the newly described posterior component separation with transversus abdominus release.[9] This technique involves dividing the transversus abdominal muscle medial to the linea semilunaris, allowing mesh to be placed laterally in the position between the transversalis fascia and the lateral edge of the divided transversus abdominus muscle.[9]

Closure of retromuscular tissue

- After the preperitoneal or retrorectus dissection has been completed and holes or fenestrations closed with absorbable suture, the tissue is closed in the midline using absorbable suture (we use a 0 Vicryl suture).
- Before closure, make sure the needle, sponge, and instrument count is correct and there are no problems in the abdomen, because closure excludes the abdominal cavity to the surgeon for the rest of the operation.
- After the peritoneum or posterior rectus sheath is closed, the space available for mesh placement can be measured.

Mesh choice/placement

- Because the mesh has been excluded from the abdominal cavity, a mesh with adhesion barriers is usually not needed (unless there are fenestrations or holes in the tissue allowing mesh to contact bowel). Synthetic meshes are preferred unless not clinically appropriate. We prefer large, macroporous, reduced-weight polypropylene mesh.
- After the mesh is chosen, it is placed in the sublay/retromuscular position.

Mesh fixation

- The inferior of the mesh is fixed to the pubis and Cooper ligament with monofilament sutures. This can be achieved by suturing the mesh directly onto the pubis and Cooper ligament or by bringing out transfascial sutures just above the pubis.
- The most likely area of recurrence in suprapubic hernias is inferiorly, so adequate fixation in this area is crucial. Depending on the size of the defect, 1 to 5 sutures are placed in this area with tack fixation if needed.
- Additional full-thickness, transfascial sutures are placed using a suture passer or Reverdine needle. The number of sutures needed varies based on the defect size and amount of mesh overlap obtained (usually 1–3 sutures for the superior portion of the mesh and 1–2 on the right and left side of the mesh).
- Mesh fixation should be taut, because the mesh buckles with anterior fascial closure, which should be attempted in all cases.

- One or 2 closed suction drains are placed above the mesh, below the fascial closure. These drains are usually left in for several days until the output is less than 30 mL/d.

Fascial closure

- After the mesh is secure, anterior fascial closure should be attempted in all cases. This is achieved with a slowly absorbing running or interrupted suture. This technique allows for medicalization of the rectus muscle and coverage of the mesh, protecting it from exposure in the event of wound infection if wound opening is required.
- If the fascia cannot be closed, the hernia sac is closed over the mesh to provide coverage.
- In suprapubic hernias, because of the location of the defect, fascial closure with the aid of a component separation is not an option (for the suprapubic part of the fascia).
- If the defect is large and obtaining fascial closure is impossible, every effort should be made to preserve the hernia sac during the initial dissection.

Closure/postoperative care

- The wounds are irrigated, drains sutured in, and skin approximated with skin staples.
- Patients usually require hospital admission for pain control and return of bowel function. Routine postoperative care includes slow advancement of diet and activity and monitoring of the wound and drain output.

Laparoscopic approach

The laparoscopic approach to the suprapubic hernia is an excellent option for repair in some patients. Laparoscopic repair for the suprapubic hernia follows the same initial steps as that for any other midline ventral hernia.

Positioning/draping

- The patient is placed supine with bilateral arms tucked. We typically use an Ioban-type drape, although these have not been shown to decrease mesh infections.[10]

Obtain safe laparoscopic access

- Although obtaining safe laparoscopic access can be straightforward, it can also be complicated in patients with many previous operations, which in some cases can preclude using the laparoscopic approach.
- In general, the surgeon should use the access technique that they are most skilled with.

Port placement

- Three to 5 trocars are used for laparoscopic repair based on the complexity of the case. One of the trocars should be an 11-mm or 12-mm trocar to help with mesh placement and facilitate a 10-mm camera if better visualization is needed for difficult adhesiolysis.
- The ports are usually placed on the lateral right and left abdomen but can be placed in a semicircular configuration depending on the size of the hernia.
- It is helpful to have at least 2 ports on each side of the abdomen to assist when tacking the mesh, which provides visualization from all angles.

Diagnostic laparoscopy and laparoscopic lysis of adhesions

- Diagnostic laparoscopy and laparoscopic lysis of adhesion is one of the most critical portions of the operation and can result in complications such as bleeding or enterotomy if not approached carefully. It can also be straightforward or challenging depending on the tenacity and extent of adhesions.
- In general, lysis of adhesion is performed sharply with laparoscopic scissors. When the surgeon is certain that the adhesions contain only omentum and no bowel, energy sources can be used with caution.
- Complete lysis of all abdominal adhesions is generally recommended but depends on the size of the defect and size of mesh used.
- After lysis of adhesions, inspect the omentum and bowel for bleeding and occult bowel injury.

Laparoscopic takedown of the bladder

- This part of the procedure is unique to the laparoscopic repair of suprapubic hernias. This bladder takedown is greatly aided by the use of a 3-way Foley catheter placed at the beginning of the operation.
- When preparing to take down the bladder, the drainage part of the Foley catheter is clamped, and approximately 300 mL of sterile normal saline is introduced into the bladder until it is identified (**Figs. 4** and **5**).
- The peritoneum is incised in the midline, and flaps are extended laterally. This procedure is often bloody, so scissors with cautery or energy devices are helpful.
- The plane is developed all the way to the pubic bone bilaterally, keeping the distended bladder inferior to the dissection (**Fig. 6**).

Measuring the hernia defect

- After all the adhesions and bladder have been taken down, intracorporeal measurement of the hernia defect is recommended. This measurement can be made using spinal needles and a suture or a ruler.
- The longitudinal and transverse diameter of the defect are measured and documented.

Mesh choice

- Several factors including surgeon preference contribute to the choice of mesh.

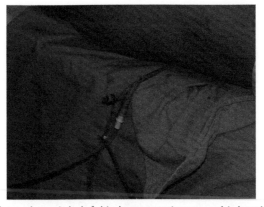

Fig. 4. A 3-way Foley catheter is helpful in laparoscopic suprapubic hernia repair. The Foley catheter is instilled with saline and clamped to allow for the bladder to distend, which allows intraoperative visualization.

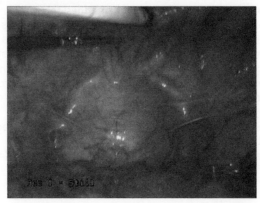

Fig. 5. With instillation of the bladder with saline, the bladder is easily visualized, making dissection easier.

- Because the mesh used in the laparoscopic repair has contact with the abdominal viscera, use a coated polypropylene or polyester mesh or a Gore-Tex-based mesh, either alone or as a composite-type mesh, with the Gore-Tex side placed toward the viscera.
- Mesh size should be based on the size of the hernia; however, at least a 4-cm overlap on each side is recommended.

Mesh preparation/placement
- Although there are many techniques for mesh placement and fixation, 1 common technique involves placing 4 sutures at the periphery of the mesh at the midpoint of the superior, inferior, and right and left lateral side.
- With a low suprapubic hernia, place the inferior stitch 2 to 4 cm off the periphery of the mesh. This strategy provides an extra 2 to 4 cm of mesh overlap on the pubic bone for tack fixation on the pubis.
- The mesh is then rolled as a scroll and placed through 1 of the large 11-mm or 12-mm trocars. Except for extremely large pieces of meshes, most can be placed through 1 of the larger trocars.

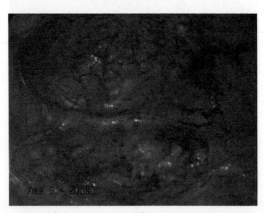

Fig. 6. Suprapubic hernia with large central defect requiring laparoscopic takedown of the bladder to facilitate mesh placement and fixation to the pubic bone and Cooper ligament.

- One technique is to place a grasper from the opposite side of the abdomen through the 11-mm or 12-mm trocar and remove the head of the trocar (or entire trocar). Pull the mesh in by twisting and constant pressure.
- After the mesh is inside the abdomen, orient it correctly so the appropriate side of the mesh is facing the viscera (if applicable). The 4 sutures are then brought up through the abdominal wall using a suture passer.
- For suprapubic hernias, it is important to pull up the inferior stitch, which should be brought up at the pubic bone or right above, first. Doing so ensures that the mesh is placed appropriately.

Mesh fixation

- Controversy about mesh fixation relates to whether suture fixation is needed for adequate fixation, and there is no consensus on this issue.[11]
- The 2 most common techniques for fixation are a combination of suture and tack fixation and the double-crown technique of placing 2 rows of tacks only for fixation.[12,13]
- Whichever technique is chosen, recurrence is most likely in the inferior/pubic region. Additional suture fixation is warranted in this area.
- In addition, to avoid neurovascular injuries when placing tacks in the suprapubic region, bimanually palpate the tip of the tacker externally to ensure that the tacks are placed above the iliopubic tract.
- The mesh should be adequately fixed and taut, because it relaxes when the pneumoperitoneum is removed (**Figs. 7** and **8**).

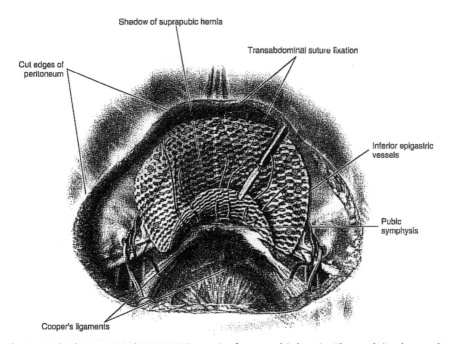

Fig. 7. Mesh placement in laparoscopic repair of suprapubic hernia. The mesh is adequately fixed to the pubic bone with transabdominal sutures and tacks. (*From* Polouse BK. Laparoscopic repair of atypical hernias. In: Rosen M, editor. Atlas of abdominal wall reconstruction. New York: Elsevier; 2011; with permission.)

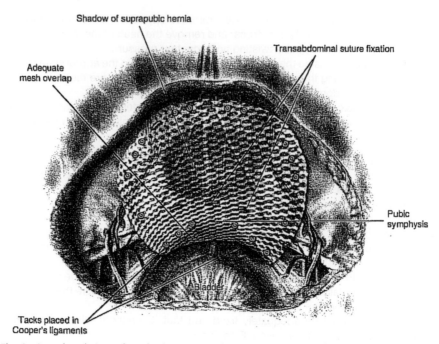

Shadow of suprapubic hernia

Transabdominal suture fixation

Adequate
mesh overlap

Pubic
symphysis

Bladder

Tacks placed in
Cooper's ligaments

Fig. 8. Completed view of mesh placement in laparoscopic repair of suprapubic hernia with suture and tack fixation. (*From* Polouse BK. Laparoscopic repair of atypical hernias. In: Rosen M, editor. Atlas of abdominal wall reconstruction. New York: Elsevier; 2011; with permission.)

- The 2 main options for tack fixation involve permanent and absorbable tacks. Although some animal studies have compared different types of tack fixation, there is no strong clinical evidence that shows the superiority of either type of tack fixation, so this is left to the surgeon's discretion.[14,15]

Closure
- After mesh placement, the omentum and bowel are examined again to rule out bleeding or occult bowel injury.
- Ports larger than 5 mm are closed using an open or laparoscopic technique.
- Ports should be removed under direct vision and incisions closed.

Postoperative care/considerations
- Most patients require admission to the hospital for pain control and observation. Patient-controlled analgesia pumps can be used, depending on the clinical situation.
- Because postoperative pain can be a difficult problem, we use several preoperative and postoperative adjuncts, including placing local anesthesia before port and transfascial suture placement and using nonsteroidal antiinflammatory medications.
- Depending on the amount of adhesiolysis, patients can develop an ileus, which is managed with ambulation, bowel rest, and time.
- Because of the nature of the laparoscopic repair, many patients with large hernia defects develop a postoperative seroma. Although these are seldom problematic, patients should be aware of this possibility preoperatively.

Subxiphoid hernia Subxiphoid hernias are most often encountered as incisional hernias after upper midline surgery, cardiac surgery, and occasionally recurrent hernias above a previously placed mesh. These hernias are difficult, because of the limit of the coastal margin and xiphoid process for transfascial fixation. Laparoscopic and open approaches are successfully used for repair of these difficult hernias.

Open approach
Preoperative planning
- Patients undergo standard evaluation for hernia surgery with CT scanning.
- Patients should be appropriate candidates for repair and understand the goals of the surgery.

Positioning
- The patient is positioned supine with arms to the side.
- A Foley catheter is placed, and appropriate antibiotics and deep vein thrombosis prophylaxis are given.

Abdominal access
- An upper midline incision is used and can be extended inferiorly to the umbilicus depending on the size of the hernia.
- A large scar from previous surgery can be excised.
- Careful abdominal access must be gained to avoid injury to abdominal contents, which can be present in the hernia.

Lysis of adhesions
- Complete abdominal wall adhesiolysis should be performed and the abdomen explored to rule out disease/abnormalities.

Retromuscular dissection/closure
- Although an onlay-type open repair of a subxiphoid hernia is feasible, getting into the preperitoneal or retrorectus space likely facilitates more mesh overlap.
- Depending on the size of the defect and the surgeon's preference, either a preperitoneal or retrorectus repair is chosen.
- A retrorectus dissection usually allows adequate mesh overlap, except in large hernias.
- The most difficult location for mesh overlap and fixation is at the xiphoid. Fascial defects going all the way to the xiphoid can be challenging to repair.
- After the preperitoneal space or retrorectus space has been dissected (as previously described), the tissue is closed in the midline. Even in difficult subxiphoid hernias, several centimeters of mesh overlap underneath the xiphoid should be possible (**Fig. 9**).
- Place suture fixation on the lateral borders of the xiphoid, if needed.

Mesh choice/placement
- Because the mesh is excluded in this type of repair, an uncoated polypropylene or polyester mesh can be used. We recommend a large, macroporous, reduced-weight mesh.

Mesh fixation
- Mesh fixation can be difficult in subxiphoid hernias. The mesh can be fixed just below the xiphoid or sutures brought up on the lateral side of the xiphoid, using suture passers.

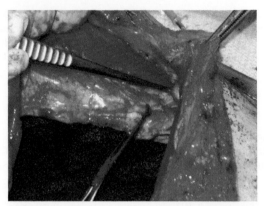

Fig. 9. Retrorectus dissection performed up to and underneath the xiphoid. The forceps are pointing to the xiphoid process. This procedure allows mesh placement up to and under the xiphoid process, and the mesh can be fixed at this point.

- The upper edges of the mesh should overlap the ribs, and transfascial sutures can be placed just below the coastal margin. This technique usually provides adequate fixation.
- The superior portion around the xiphoid and costal margin are fixed first, then the inferior and lateral portions of the mesh.
- Four to 8 transfascial sutures are usually required, depending on the size of the defect.

Fascial closure
- Fascial closure should be per the surgeon's preference.
- Because external component separation imparts little advantage in the upper-most fascia/subxiphoid region, this technique is seldom required, unless there is a large hernia low in the abdomen.
- Fascial closure can be difficult just below the xiphoid. A standard running closure with slowly absorbing suture is recommended.[16,17]
- Before fascial closure, 1 to 2 closed suction drains can be placed to lie above the mesh.

Closure/postoperative care
- Wounds are irrigated, drains sutured in, and skin approximated with skin staples.
- Transfascial suture sites can be covered with a surgical glue, Steri-Strips, or other dressing.
- Patients usually require hospital admission for pain control and return of bowel function.
- Routine postoperative care includes slow advancement of diet and activity and monitoring of the wound and drain output.

Laparoscopic approach
Patient positioning/draping
- The patient is placed supine with both arms tucked and padded. Ioban drapes are used per the surgeon's preference.

Laparoscopic access
- Laparoscopic access uses either an open or closed technique. Subxiphoid her-nias usually occur in patients with previous surgery, so laparoscopic access should be gained cautiously.

- Avoid entering the abdomen at previous incision sites, because of the likelihood of adhesions.

Port placement
- Three to 5 trocars are used based on the complexity of the case, with 1 trocar being 11 mm or 12 mm. Three trocars are usually placed on the left lateral abdomen and 1 or 2 on the right lateral abdomen, depending on the hernia size.
- If the hernia is confined to the upper abdomen, the inferior trocars are brought in medially in a semicircular configuration. However, in general, trocars should be placed as lateral on the abdominal wall as possible to facilitate range of motion of instruments and allow wide mesh overlap and visibility.

Diagnostic laparoscopy and laparoscopic lysis of adhesions
- Diagnostic laparoscopy should be performed to identify adhesions and associated abdominal disease.
- Depending on the amount and tenacity of adhesions, it is sometimes prudent to convert to an open operation early to save time and avoid the possibility of iatrogenic enterotomy.
- Careful, sharp lysis of adhesions is then pursued.

Laparoscopic takedown of the falciform This part of the procedure is unique to laparoscopic repair of subxiphoid hernias.

- Takedown of the falciform ligament is mandatory in most subxiphoid hernias to allow for adequate mesh overlap.
- After the abdominal wall is cleared of adhesions and the hernia is visualized, the falciform should be taken down using cautery and scissors all the way up to the diaphragm (**Fig. 10**).
- Energy devices can be used, because hemostasis is crucial, and bleeding often occurs at the beginning of the dissection.
- Part of the falciform can be within the hernia defect, so every effort should be made to reduce this and take the ligament down close to the abdominal wall.

Measuring the hernia defect
- The hernia defect is measured intracorporeally, as described earlier, obtaining a transverse and longitudinal measurement.

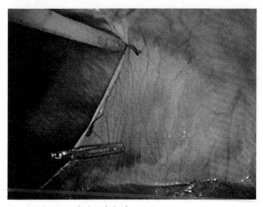

Fig. 10. Laparoscopic takedown of the falciform ligament is mandatory in repairing subxiphoid hernias to allow adequate mesh overlap. This takedown can be achieved with energy devices or scissors with electrocautery.

Mesh choice

- Several mesh types are used for this repair, but the mesh should be appropriate for intra-abdominal placement. This mesh is usually an absorbable coated polyester or polypropylene, composite mesh with polypropylene and Gore-Tex, or plain Gore-Tex mesh.

Mesh preparation/placement

- Mesh preparation and placement are similar to suprapubic hernias, as described earlier. However, for subxiphoid hernias, the superior-most stitch placed in the mesh often must be brought down several centimeters so that it can be brought out just below the xiphoid.
- Placing the stitch several centimeters below this position facilitates mesh overlap above the xiphoid, which is key for a successful repair (**Fig. 11**).
- After 4 sutures are placed, the mesh is rolled as a scroll and pushed or pulled through one of the 11-mm or 12-mm port sites.

Mesh fixation

- Mesh fixation follows the same principles as for the suprapubic hernia repair, with a few caveats.
- In subxiphoid hernia repair, fixation above the coastal margins is generally not recommended, because fixation in this area can cause chronic pain, and tack fixation can cause pericardial injury.[18]
- For subxiphoid hernias, tacks are placed at the costal margin, and, if warranted, additional transfascial suture fixation can be placed just below the costal margin.
- An important key to successful laparoscopic repair is to ensure adequate mesh overlap up to the diaphragm, even if it cannot be adequately fixed. This mesh is pushed up by the liver and allows for wide overlap of the hernia. Alternatively, the excess mesh above the costal margin and xiphoid can be glued to the abdominal wall.

Closure

- After mesh placement, the omentum and bowel are examined for possible bleeding or occult bowel injury.

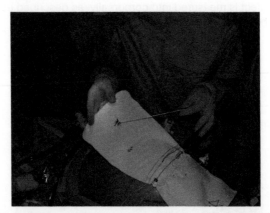

Fig. 11. Placing the initial transfascial suture several centimeters below the cephalad portion of the mesh allows mesh overlap above the xiphoid and costal margin. This upper portion of the mesh can be fixed with fibrin sealant or the liver can hold the mesh in place. (*From* Polouse BK. Laparoscopic repair of atypical hernias. In: Rosen M, editor. Atlas of abdominal wall reconstruction. New York: Elsevier; 2011; with permission.)

- Ports larger than 5 mm are closed using an open or laparoscopic technique, and ports should be removed under direct vision.
- The incisions are closed per the surgeon's preference.

Postoperative care/considerations
- Routine postoperative care is used, and most patients require admission to the hospital for observation and pain control.
- Depending on the size of the hernia, patients often develop seromas at the site of the hernia.
- These seromas are usually asymptomatic and require no intervention.
- The possibility of seroma development should be discussed with the patient preoperatively to alleviate anxiety after surgery.

Flank hernia Flank hernias are a challenge, because they are bordered by several bony structures and sometimes provide limited tissue to work with. Incisional hernias from iliac bone harvest, trauma, and retroperitoneal surgery for aortic disease, urologic/kidney disease, or spine exposure are the most commonly encountered flank hernias; however, there are some congenital flank hernias that warrant mentioning. The congenital or lumbar-type hernias can be subclassified into superior triangle (Grynfeltt) or inferior triangle (Petit) defects. The proximity of many of these hernias to bony structures, such as the iliac crest and 12th rib, make them especially challenging to fix. Laparoscopic and open approaches to these difficult hernias are discussed, including the importance of wide mesh overlap with appropriate fixation for durable repair.

Open approach
Preoperative planning
- CT scanning is recommended to help determine the size and location of the hernia and previous mesh or foreign material, which may be encountered at the time of surgery.
- The CT scan also helps distinguish a true hernia from laxity of the flank region, which can occur from denervation of the thoracic nerves.
- Because these repairs often require large incisions and dissections, postoperative pain management can be problematic. Placement of epidural catheters or other pain management adjuncts is advised in these cases.
- Appropriate preoperative antibiotics and deep vein thrombosis prophylaxis should be administered.

Patient positioning/preparing
- Patients are placed in the lateral decubitus position using a beanbag or roll.
- The approximate degree of laterality should be determined by the size and location of the hernia.
- The patient is padded and secured to the bed with an axillary roll.
- A wide preparation including the midline of the abdomen is recommended. Ioban-type dressings may be used to assist in draping.

Incision/abdominal access
- For flank incisional hernias, the incision is typically made overlying the previous incision, and the scar can be excised if unsightly or per the patient's preference.

Dissection/adhesiolysis
- Dissection is carried down through the Camper and Scarpa fascia to identify the musculature of the abdominal wall.

- If the hernia sac is encountered, this can be carefully opened or left intact and dissected laterally to the fascial edges. It is preferable to leave the hernia sac intact and use it to dissect into the preperitoneal space without having to enter the abdomen.
- If the abdominal cavity is entered, careful adhesiolysis is needed.
- If the hernia sac cannot be located, the layers of the abdominal wall are divided, including the external oblique, internal oblique, and transversus abdominis.
- The preperitoneal plane is the ideal plane to place the mesh in flank hernias, because it allows large overlap of a mesh prosthetic. This preperitoneal plane can be dissected at the fascial edges if the abdominal cavity/hernia sac is entered or by dissecting the hernia sac to the lateral edges of the fascia.
- After the preperitoneal space is entered, it is bluntly dissected to allow for a large area for mesh placement. It can be dissected to the diaphragm superiorly, posteriorly to the psoas muscle, medially to the rectus sheath or linea alba, and inferiorly to the Cooper ligament and the pelvis (**Fig. 12**).
- The peritoneum is closed if it was entered and all holes closed with an absorbable suture, excluding the space from abdominal viscera.

Mesh placement
- The preperitoneal space is measured to choose the appropriate size of mesh.
- The mesh is oriented and placed in the space to gauge the appropriate size.
- Cutting mesh is not usually recommended; however, most meshes can be cut to size without damaging the mesh to achieve an appropriately taut and well-fitted mesh.
- The mesh is fixed posteriorly first with transfascial sutures using a suture passer under direct vision. The amount of space available to place transfascial sutures is limited by the iliac crest and other structures.
- Several approaches can be used to achieve adequate fixation. Bone anchor fixation has been described.[19,20]
- Alternatively, mesh can be fixed at the edge of the iliac crest, and the mesh can overlap into the preperitoneal space. This excessive mesh without suture fixation can be glued into place using commercially available surgical glues.
- The recommended method of fixation starts posteriorly, then medially, then inferiorly, and superiorly, but this can be based on the surgeon's preference (**Fig. 13**).
- The important point is wide overlap with adequate fixation and for the mesh to be under physiologic tension.
- It is helpful to be sure that the bed is neutral and not flexed (if this was used to expose this area at the beginning of the operation).

Closure
- After suture fixation of the mesh, closed suction drains are placed above the mesh, depending on the amount of dissection.
- The area is irrigated, and the fascia closed using a slowly absorbing monofilament running suture.

Postoperative care
- Routine postoperative care is used, with a special emphasis on pain control. Abdominal binders are useful for patient comfort and for a feeling of stability. Closed suction drains are left until the output is less than 30 mL/d.

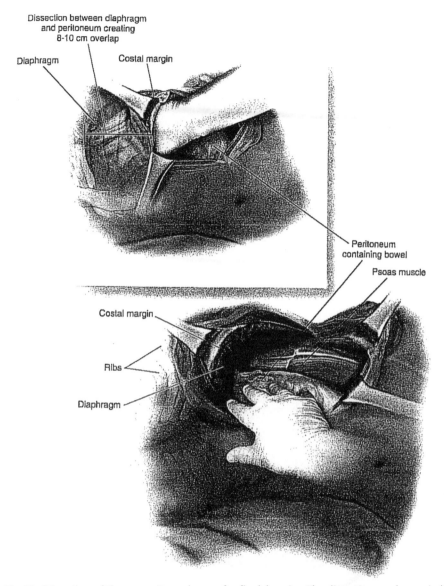

Fig. 12. Dissection of the preperitoneal space for flank hernias. The dissection can be carried out toward the diaphragm superiorly, posteriorly to the psoas muscle and spine, medially to the linea alba, and inferiorly to the Cooper ligament. (*From* Philips MS, Rosen MJ. Open flank hernia repair. In: Rosen M, editor. Atlas of abdominal wall reconstruction. New York: Elsevier; 2011; with permission.)

Laparoscopic approach

Flank hernias can be successfully repaired laparoscopically, but to be safely performed, this requires advanced laparoscopic and dissection skills and knowledge of the details of the retroperitoneal anatomy.

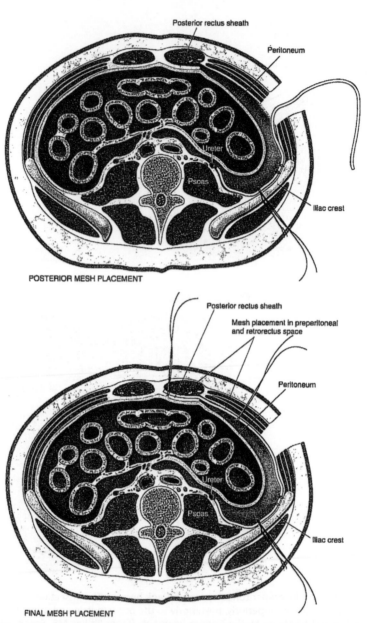

Fig. 13. The mesh placement for open flank hernia repair with the mesh being placed and fixed in the preperitoneal space. (*From* Philips MS, Rosen MJ. Open flank hernia repair. In: Rosen M, editor. Atlas of abdominal wall reconstruction. New York: Elsevier; 2011; with permission.)

Preoperative planning

- CT scanning is recommended, because of the complexity and operative planning required to repair this hernia (**Fig. 14**).
- Appropriate preoperative antibiotics and deep vein thrombosis prophylaxis should be administered.

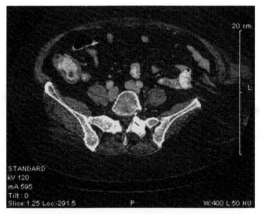

Fig. 14. CT scan in a patient with a flank incisional hernia. Flank hernia seen on the right side of the CT scan (*patient's left*) above the iliac crest. CT scans can help define anatomy and help in surgical planning.

Patient positioning/prepping
- Patients are placed in a semilateral or full lateral decubitus position depending on the size and location of the hernia defect, which can be assessed with CT scanning and clinical examination.
- This positioning can be achieved with either a beanbag or a roll.
- The patient should be adequately secured and padded with an axillary roll. Ioban or similar dressings are helpful in preparing and facilitating easy marking on the patient.

Laparoscopic access
- Laparoscopic access is obtained using an open or closed technique per the surgeon's preference.
- Access can be difficult, because the patient is not supine, and landmarks used for safe access are not available.
- Safe laparoscopic access is essential and should be performed with caution, especially in the reoperative abdomen.

Port placement
- Three to 5 trocars arranged in a semicircular configuration are placed opposite the hernia.
- One port should be an 11-mm or 12-mm port to facilitate easy mesh placement, but can vary based on mesh type used and hernia size.
- Ports are placed to facilitate good triangulation, visualization of the hernia defect, and dissection of the colon.

Diagnostic laparoscopy and laparoscopic lysis of adhesions
- Diagnostic laparoscopy can rule out occult hernias or disease not identified on CT scanning. It also shows the surgeon the anatomy around the hernia and in the lateral position.
- As always, safe adhesiolysis with laparoscopic scissors is performed to clear the entire abdominal wall of adhesions.

Laparoscopic mobilization of colon
- Depending on the size and location of the hernia, the right or left colon likely needs to be partially or fully mobilized to permit adequate visualization and fixation of the hernia.
- This procedure is similar to open and laparoscopic colon mobilization and is aided by having the patient in the lateral position.
- Dissection ensues along the white line of Toldt up to the splenic or hepatic flexure, depending on how much of the colon needs to be mobilized.

Taking down peritoneum
- Although not mandatory, taking down the peritoneum at the level of the hernia posteriorly provides a pocket for the mesh and a way for the mesh to be partially covered by the peritoneum.
- Taking down the peritoneum is similar to a transabdominal preperitoneal repair.
- The surgeon grabs the thin peritoneum and blunt dissects posteriorly toward the psoas muscle. This dissection is performed as much as needed to provide mesh overlap posteriorly and laterally.
- Although laparoscopic repair of the flank hernia does not mandate taking down the peritoneum and the mesh can be placed totally intra-abdominally as in a standard laparoscopic hernia repair, taking down the peritoneum allows wider mesh overlap and reduces the amount of fixation necessary.

Hernia measurement
- The hernia defect is measured intracorporeally as described earlier, obtaining a transverse and longitudinal measurement. This measurement is used to choose the size of the mesh.

Mesh preparation/placement
- The correct size and type of mesh are chosen (mesh compatible with intra-abdominal placement must be used). This type is usually barrier mesh, using either an absorbable or permanent barrier, or Gore-Tex mesh.
- Four nonabsorbable sutures are placed at the midpoint of the superior, inferior, left and right lateral portion of the mesh, and it is rolled as a scroll to be placed in the abdomen.
- The mesh can be pulled or pushed into the abdomen, usually through the 11-mm or 12-mm trocar.
- The mesh is unrolled inside the abdomen. The 4 sutures are then pulled up through the abdominal wall using a suture passer.
- If the mesh overlaps the iliac crest or ribs on the superior or inferior portion of the mesh and transfascial suture fixation is impossible, the options are to place the sutures off the periphery of the mesh, where the suture can be brought out through tissue and fascia, or to use bone anchors to secure the mesh.
- If a large preperitoneal space has been created superiorly and inferiorly, a third option is to tuck the mesh in this space and use surgical glue for fixation.

Mesh fixation
- The mesh can be fixed with additional transfascial sutures if the surgeon prefers and there is adequate fascia and soft tissue to place additional sutures.
- The mesh can also be tacked to the abdominal wall and peritoneum using permanent or absorbable tacks.
- Tacks should not be placed where the adjacent soft tissue with bimanual palpation cannot be felt or in areas where neurovascular bundles run.

- Careful attention to the anatomy is crucial to avoid neurovascular injuries or chronic pain from a misplaced tack or suture.

Closure

- After mesh fixation, the peritoneum, if dissected, is tacked or glued to partially cover the posterior portion of the mesh.
- The abdominal contents are again evaluated for occult bowel injury and bleeding, and the ports are removed under direct vision, making sure to close trocar sites greater than 10 mm.

Postoperative care/considerations

- Most patients require hospital admission for pain control and observation.
- Routine postoperative care is administered, with an emphasis on pain control and early ambulation.

Clinical Results in the Literature

Although atypical hernias are not rare, there are few reports specifically related to outcomes of these, because they are often grouped with other midline hernias. Several series have been published on atypical hernias and the unique problems associated with their repair. Less has been published on open repair of atypical hernias, especially the suprapubic and subxiphoid hernias, because again these are often grouped with all open ventral hernia repairs.

Several series (**Table 1**) have examined the laparoscopic approach to the suprapubic hernia. Although their outcomes are similar, variations in techniques and types of mesh must be accounted for when evaluating the data. In a series by Carbonell and colleagues,[21] all patients underwent laparoscopic repair with expanded polytetrarfluorethyelene mesh; however, over the period of the study and in response to some recurrences early in the series, the repair evolved to include transabdominal suture fixation to the pubic bone, Cooper ligament, and above the iliopubic tract. Palanivelu and colleagues[22] used laparoscopic repair with Parietex mesh (Covidien, Mansfield, MA) in all cases, transabdominal suture fixation, and intracorporeal suture closure of the hernia defect. Varnell and colleagues[23] reported a series from several surgeons using various meshes, including Gore-Tex Dual Mesh (Gore WL, Flagstaff, AZ), Proceed (Johnson & Johnson, Cincinnati, OH), and Parietex Composite (Covidien, Mansfield, MA), and transabdominal suture fixation. Sharma and colleagues[24] reported the largest and most recent series using a transabdominal partial extraperitoneal technique using Proceed and transabdominal suture fixation. Jenkins and colleagues[25] reported on clinical predictors of complexity in laparoscopic ventral hernia showing suprapubic hernias to be one of many predictors of longer placement time of adhesiolysis mesh.

For subxiphoid hernias, there is literature related to the natural history and incidence after certain procedures, outcome data on the open and laparoscopic repair, and a review article. Kim and colleagues[26] evaluated the incidence and risk factors of developing subxiphoid hernias after coronary bypass grafting in 1656 patients with a mean follow-up of 49.5 months. These investigators reported an incisional hernia rate requiring operation of 0.8% and risk factors for occurrence being female gender and low cardiac output syndromes.[26] Another study by Barner[27] reported a technique of a modified median sternotomy in 2500 patients that resulted in a 0 incidence of subxiphoid incisional hernia. Outcome data for published series of open and laparoscopic repair specific to subxiphoid hernia are presented in **Table 2**. The data are from small series with limited follow-up and are all retrospective. The largest series by Mackey

Table 1
Published series on laparoscopic repair of suprapubic hernias

Author/Year	Number of Patients	Mean Follow-Up (mo)	Operating Room Time (min)	Length of Hospital Stay (d)	Conversion to Open (%)	Complication Rate (%)	Recurrence Rate (%)
Carbonell et al,[19,21] 2005	36	21.1	178.7	2.4	2.7	16.6	5.5
Palanivelu et al,[22] 2008	17	9	95	1.5	0	29.4	5.8
Varnell et al,[23] 2008	47	2.6	130	3	2.1	38	6.3
Sharma et al,[24] 2011	72	57.6	116	2.2	0	27.8	6.9

Data from Refs.[21-24]

Table 2
Published series on open and laparoscopic repair of subxiphoid hernias

Author/Year	Technique of Repair	Number of Patients	Mean Follow-Up (mo)	Operating Room Time (min)	Length of Hospital Stay (d)	Complication Rate (%)	Recurrence Rate (%)
Cohen & Starling,[32] 1985	Polypropylene onlay	14	4–36	NR	NR	0	0
Davidson & Bailey,[33] 1987	Open primary repair	8	22	NR	NR	NR	0
Bouillot et al,[34] 1997	Retromuscular repair with polypropylene mesh	23	1–5 y	NR	NR	NR	0
Muscarella et al,[35] 2000	Laparoscopic	1	6	NR	NR	NR	0
Landau et al,[36] 2001	Laparoscopic	10	—	55	—	30	10
Mackey et al,[28] 2005	Open and laparoscopic primary and mesh repair	45	48	NR	NR	NR	36
Eisenberg et al,[37] 2008	Laparoscopic	4	NR	122	6.5	50%	NR
Carbonell et al,[38] 2011	Open double-mesh technique	35	4–80	NR	NR	20	0

Abbreviation: NR, not recorded.
Data from Refs.[28,32–38]

Table 3
Published series on open and laparoscopic repair of flank hernias

Author/Year	Technique of Repair	Number of Patients	Mean Follow-Up (mo)	Operating Room Time (min)	Length of Hospital Stay (d)	Complication Rate (%)	Recurrence Rate (%)
Shekarriz et al,[39] 2001	Laparoscopic	3	12	138	2	0	0
Petersen et al,[40] 2002	Open retromuscular	4	33	208	15	0	0
Zieren et al,[41] 2007	Open retromuscular and onlay	15	60	101	NR	NR	13
Edwards et al,[42] 2009	Laparoscopic	27	3.6	144	3.1	3.7	0
Fei & Li,[43] 2010	Open retromuscular	23	24.5	NR	NR	13	13
	Open extended retromuscular	18	26.2	NR	NR	27.8	0
Veyrie et al,[44] 2012	Open retromuscular	61	47	136	7	18	4.9
Phillips et al,[45] 2012	Open retromuscular	16	16.8	178	6.3	19	0

Abbreviation: NR, not recorded.
Data from Refs.[39-45]

and colleagues[28] evaluated a few patients undergoing primary repair (14), laparoscopic repair with mesh (10), and open repair with mesh (21), with recurrence rates of 43%, 30%, and 33%, respectively. These investigators also reported that previous sternal wound infection was a risk factor for recurrent hernias after repair, with 6 of 16 patients with recurrences also having a previous sternal wound infection.[28]

Data related to incidence and outcomes of flank hernias, resulting mostly from traumatic injuries and incisions, are also a mixture of open and laparoscopic cases. Although not true hernias, there are data related to the incidence of flank bulging after retroperitoneal incisions and possible mechanism of this occurrence. Chatterjee and colleagues[29] evaluated 70 patients undergoing flank incisions for nephrectomy and reported 49% of patients complaining of flank bulging. Gardner and colleagues[30] performed an analysis of flank bulge using neurophysiologic testing, cadaver dissection, and clinical data on 63 patients. These investigators reported an 11% incidence of flank bulge and showed that this phenomenon is related to intercostal nerve injury with subsequent paralysis of the abdominal wall musculature. Data from series (>1 patient) on open and laparoscopic repair of flank hernias are shown in **Table 3**. In general, these series report on standard techniques of the open and laparoscopic repair of the flank hernia, adhering to the principles of wide overlap of mesh with appropriate fixation. However, because of patient factors, slight differences in techniques, and use of mesh, there is some variability in the outcomes.

A few other published reports on the topic of atypical hernia repair deserve mention, although they do not fit specifically into 1 category of hernia repair. Ferrari and colleagues[31] reported on a series of 39 patients undergoing laparoscopic repair of suprapubic (18), subxiphoid (15), and lateral hernias (6). These investigators showed acceptable outcomes, with a 3% conversion rate, 18% complication rate, mean hospital stay of 5.1 days, and at a mean follow-up of 38 months, a 7.7% recurrence rate. There are also 2 reports on the use of bone anchor fixation for atypical hernias. Carbonell and colleagues[19] reported on 10 patients undergoing open retromuscular repair of lumbar hernias with the use of bone anchors for fixation. These investigators reported excellent outcomes, with a mean hospital length of stay of 5.2 days, no postoperative complications, and at a mean follow-up of 40 months, no recurrences.[19] Yee and colleagues[20] evaluated bone anchor fixation in laparoscopic repairs in 30 patients, with 17 suprapubic, and 13 lateral. These investigators reported an average length of hospital stay of 5.2 days, 23.3% complication rate, 3.3% mortality, and a 6.7% recurrence rate at a mean follow-up of 13.2 months.

SUMMARY

Atypical hernias or hernias located at the abdominal borders can be challenging to repair. Thorough knowledge of anatomy, appropriate preoperative planning, and reliance on the principles of hernia repair, including wide mesh overlap and fixation, ensure successful outcomes. Many options for repair, including technique and mesh choice, are available for the surgeon. The hernia surgeon should be well versed in the open and laparoscopic approaches and apply them based on the individual clinical presentation. Long-term outcomes related to suprapubic, subxiphoid, and lateral hernia repairs are limited; however, open and laparoscopic repairs using wide mesh overlap and adequate fixation have acceptable outcomes and recurrence rates. Future research will likely focus on comparative studies based on patient factors, techniques, mesh, and cost to help surgeons choose the appropriate repairs for individual patients.

REFERENCES

1. Burger JW, Luijendijk RW, Hop WC, et al. Long-term follow-up of a randomized controlled trial of suture versus mesh repair of incisional hernia. Ann Surg 2004;240:578–83 [discussion: 83–5].
2. Luijendijk RW, Hop WC, van den Tol MP, et al. A comparison of suture repair with mesh repair for incisional hernia. N Engl J Med 2000;343:392–8.
3. Rosen MJ. Biologic mesh for abdominal wall reconstruction: a critical appraisal. Am Surg 2010;76:1–6.
4. Bachman S, Ramshaw B. Prosthetic material in ventral hernia repair: how do I choose? Surg Clin North Am 2008;88:101–12, ix.
5. Shell DH, de la Torre J, Andrades P, et al. Open repair of ventral incisional hernias. Surg Clin North Am 2008;88:61–83, viii.
6. Finan KR, Vick CC, Kiefe CI, et al. Predictors of wound infection in ventral hernia repair. Am J Surg 2005;190:676–81.
7. Conze J, Binnebosel M, Junge K, et al. Incisional hernia–how do I do it? Standard surgical approach. Chirurg 2010;81:192–200 [in German].
8. Voeller GR, Ramshaw B, Park AE, et al. Incisional hernia. J Am Coll Surg 1999; 189:635–7.
9. Novitsky YW, Elliott HL, Orenstein SB, et al. Transversus abdominis muscle release: a novel approach to posterior component separation during complex abdominal wall reconstruction. Am J Surg 2012;204:709–16.
10. Swenson BR, Camp TR, Mulloy DP, et al. Antimicrobial-impregnated surgical incise drapes in the prevention of mesh infection after ventral hernia repair. Surg Infect (Larchmt) 2008;9:23–32.
11. LeBlanc KA. Laparoscopic incisional hernia repair: are transfascial sutures necessary? A review of the literature. Surg Endosc 2007;21:508–13.
12. Heniford BT, Park A, Ramshaw BJ, et al. Laparoscopic repair of ventral hernias: nine years' experience with 850 consecutive hernias. Ann Surg 2003;238:391–9 [discussion: 399–400].
13. Morales-Conde S, Cadet H, Cano A, et al. Laparoscopic ventral hernia repair without sutures–double crown technique: our experience after 140 cases with a mean follow-up of 40 months. Int Surg 2005;90:S56–62.
14. Byrd JF, Agee N, Swan RZ, et al. Evaluation of absorbable and permanent mesh fixation devices: adhesion formation and mechanical strength. Hernia 2011;15: 553–8.
15. Reynvoet E, Berrevoet F, De Somer F, et al. Tensile strength testing for resorbable mesh fixation systems in laparoscopic ventral hernia repair. Surg Endosc 2012; 26:2513–20.
16. van 't Riet M, Steyerberg EW, Nellensteyn J, et al. Meta-analysis of techniques for closure of midline abdominal incisions. Br J Surg 2002;89:1350–6.
17. O'Dwyer PJ, Courtney CA. Factors involved in abdominal wall closure and subsequent incisional hernia. Surgeon 2003;1:17–22.
18. Frantzides CT, Welle SN. Cardiac tamponade as a life-threatening complication in hernia repair. Surgery 2012;152:133–5.
19. Carbonell AM, Kercher KW, Sigmon L, et al. A novel technique of lumbar hernia repair using bone anchor fixation. Hernia 2005;9:22–5.
20. Yee JA, Harold KL, Cobb WS, et al. Bone anchor mesh fixation for complex laparoscopic ventral hernia repair. Surg Innov 2008;15:292–6.
21. Carbonell AM, Kercher KW, Matthews BD, et al. The laparoscopic repair of suprapubic ventral hernias. Surg Endosc 2005;19:174–7.

22. Palanivelu C, Rangarajan M, Parthasarathi R, et al. Laparoscopic repair of suprapubic incisional hernias: suturing and intraperitoneal composite mesh onlay. A retrospective study. Hernia 2008;12:251–6.
23. Varnell B, Bachman S, Quick J, et al. Morbidity associated with laparoscopic repair of suprapubic hernias. Am J Surg 2008;196:983–7 [discussion: 87–8].
24. Sharma A, Dey A, Khullar R, et al. Laparoscopic repair of suprapubic hernias: transabdominal partial extraperitoneal (TAPE) technique. Surg Endosc 2011;25: 2147–52.
25. Jenkins ED, Yom VH, Melman L, et al. Clinical predictors of operative complexity in laparoscopic ventral hernia repair: a prospective study. Surg Endosc 2010;24: 1872–7.
26. Kim HS, Kim KB, Hwang HY, et al. Subxiphoid incisional hernia development after coronary artery bypass grafting. Korean J Thorac Cardiovasc Surg 2012;45: 161–5.
27. Barner HB. A technical modification of median sternotomy to eliminate subxiphoid incisional hernias. Arch Surg 1987;122:843.
28. Mackey RA, Brody FJ, Berber E, et al. Subxiphoid incisional hernias after median sternotomy. J Am Coll Surg 2005;201:71–6.
29. Chatterjee S, Nam R, Fleshner N, et al. Permanent flank bulge is a consequence of flank incision for radical nephrectomy in one half of patients. Urol Oncol 2004; 22:36–9.
30. Gardner GP, Josephs LG, Rosca M, et al. The retroperitoneal incision. An evaluation of postoperative flank 'bulge'. Arch Surg 1994;129:753–6.
31. Ferrari GC, Miranda A, Sansonna F, et al. Laparoscopic repair of incisional hernias located on the abdominal borders: a retrospective critical review. Surg Laparosc Endosc Percutan Tech 2009;19:348–52.
32. Cohen MJ, Starling JR. Repair of subxiphoid incisional hernias with Marlex mesh after median sternotomy. Arch Surg 1985;120:1270–1.
33. Davidson BR, Bailey JS. Repair of incisional hernia after median sternotomy. Thorax 1987;42:549–50.
34. Bouillot J, Badawy A, Alexandre J. Incisional abdominal hernia after median sternotomy. Repair with the use of Dacron mesh. Hernia 1997;1:129–30.
35. Muscarella P, Needleman B, Goldstein A, et al. Laparoscopic repair of a subxiphoid incisional hernia following median sternotomy. Surg Rounds 2000;23: 605–11.
36. Landau O, Raziel A, Matz A, et al. Laparoscopic repair of poststernotomy subxiphoid epigastric hernia. Surg Endosc 2001;15:1313–4.
37. Eisenberg D, Popescu WM, Duffy AJ, et al. Laparoscopic treatment of subxiphoid incisional hernias in cardiac transplant patients. JSLS 2008;12:262–6.
38. Carbonell Tatay F, Garcia Pastor P, Bueno Lledo J, et al. Subxiphoid incisional hernia treatment: a technique using a double mesh adjusted to the defect. Cir Esp 2011;89:370–8.
39. Shekarriz B, Graziottin TM, Gholami S, et al. Transperitoneal preperitoneal laparoscopic lumbar incisional herniorrhaphy. J Urol 2001;166:1267–9.
40. Petersen S, Schuster F, Steinbach F, et al. Sublay prosthetic repair for incisional hernia of the flank. J Urol 2002;168:2461–3.
41. Zieren J, Menenakos C, Taymoorian K, et al. Flank hernia and bulging after open nephrectomy: mesh repair by flank or median approach? Report of a novel technique. Int Urol Nephrol 2007;39:989–93.
42. Edwards C, Geiger T, Bartow K, et al. Laparoscopic transperitoneal repair of flank hernias: a retrospective review of 27 patients. Surg Endosc 2009;23:2692–6.

43. Fei Y, Li L. Comparison of two repairing procedures for abdominal wall reconstruction in patients with flank hernia. Zhongguo Xiu Fu Chong Jian Wai Ke Za Zhi 2010;24:1506–9 [in Chinese].
44. Veyrie N, Poghosyan T, Corigliano N, et al. Lateral incisional hernia repair by the retromuscular approach with polyester standard mesh: topographic considerations and long-term follow-up of 61 consecutive patients. World J Surg 2013; 37(3):538–44.
45. Phillips MS, Krpata DM, Blatnik JA, et al. Retromuscular preperitoneal repair of flank hernias. J Gastrointest Surg 2012;16:1548–53.

Takedown of Enterocutaneous Fistula and Complex Abdominal Wall Reconstruction

Dominic Alexander James Slade, MB ChB, FRCS,
Gordon Lawrence Carlson, BSc, MD, FRCS*

KEYWORDS

• Intestinal failure • Open abdomen • Sepsis • Stoma • Separation of components

KEY POINTS

- Reconstruction of the gastrointestinal tract and an associated abdominal wall defect is not an operation to be undertaken on an occasional basis.
- Patients with enterocutaneous fistulas have complex physical and psychological health problems, which need to be fully addressed preoperatively by a multidisciplinary team.
- Definitive reconstructive surgery should never be undertaken until the patient's condition has been optimized, with particular regard paid to eradicating sepsis and restoration of nutritional status.
- Preoperative assessment of the gastrointestinal tract and abdominal wall should be undertaken, to enable a detailed plan to be devised for reconstruction of both.
- Definitive reconstructive surgery may require several, staged procedures.
- Large complex abdominal wall defects continue to present exceptionally challenging problems and may be best addressed by plastic surgical reconstruction and staged reconstruction of the gastrointestinal tract.
- Newer approaches, including biologic implants, may offer alternatives for reconstruction of large contaminated abdominal wall defects in patients with enterocutaneous fistulas but have not yet been adequately evaluated.

INTRODUCTION

Reconstruction of a large contaminated abdominal wall defect represents a significant challenge, even for the experienced surgeon. Perhaps the most extreme example of the difficulties and complexities associated with these procedures is that of the large abdominal wall defect associated with an enterocutaneous fistula. The surgical

Department of Surgery, National Intestinal Failure Centre, Salford Royal NHS Foundation Trust, Eccles Old Road, Salford, Manchester M6 8HD, UK
* Corresponding author.
E-mail address: gordon.carlson@srft.nhs.uk

Surg Clin N Am 93 (2013) 1163–1183
http://dx.doi.org/10.1016/j.suc.2013.06.006
0039-6109/13/$ – see front matter © 2013 Elsevier Inc. All rights reserved.

management of a complex abdominal wall defect in the setting of enterocutaneous fistulation involves a series of important issues, including the following:

- Management of abdominal sepsis
- Optimization of nutritional status, to facilitate definitive reconstructive surgery and postoperative healing
- Detailed assessment of intestinal anatomy
- Control of underlying medical disease (especially inflammatory bowel disease)
- Preservation of intestinal length and avoidance of short bowel syndrome after reconstructive surgery
- Creation of (often multiple) bowel anastomoses or stomas
- Absence of abdominal musculature and skin cover as a result of fistula-related wound infection and necrosis
- Significant contamination of the operative field with enteric organisms and their associated biofilm
- Loss of abdominal domain and the potential for abdominal hypertension after abdominal wall reconstruction
- Inability to use many prosthetic materials because of the degree of contamination, and unproven efficacy of those materials that are available
- Psychological support, especially for patients with enteroatmospheric fistulation and prolonged hospitalization

Surgery to take down enterocutaneous fistulas and reconstruct sizable complex abdominal wall defects is technically challenging and relatively high risk, even in expert hands. Attention to detail is vital if acceptable results are to be obtained, and the complex, multifaceted nature of the care lends itself to a multidisciplinary team approach. Awareness of these issues in the United Kingdom has led to the establishment of nationally designated acute intestinal failure units, offering specialized treatment of patients with enterocutaneous fistulas.

ACUTE INTESTINAL FAILURE AND ENTEROCUTANEOUS FISTULATION

Many patients with enterocutaneous fistulas have intestinal failure, a condition characterized by dependence on the parenteral provision of fluids/electrolytes or nutrition for the maintenance of health (**Table 1**).[1]

Acute intestinal failure, which is reversible, is distinguished from chronic intestinal failure (short bowel syndrome), which is not.[2] Acute intestinal failure is usually further subclassified into type 1 (which is self-limiting, usually within 14 days) and type 2 intestinal failure, which is also capable of resolution, but over a longer time course. Most patients with type 1 intestinal failure have simple ileus or postoperative intestinal obstruction, whereas intestinal failure occurring in patients with enterocutaneous fistulas is usually type 2 intestinal failure, requiring many months of treatment and, frequently, major reconstructive surgery before nutritional autonomy is restored.[1] Management of patients with type 2 intestinal failure is best undertaken by dedicated teams of health professionals, comprising surgeons, physicians, nurses, enterostomal therapists, dieticians, pharmacists, clinical biochemists, and psychologists.[2,3]

CAUSE AND CLASSIFICATION

An intestinal fistula is an abnormal communication between the intestinal tract and another epithelialized surface, usually the skin. Intestinal fistulas can be internal, communicating with other loops of bowel or another hollow viscus (eg, bladder or vagina) or external, communicating with the skin (enterocutaneous). When fistulation

Table 1 Classification of intestinal failure		
Classification	**Clinical Behavior and Therapy**	**Cause**
Type 1	Self-limiting Duration <14 d TPN	Usually postoperative (eg, ileus, small bowel obstruction)
Type 2	Medium-term Duration 14 d–6 mo Likely to require surgery TPN/fistuloclysis	Intestinal fistula, high-output stoma Postoperative septic and metabolic complications
Type 3	Long-term TPN Usually permanent May require intestinal lengthening/transplantation	Short bowel syndrome after multiple resections or severe intrinsic disease

Abbreviation: TPN, total parenteral nutrition.
From Lal S, Teubner A, Shaffer JL. Review article: intestinal failure. Aliment Pharmacol Ther 2006;24(1):19–31; with permission.

occurs in an open abdomen, leaving open loops of bowel exposed within the wound, the fistula is said to be enteroatmospheric (**Fig. 1**). Simple fistulas open directly onto the skin surface, whereas complex fistulas involve abscess cavities or another viscus.

Enterocutaneous fistulas are often classified according to the daily volume of intestinal effluent. High-output intestinal fistulas produce greater than 500 mL of fluid per day, and treatment usually requires parenteral nutrition.

Intestinal fistulation may result from intrinsic disease of the gastrointestinal tract or as a consequence of complications of abdominal surgery (**Table 2**).[4]

Any operation in which dissection of the small intestine occurs may result in postoperative intestinal fistulation. More than three-quarters of enterocutaneous fistulas develop as a consequence of surgery, usually because of breakdown of an intestinal anastomosis or an enteric injury.[4] Up to half of postoperative small bowel fistulas occur after surgery in which no resection or anastomosis has been performed. Division of abdominal adhesions, resulting in unplanned enterotomy and postoperative enteric leakage, either as result of unrecognized small bowel injury, or from an enterotomy repair, account for many of these cases. Avoiding accidental bowel injury is therefore crucially important when undertaking reconstructive surgery (see later discussion).

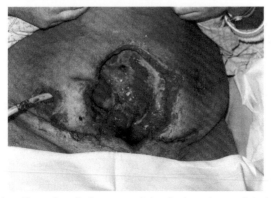

Fig. 1. Obliterated peritoneal cavity in severe abdominal sepsis associated with fistulation in the open abdomen.

Table 2	
Cause of small bowel fistula	
No Intrinsic Small Bowel Disease **>75%**	**Intrinsic Small Bowel Disease** **<25%**
Enterotomy/resection	Crohn's disease
Adhesiolysis	Diverticulosis
Injury to small bowel exposed in open abdomen	Carcinoma
	Lymphoma
	Radiation enteritis
	Appendicitis
	Vasculitis/ischemia
	Trauma
	Pancreatitis
	Tuberculosis

Data from Berry SM, Fischer JE. Classification and pathophysiology of enterocutaneous fistulas. Surg Clin North Am 1996;76(5):1009–18.

Enteroatmospheric fistulation almost always results from management of the open abdomen. Although open abdominal management as part of damage control laparotomy for trauma and severe abdominal sepsis has been reported to be beneficial,[5–7] allowing improved sepsis control, facilitating inspection of the abdominal contents, and avoiding abdominal hypertension, a potentially disastrous consequence of open abdominal management is the danger of injury to the exposed viscera. The open abdomen seems to be an inherently fistulogenic environment,[8] especially in the setting of abdominal sepsis. Although negative pressure wound therapy (NPWT) seems to be safe when used for short-term wound care after damage control laparotomy, with fistulation reported in 5% or less of patients,[6,9–13] fistulation seems to be considerably more common when NPWT is used for the management of abdominal sepsis,[14–17] with an incidence varying between 10% and 21%. Fistulation in the open abdomen is particularly difficult to manage and significantly increases mortality.[14]

PREOPERATIVE MANAGEMENT

Reconstructive surgery for a patient with an enterocutaneous fistula should not be undertaken until the patient's condition is optimized. This optimization requires a detailed appraisal of the patient's fitness for surgery, eradication of sepsis, correction of nutritional depletion, and assessment of local, abdominal conditions that are likely to determine the timing of, and techniques used for, reconstructive surgery. It is helpful to deal with issues that limit the patient's suitability for surgery in order of their importance with regard to threat to life. These management principles may be usefully summarized with the acronym SNAP:

- Sepsis: elimination of sepsis and provision of skin care
- Nutrition: appropriate, effective, and uncomplicated nutritional support
- Anatomy: definition of the anatomy of fistulas, proximal and distal gastrointestinal tract, and the abdominal wall
- Procedure: planning and undertaking the surgical procedure to take down the fistula and close the associated abdominal wall defect (where appropriate)

DIAGNOSIS AND MANAGEMENT OF ABDOMINAL SEPSIS

Sepsis remains as important a negative prognostic factor in patients with intestinal fistulas[18] as it was when described in 1978.[19] Inadequately treated abdominal sepsis leads to progressive impairment of organ function and death from multiple organ failure syndrome. Low-grade abdominal and pelvic infection (eg, a pelvic abscess associated with a complex fistula) may also be present without sepsis, but may result in a state of chronic catabolism, resulting in failure to respond to nutritional support. The classic features of sepsis, including swinging pyrexia, tachycardia, tachypnea, and leukocytosis may be absent, particularly in the patient with long-standing, walled-off infection. Hypoalbuminemia, hyponatremia, or unexplained jaundice may be more subtle signs of abdominal infection and should initiate a careful search for a septic focus. The abdomen is usually the focus of infection in patients who have undergone abdominal surgery, but other sources such as urinary, respiratory, or catheter-related bloodstream sepsis may also need to be excluded.

Abdominal infection should be investigated with contrast-enhanced computed tomography (CT), which has a diagnostic accuracy of greater than 97% in experienced hands. When combined with oral contrast, it is possible to distinguish an intra-abdominal or pelvic abscess from immotile, fluid-filled loops of bowel. Alternative techniques, including ultrasonography, magnetic resonance imaging, and labeled leukocyte scanning, may be of value in some patients, but have not been shown to be superior to CT. Ultrasonography may be of value in the detection of subphrenic or pelvic collections but may be difficult to perform and interpret in the postoperative patient, in whom the presence of drains or stomas makes scanning the patient technically difficult, and gaseous distention of the abdomen degrades quality. Radiolabeled leukocyte scanning usually takes too long to organize and perform to be satisfactory and also has a lower specificity than CT. However, it may be of particular value in cases in which an abnormality is suspected and may allow more detailed, focused imaging with CT or magnetic resonance imaging at the site of a suspected hot spot. It is important to emphasize that it may (rarely) be necessary to undertake a laparotomy if the clinical features of abdominal infection are convincing despite negative imaging, and the patient is deteriorating.

Identification of a focus of abdominal infection must be dealt with promptly. Antibiotic therapy alone may be of value but does not usually allow complete resolution of abdominal sepsis if there is an established abscess cavity. Percutaneous drainage under radiologic guidance is possible in many cases, because enlarging abscesses tend to assume a globular shape and push neighboring structures aside. Percutaneous drainage may avoid the morbidity and mortality of the second hit associated with surgical trauma in a patient with abdominal sepsis. In addition, large drains (8–10 French) can be inserted into abscess cavities under local anesthetic, and if several drains are inserted simultaneously, the cavity can be irrigated regularly, ensuring adequate and prolonged drainage. Drains are usually kept in place and a contrast study performed through one of them to ensure that the abscess cavity has collapsed, before drain removal.

Sometimes, this approach may be ineffective, particularly if the CT scan shows multiple interloop abscesses, or when the pus is of a particularly thick consistency (eg, in infected pancreatic necrosis). In such cases and in sepsis associated with complete anastomotic dehiscence, surgical exploration is required. Adequate source control of sepsis in complete anastomotic dehiscence usually requires exteriorization of the relevant bowel segments.

WOUND AND FISTULA CARE

Maintenance of skin integrity is of the upmost importance in the presence of an intestinal fistula. Inadequate care and protection of the skin around enteroatmospheric fistulas may lead to painful and progressive digestion with secondary infection, particularly in the presence of high-output proximal gastrointestinal fistulas. Early involvement of a specialist nurse or enterostomal therapist is essential for physical and psychological well-being. Large Eakin bags can be cut to suit the shape of the abdominal wall and, when combined with suction catheters and adhesive paste, control most fistulas. However, in certain cases, it may be almost impossible to adequately control the output of a fistula. This situation may occur when a high-output fistula has developed in the base of a deep or irregularly shaped wound. In these circumstances, repeated failed attempts to keep a bag on a fistula may be demoralizing, and it may be preferable to fashion a loop jejunostomy in the left upper quadrant.[2] The region of the duodenojejunal junction is usually soft and accessible, even in patients who have had repeated laparotomies, and it may be possible to safely exteriorize a segment of very proximal small bowel in the left upper abdomen, however hostile the remaining peritoneal cavity. Although this strategy produces a very-high-output proximal stoma, it is at least possible to control the output with a stoma bag, which is preferable to an uncontrolled fistula with extensive skin excoriation.

NUTRITIONAL SUPPORT

A detailed discussion regarding nutritional support for patients with enterocutaneous fistulas is beyond the scope of this article but has recently been extensively reviewed elsewhere.[20] The aim of nutritional support for the patient with an enterocutaneous fistula is to maintain adequate nutritional status until the fistula has healed or has been surgically corrected. Many patients with enterocutaneous fistulas are nutritionally depleted, and nutritional support in these patients is required for restoration of lean body mass and to optimize recovery from surgical treatment.

Patients with low-output enterocutaneous fistulas may require little or no additional nutritional attention, provided they are able to maintain satisfactory dietary intake. Simple nutritional supplements may be helpful in ensuring that nutritional requirements are met. Patients with acute intestinal failure (usually corresponding to a high-output fistula) generally require parenteral nutrition, and the ability to provide this with minimal risk of complications is one of the defining features of specialized centers in the United Kingdom. In patients with mucocutaneous continuity, the ability to cannulate the gut distal to the fistula enables nutritional support by feeding directly downstream of the fistula (fistuloclycis).[21] Fistuloclycis is safe and considerably less expensive than parenteral nutrition. Provided there is sufficient healthy small intestine distal to the fistula, fistuloclycis, even without reinfusion of chyme, can allow weaning from parenteral nutrition and prevent or reverse the atrophy associated with defunctioning of the gut distal to the fistula, facilitating subsequent surgical adhesiolysis and intestinal reanastomosis.

PSYCHOLOGICAL SUPPORT

Many patients with enterocutaneous fistulas have had multiple and prolonged hospital admissions as well as failed surgical procedures. They frequently have fistulas or stomas in unplanned and unacceptably intrusive positions. There may be significant problems with stoma and wound care, leading to concerns regarding odor, personal hygiene, and body image. Patients with enterocutaneous fistulas consequently have complex emotional, psychological, social, and financial needs. Depression and anxiety are common, yet commonly overlooked, and they require aggressive, expert treatment. Drug treatment may be compromised by poor enteral absorption of psychotropic medication. Chronic pain and narcotic dependence are also common, and efforts should be made to eliminate or substantially reduce the use of narcotic analgesics, especially before surgery, because of the difficulties this causes for postoperative pain management. An appreciation of the patient's psychological well-being and the support of a clinical psychologist are vital if effective, holistic care is to be provided.[3]

PRINCIPLES OF DEFINITIVE SURGICAL RECONSTRUCTION

Surgical reconstruction of an intestinal fistula, and associated abdominal wall defect, is complex, technically demanding surgery, with considerable associated morbidity, even in expert hands. This description is particularly true of enteroatmospheric fistulation, which was shown to have a mortality of 60% as recently as 1990.[22] More recent studies from specialized centers reporting the outcome of complex reconstruction of the gastrointestinal tract and abdominal wall in selected patients deemed suitable for reconstructive surgery and subjected to optimal preoperative preparation and perioperative care have reported surgical site infection in more than 30% of cases, mortality of up to 5%, and refistulation and incisional hernia rates of 11% and 29%, respectively.[23] It is therefore essential that, before an attempt is made to take down the fistula and reconstruct the abdominal wall, the patient is judged to have recovered both physically and, as far as possible, psychologically from the period of acute illness associated with the development of the fistula.[24]

Specific goals, before undertaking reconstructive surgery, should be to ensure that both systemic and local conditions are suitable for surgical reconstruction. Patients should be free from sepsis and adequately nourished, and the abdomen should be as soft and supple as possible. It is important that sufficient time has elapsed after the previous operation to enable entry into the abdomen to be as safe and uncomplicated as possible.

Inadvertent enterotomy is particularly problematic in complex reconstructive abdominal surgery. It may complicate more than 50% of cases in which 4 or more previous laparotomies have been undertaken and has been shown to be strongly predictive of postoperative complications, especially the need for urgent reoperation, intensive care admission, and acute intestinal failure.[25,26] It is therefore important that the strategy for entry into the abdomen is thought through carefully before undertaking surgery. Conditions within the peritoneal cavity are likely to be suitable when re-epithelialization of the abdominal defect (with or without the aid of a split skin graft) is complete, and there has been neoperitonealization of the previously obliterated peritoneal cavity. This process is gradual, probably associated with the movement of peritoneal stem cells into the peritoneal compartment. It may take more than 6 months for favorable operating conditions to be established in patients with enteroatmospheric fistulation.[2,27,28] Before this time, a solid block of vascularized granulation tissue covers the surface of multiple loops of bowel and the fistulating segments, which are usually indistinguishable from each other (see **Fig. 1**; **Figs. 2** and **3**).[29] This situation makes an attempt to undertake surgical reconstruction unacceptably hazardous.

In some circumstances, notably after abdominal radiotherapy,[30] and in some collagen disorders such as Ehlers-Danlos syndrome, there may be little or no effective neoperitonealization, even after lengthy delay, making an attempt to deal with an intestinal fistula in such cases uniquely challenging.

The axiom that it is "impossible to undertake reconstructive surgery for an enterocutaneous fistula too late; only too early"[31] is generally sound advice. However, the deleterious impact of an open abdomen with multiple fistulas and type 2 intestinal failure on the quality of life of the affected patients and their family may lead to

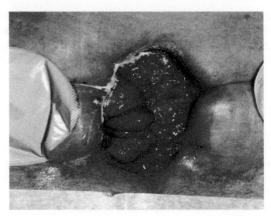

Fig. 2. Abdomen at 3 months, showing beginning of bowel prolapsing and small defect filled with granulation tissue.

considerable pressure being applied on the surgeon to undertake an early operation. The availability of a multidisciplinary team, expert nutritional and psychological support, and, above all, excellent communication and rapport between the medical team and the patient and their family are essential if overtures for inappropriately timed surgery are to be avoided.[3] Conversely, excessive delay in undertaking definitive reconstructive surgery may lead to loss of abdominal domain as a result of retraction of the abdominal wall, resulting in a more difficult abdominal wall reconstruction and a higher rate of subsequent incisional hernia formation.[32,33]

The presence of suitable local conditions for reconstructive surgery is indicated by the ability to pinch up the skin that has grown over (or been grafted over) previously exposed loops of bowel,[32] as is prolapse of bowel loops at the fistula site (**Fig. 4**).[24]

Before planning reconstructive surgery, it is important to have a clear understanding of the anatomy of the intestinal fistulation. The segments of the gastrointestinal tract involved in fistulation should be delineated as clearly as possible, as well as the intact gastrointestinal tract proximal and distal to them. It is particularly important to exclude stricturing in the gastrointestinal tract distal to fistulas, especially in patients whose distal gut has not been used for fistuloclycis, and, which therefore remains untested.

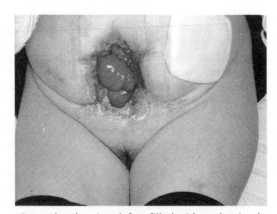

Fig. 3. Abdomen at 6 months, showing defect filled with prolapsing bowel.

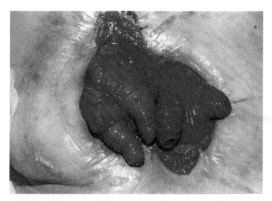

Fig. 4. Prolapse of bowel at the site of an enteroatmospheric fistula.

A combination of contrast radiologic investigations, including fistulography, barium enema, and follow-through examinations and cross-sectional imaging is usually appropriate, although assessment of the biliary tract (endoscopic retrograde cholangiopancreatography, magnetic resonance cholangiopancreatography) and the urinary tract (cystoscopy, intravenous urography) may also be needed.

Wherever possible, a strategy for abdominal wall reconstruction should have been made before commencing the gastrointestinal reconstruction. This strategy may require detailed assessment of the size and nature of the abdominal defect using cross-sectional imaging, as well as a plastic surgery opinion regarding the possibility of flap reconstruction, should this prove necessary.

OPERATIVE TECHNIQUE
Positioning and Immediate Preoperative Preparation

The anesthetized patient may be placed in the supine or Lloyd-Davies position, depending on the position of the fistula and whether or not the patient has previously undergone pelvic surgery. If there is a likelihood of a significant pelvic dissection being required, then the Lloyd-Davies position (which gives better access to the pelvis) is preferred. In such cases, and especially when fistulation secondarily involves the urinary tract, consideration should also be given to insertion of ureteric stents before abdominal surgery, to aid identification of the ureters.[34]

Before undertaking the abdominal incision, the patient is given suitable antibiotic prophylaxis (a second-generation cephalosporin and metronidazole is an appropriate combination), and the abdominal wall is swabbed and draped aseptically. The presence of a discharging fistula may make this difficult to achieve. Our preference is to attempt to seal the area of the fistula initially using a gauze swab and an adherent occlusive dressing. Although the dressing is removed later in the operation when the fistula is taken down, the inevitable contamination of the remainder of the abdominal wound can be minimized.

Gaining Entry to the Abdomen and Taking Down the Fistula

Successful local management of small, bud enterocutaneous fistulas, in which a modest pouting of mucosa occurs, has been described, using local extraperitoneal repair.[35,36] Although an advantage of this approach is that the need for further, extensive exploration of a hostile abdomen might be avoided, the results are generally poor, with a failure rate as high as 50%.[36] It has been suggested that reinforcing the suture line with biological material such as cadaveric or porcine collagen matrix, together with the use of tissue adhesives, might improve the success rate.[31] Similarly, although local repair and wedge resection of fistulas can be safely undertaken, these techniques are associated with a refistulation rate almost 3-fold higher than formal laparotomy and fistula resection[28]

Our preference, therefore, is to formally explore the abdomen and resect the fistula. This strategy allows the underlying intestinal disorder (when relevant) to be addressed, as well as the opportunity to correct the abdominal wall defect that commonly accompanies the fistula. With careful attention to detail and meticulous operative technique, refistulation rates of approximately 10% can be obtained, even in the most complex of cases.[23]

Careful entry into the neoperitoneal cavity is made through the intact abdominal wall above or below the fistula(s), and the abdominal wall is retracted vertically, allowing adherent loops of bowel to be separated from the back of the abdominal wall by sharp dissection.[37] Strong, toothed instruments such as Kocher forceps are particularly useful for this procedure, especially if the abdominal wall is indurated. Once the neoperitoneal cavity has been entered above or below the fistulating segments of bowel (**Fig. 5**), a painstaking dissection is undertaken, aimed at freeing up all of the small and large intestine. In most cases, the left upper quadrant of the abdomen is relatively free, and an early goal of surgery should be to identify and protect the duodenojejunal junction, then proceed distally, preserving as much intact bowel as possible.

Damage to the gastrointestinal tract during reconstructive surgery is responsible for much chronic intestinal failure in patients with intestinal fistulas and has been shown to be the major cause of short bowel syndrome in Crohn's disease.[38] Most bowel injuries during reconstructive surgery are caused by excessive traction, and therefore knife dissection, although seemingly more hazardous, results in a lower rate of bowel injury. Meticulous and unrushed knife dissection of adhesions is therefore undertaken (**Fig. 6**) until the fistula is isolated, by circumcising the skin around it (**Fig. 7**), and then taken down (**Fig. 8**). When fistulation is associated with an abscess cavity, the pus should be sent for culture and granulation tissue and foreign material removed. Fistulating segments of bowel should be resected and the segments of bowel proximal and distal to them marked with suture material so that they can be easily identified for reconstructive surgery. When fistulation has occurred in association with prosthetic material, it is essential that all visible traces of the foreign material (which is usually densely adherent to the fistulating bowel) is resected, to prevent the remaining nidus of chronically infected material acting as a focal point of further gastrointestinal adhesion and refistulation.

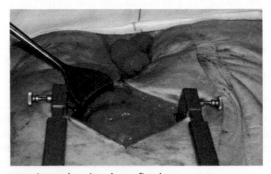

Fig. 5. Entry into neoperitoneal cavity above fistula.

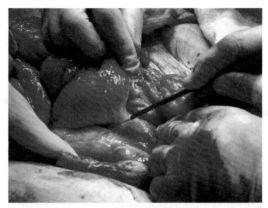

Fig. 6. Sharp knife dissection of dense intraperitoneal adhesions.

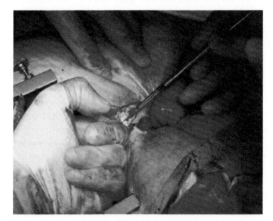

Fig. 7. Isolation and circumcision of the fistulating bowel.

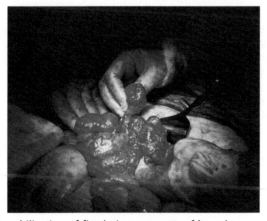

Fig. 8. Completed mobilization of fistulating segments of bowel.

Restoration of Gastrointestinal Continuity

The strategy for restoration of intestinal continuity should ideally have been made before surgery is undertaken, and discussed fully with the patient. The general principles are more important than the specific anastomotic technique used. Intestinal anastomosis should be undertaken only if the patient is well nourished and free from sepsis. In the absence of conditions causing protein loss (such as nephrotic syndrome or protein-losing enteropathy), a preoperative serum albumin level greater than 32 g/L is a useful indicator of the likelihood of satisfactory anastomotic healing. However, bowel should be anastomosed only if it seems healthy and distal patency has been confirmed. An anastomosis should not be constructed within an existing abscess cavity. Although any competently undertaken anastomotic technique is acceptable, an end-to-end anastomosis may be preferable in patients in whom a significant amount of small intestine has been resected, to maximize the remaining absorptive surface. The bowel distal to a fistula may be of small caliber and atrophic, especially if fistuloclycis has not been undertaken. The resulting disparity may create technical challenges for an intestinal anastomosis, and if several, difficult, small-caliber anastomoses are needed in thin-walled bowel that has been defunctioned for several months, it may be preferable to undertake a staged reconstruction, with a proximal defunctioning loop jejunostomy,[39,40] which can be closed subsequently when downstream anastomotic healing has been confirmed radiologically, and distal feeding successfully undertaken.

A defunctioning tube gastrostomy may also be of value in cases in which a proximal small bowel anastomosis has been undertaken at the site of fistula resection but the bowel downstream is atrophic. Under these circumstances, a lengthy period of postoperative small bowel obstruction and delayed return of gastrointestinal function are common. A gastrostomy may allow the patient to avoid prolonged nasogastric intubation and dieticians to gradually introduce enteral feeding via the gastrostomy tube.

Closure of the Abdominal Wall After Fistula Takedown

Closure of the abdominal wall defect is a vital component of takedown of enterocutaneous fistulas. The goal of abdominal wall reconstruction in such cases is to provide effective cover for the reconstructed gastrointestinal tract with healthy, mechanically strong material, which, as nearly as possible, replicates the dynamic properties of an intact, native abdominal wall. It is becoming increasingly clear that, as well as functional and cosmetic considerations, the outcome of a successful takedown of the fistula in terms of refistulation may also depend heavily on the technique used for abdominal wall reconstruction.[23,37,41] The nature of the challenge posed by the abdominal wall varies enormously, from cases in which a fistula can simply be pinched off the otherwise intact abdominal wall, to cases in which the abdominal wall is almost completely absent.

Larger abdominal wall defects may require a staged approach to reconstruction. There is no clear evidence to support a single-stage versus multiple-staged approach to abdominal wall reconstruction in this setting, and the ideal solution depends on several factors, including the size and nature of the abdominal wall defect, the fitness of the patient, and the locally available expertise and resources. Both single-stage and multiple-staged approaches have advantages and disadvantages.

Single-Stage Versus Multiple-Staged Approaches

A single-stage approach to reconstruction of the abdominal wall after resection of the intestinal fistula is ideal for those fistulas in which there has been minimal loss of abdominal wall. It is frequently possible in such cases simply to curette the fistula track and close the abdomen again in the midline, leaving the cutaneous opening of the fistula packed to heal by secondary intention. In cases with larger abdominal wall defects, it may be possible, depending on the loss of abdominal wall and the degree of fibrosis, simply to undertake a limited mobilization of the abdominal wall and then close the abdomen with near and far sutures.[42] It is important that all chronically infected synthetic material is excised back to healthy, native abdominal wall if postoperative chronic sinus formation in the abdominal wall is to be avoided.

When the abdominal wall defect is completely occupied by a mass of fistulating small intestine (**Fig. 9**), there may be little or no native abdominal wall left to reconstruct once the fistulas have been resected (**Fig. 10**) but the figure showing a large abdominal wall defect after resection of mass. These larger defects may require more complex procedures to repair them, ranging from separation of components to the use of biological implants and plastic surgical flaps, or a combination of these techniques. There is controversy in these cases regarding the use of single-stage versus multiple-staged procedures.[33,43] Although undertaking a single-stage approach to the reconstruction of the abdominal wall in patients with enterocutaneous fistulas may return the patient to normal more quickly avoiding the cost and physical and psychological morbidity associated with additional procedures, a 1-stage reconstruction policy of separation of components to close the abdominal wall defect in patients with enterocutaneous fistulation resulted in recurrent fistulation in 26% and incisional hernia formation in 21% within 2 years of follow-up.[44] Even allowing for these poor results, adding a definitive abdominal wall reconstruction to takedown of a fistula results in considerable extension of the operation, in a patient who may already have been on the operating table for more than 8 hours before abdominal wall reconstruction begins, and this may contribute significantly to postoperative morbidity in such cases.

In order to ensure that surgical decision making regarding abdominal wall reconstruction is not adversely influenced by fatigue among the surgical team, such procedures are best planned by a multidisciplinary surgical team, including gastrointestinal, hernia, and plastic surgeons, with separate teams undertaking the intestinal and abdominal wall phases of the procedure when a single-stage procedure is planned.

Multiple-staged procedures may allow abdominal wall reconstruction to be undertaken after closure of the intestinal fistula, in an uncontaminated abdominal wound. However, this strategy does require the patient to undergo multiple procedures, which many patients may find less desirable. These procedures also expose the patient to the additional risks associated with the subsequent stages of reconstruction. In

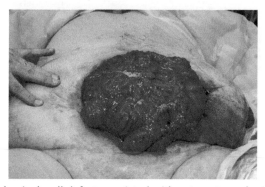

Fig. 9. Massive abdominal wall defect associated with enteroatmospheric fistulation.

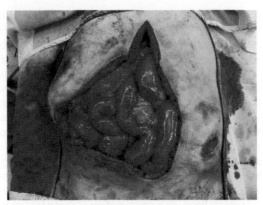

Fig. 10. Massive abdominal wall defect after takedown of fistula.

particular, repeat contamination of the abdominal wall by creation of a further enterotomy during the subsequent clean surgery would be a catastrophic outcome of such a strategy.

However, staged procedures are ideally suited to patients who are becoming unstable after prolonged abdominal surgery, in which it would be advantageous to curtail the operative procedure and stabilize the patient in an appropriate postoperative critical care environment. In such cases, closing the abdominal wall defect, with an absorbable polyglactin mesh, at the time of the gastrointestinal reconstruction may be the safest option (**Fig. 11**).[45] Although the polyglactin is hydrolyzed and disappears over the following months, leaving hernias in most patients,[23,45] the hernia is usually preferable to an intestinal fistula. Should the skin break down, the mesh becomes covered with granulation tissue that rapidly epithelializes spontaneously. If there is a significant skin defect, a split skin graft can be placed directly on the polyglactin mesh.

Under some circumstances, notably when there has been a complex reconstruction of the gastrointestinal tract and abdominal wall with a plastic surgical flap, the use of a proximal diverting loop stoma may be necessary to ensure that there are no suture lines left in continuity behind the flap to protect the patient from the potentially disastrous consequences of an anastomotic leak and resulting loss of the flap.[37] In this

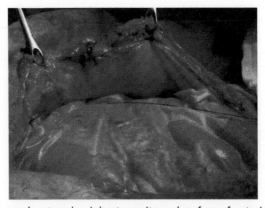

Fig. 11. Polyglactin mesh sutured as inlay to peritoneal surface of anterior abdominal wall.

strategy, it is therefore the gastrointestinal, rather than the abdominal wall, reconstruction that is staged.

Choice of Technique for Larger Abdominal Wall Defects

The precise technique to be used for reconstruction of larger abdominal wall defects in patients with enteroatmospheric fistulation, or in whom an enterocutaneous fistula coexists with a large incisional hernia, is determined by locally available expertise and personal preference. These cases occur in small numbers, even in specialized centers, and there are no randomized trials or even large cohort studies to allow an adequately evidence-based approach to be developed. However, there are some general principles that influence surgical decision making with regard to reconstruction of the largest abdominal defects in patients undergoing surgery for enterocutaneous fistulas. All abdominal wall reconstructions represent a further, major surgical undertaking and should be performed only in patients who are deemed sufficiently fit. Although polypropylene and other synthetic materials have proved to be inert and inexpensive, making them ideally suited to incisional hernia repair, the fact that the abdominal wall defect in a patient with an enterocutaneous fistula is intrinsically contaminated at the outset makes synthetic material unsuitable for abdominal wall reconstruction.

Reconstruction with Autologous Tissue

The use of autologous tissue for reconstructing the abdominal wall, after takedown of an enterocutaneous fistula, has the advantage of using native tissue in a (often heavily) contaminated field. The available techniques have been reviewed extensively[41] and include separation of components,[46] as well a variety of thigh flaps, both pedicled[37,47–49] and free[50] and combinations of the 2,[51] with or without additional biological material to facilitate closure of the abdominal wall defect with the flap.[52] Of all of the reported techniques, separation of components has probably been most widely used in abdominal wall closure for patients with enterocutaneous fistulas. Separating the rectus muscle from the posterior rectus sheath and detaching the external oblique from the internal oblique generates up to 10 cm of additional abdominal wall at the midabdomen and approximately 5 to 6 cm at the epigastrium and the suprapubic regions (where there is usually a smaller requirement for abdominal wall in reconstructive surgery anyway). When undertaken bilaterally, separation of components may therefore generate up to 20 cm of additional abdominal wall, and this may allow all but the biggest of defects to be closed.

Although this is an attractive option, and it is certainly simpler and better tolerated than plastic surgical flaps taken from the thigh, it is not without problems when used for patients who are undergoing gastrointestinal reconstruction. Wound complications are common, and significant wound morbidity was reported in 24%, and incisional hernia in 18.2%, of the 354 cases reported in the largest meta-analysis reported to date.[41] Plastic surgical reconstruction was associated with even higher wound morbidity (42%) and incisional hernia (29%). Separation of components may create particular problems when the gastrointestinal reconstruction requires creation of stomas through abdominal wall that has been weakened or distorted by the dissection required for separation of the external and internal oblique muscles. It is unclear whether this results in a significantly greater incidence of parastomal hernia, although that seems likely.

Plastic surgical flaps are probably best reserved for large defects (>200 cm^2) in fit patients. Pedicled flaps based on the lateral circumflex femoral artery, such as the subtotal lateral thigh flap,[37] are technically demanding but allow virtually the entire

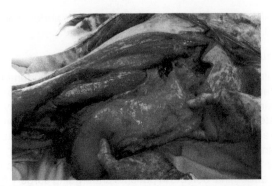

Fig. 12. Subtotal lateral thigh flap used to fill defect after fistula takedown.

abdominal wall (800 cm^2) to be replaced. This flap is a myofasciocutaneous flap and allows reconstruction of the abdominal wall skin as well as muscle, with a reasonable cosmetic result (**Figs. 12–14**). The donor site usually requires covering with a split skin graft taken from the contralateral thigh (**Fig. 15**). The complexity and high complication rates associated with such procedures probably limit their applicability to specialized centers and just a handful of suitable patients.

Reconstruction with Biological Implants

The concept underlying the use of biological materials when used to reconstruct the abdominal wall after takedown of enterocutaneous fistula is that they are being put into an operative field that is, at best, heavily contaminated and, at worse, dirty. A detailed description of these materials is beyond the scope of this article, but, in general, they are based on collagen derived from porcine, bovine, or human sources. The collagen may be derived from skin (dermis), gastrointestinal submucosa, or pericardium. The material is processed to ensure sterility, remove antigenicity, and may be

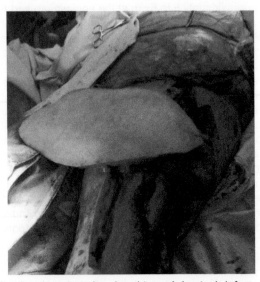

Fig. 13. Flap mobilized and ready to be placed into abdominal defect.

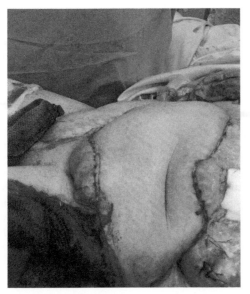

Fig. 14. Flap sutured into abdominal defect.

chemically cross-linked in an attempt to resist or delay enzymatic degradation. These products are expensive and have not been subjected to randomized controlled trials in this setting. There are no cohort studies specifically pertaining to their use in enterocutaneous fistula. A recent prospective study of a non–cross-linked porcine collagen

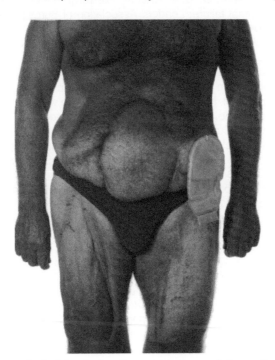

Fig. 15. Cosmetic result of abdominal wall reconstruction and donor site from right thigh.

implant used to reinforce repair of contaminated abdominal hernia wounds reported a recurrence rate of 28% at 2 years.[53]

The key issue with the use of porcine dermal collagen in reconstructing the abdominal wall after enterocutaneous fistula is where to place the material. Biological implants seem to work most effectively when interleaved between layers of vascularized host tissue, thus encouraging ingrowth of blood vessels and remodeling. They may therefore be effective when used to support an abdominal wall closed by separation of components.

Although the material might be even more useful as a bridge in cases in which separation of components leaves a sizable defect, the rate of mechanical failure of the implant in this setting seems to be so high as to make it no more effective than a (considerably less expensive) piece of polyglactin. Incisional herniation has been reported to occur in between 44% and 80% of such patients.[53,54] Placement of cross-linked porcine dermal collagen material in direct contact with intestine has been shown to be associated with a 41.7% incidence of refistulation,[23] which is clearly unacceptable. The bowel seems to become densely adherent to the implant in such cases, making further attempts to reconstruct the gastrointestinal tract especially challenging.

REFERENCES

1. Lal S, Teubner A, Shaffer JL. Review article: intestinal failure. Aliment Pharmacol Ther 2006;24(1):19–31.
2. Carlson GL, Dark P. Acute intestinal failure. Curr Opin Crit Care 2010;16(4): 347–52.
3. Carlson GL, McKee R, Gardiner K, et al. The surgical management of patients with acute intestinal failure. London: Association of Surgeons of Great Britain and Ireland; 2010.
4. Berry SM, Fischer JE. Classification and pathophysiology of enterocutaneous fistulas. Surg Clin North Am 1996;76(5):1009–18.
5. Adkins AL, Robbins J, Villalba M, et al. Open abdomen management of intra-abdominal sepsis. Am Surg 2004;70(2):137–40 [discussion: 40].
6. Barker DE, Green JM, Maxwell RA, et al. Experience with vacuum-pack temporary abdominal wound closure in 258 trauma and general and vascular surgical patients. J Am Coll Surg 2007;204(5):784–92 [discussion: 92–3].
7. MacLean AA, O'Keeffe T, Augenstein J. Management strategies for the open abdomen: survey of the American Association for the Surgery of Trauma membership. Acta Chir Belg 2008;108(2):212–8.
8. Trevelyan SL, Carlson GL. Is TNP in the open abdomen safe and effective? J Wound Care 2009;18:24–5.
9. Stonerock CE, Bynoe RP, Yost MJ, et al. Use of a vacuum-assisted device to facilitate abdominal closure. Am Surg 2003;69(12):1030–4 [discussion: 4–5].
10. Boele van Hensbroek P, Wind J, Dijkgraaf MG, et al. Temporary closure of the open abdomen: a systematic review on delayed primary fascial closure in patients with an open abdomen. World J Surg 2009;33(2):199–207.
11. Miller PR, Meredith JW, Johnson JC, et al. Prospective evaluation of vacuum-assisted fascial closure after open abdomen: planned ventral hernia rate is substantially reduced. Ann Surg 2004;239(5):608–14 [discussion: 14–6].
12. Navsaria PH, Bunting M, Omoshoro-Jones J, et al. Temporary closure of open abdominal wounds by the modified sandwich-vacuum pack technique. Br J Surg 2003;90(6):718–22.

13. Barker DE, Kaufman HJ, Smith LA, et al. Vacuum pack technique of temporary abdominal closure: a 7-year experience with 112 patients. J Trauma 2000;48(2): 201–6 [discussion: 6–7].

14. Rao M, Burke D, Finan PJ, et al. The use of vacuum-assisted closure of abdominal wounds: a word of caution. Colorectal Dis 2007;9:266–8.

15. Bosscha K, Hulstaert PF, Visser MR, et al. Open management of the abdomen and planned reoperations in severe bacterial peritonitis. Eur J Surg 2000;166(1): 44–9.

16. Subramonia S, Pankhurst S, Rowlands BJ, et al. Vacuum-assisted closure of postoperative abdominal wounds: a prospective study. World J Surg 2009; 33(5):931–7.

17. Amin AI, Shaikh IA. Topical negative pressure in managing severe peritonitis: a positive contribution? World J Gastroenterol 2009;15(27):3394–7.

18. Martinez JL, Luque-de-Leon E, Mier J, et al. Systematic management of postoperative enterocutaneous fistulas: factors related to outcomes. World J Surg 2008;32(3):436–43 [discussion: 44].

19. Reber HA, Roberts C, Way LW, et al. Management of external gastrointestinal fistulas. Ann Surg 1978;188(4):460–7.

20. Polk TM, Schwab CW. Metabolic and nutritional support of the enterocutaneous fistula patient: a three-phase approach. World J Surg 2012;36(3):524–33.

21. Teubner A, Morrison K, Ravishankar HR, et al. Fistuloclysis can successfully replace parenteral feeding in the nutritional support of patients with enterocutaneous fistula. Br J Surg 2004;91(5):625–31.

22. Schein M. Intestinal fistulas and the open management of the septic abdomen. Arch Surg 1990;125(11):1516–7.

23. Connolly PT, Teubner A, Lees NP, et al. Outcome of reconstructive surgery for intestinal fistula in the open abdomen. Ann Surg 2008;247(3):440–4.

24. Carlson GL. Surgical management of intestinal failure. Proc Nutr Soc 2003; 62(3):711–8.

25. Van Der Krabben AA, Dijkstra FR, Nieuwenhuijzen M, et al. Morbidity and mortality of inadvertent enterotomy during adhesiotomy. Br J Surg 2000;87(4): 467–71.

26. ten Broek RP, Schreinemacher MH, Jilesen AP, et al. Enterotomy risk in abdominal wall repair: a prospective study. Ann Surg 2012;256(2):280–7.

27. Scripcariu V, Carlson G, Bancewicz J, et al. Reconstructive abdominal operations after laparostomy and multiple repeat laparotomies for severe intra-abdominal infection. Br J Surg 1994;81(10):1475–8.

28. Lynch AC, Delaney CP, Senagore AJ, et al. Clinical outcome and factors predictive of recurrence after enterocutaneous fistula surgery. Ann Surg 2004;240(5): 825–31.

29. Scott BG, Feanny MA, Hirshberg A. Early definitive closure of the open abdomen: a quiet revolution. Scand J Surg 2005;94(1):9–14.

30. Girvent M, Carlson GL, Anderson I, et al. Intestinal failure after surgery for complicated radiation enteritis. Ann R Coll Surg Engl 2000;82(3):198–201.

31. Schecter WP, Hirshberg A, Chang DS, et al. Enteric fistulas: principles of management. J Am Coll Surg 2009;209(4):484–91.

32. Jernigan TW, Fabian TC, Croce MA, et al. Staged management of giant abdominal wall defects: acute and long-term results. Ann Surg 2003;238(3):349–55 [discussion: 55–7].

33. Johnson EK, Tushoski PL. Abdominal wall reconstruction in patients with digestive tract fistulas. Clin Colon Rectal Surg 2010;23(3):195–208.

34. Shackley DC, Brew CJ, Bryden AA, et al. The staged management of complex entero-urinary fistulae. BJU Int 2000;86(6):624–9.

35. Sarfeh IJ, Jakowatz JG. Surgical treatment of enteric 'bud' fistulas in contaminated wounds. A riskless extraperitoneal method using split-thickness skin grafts. Arch Surg 1992;127(9):1027–30 [discussion: 30–1].

36. Jamshidi R, Schecter WP. Biological dressings for the management of enteric fistulas in the open abdomen: a preliminary report. Arch Surg 2007;142(8): 793–6.

37. Lambe G, Russell C, West C, et al. Autologous reconstruction of massive enteroatmospheric fistulation with a pedicled subtotal lateral thigh flap. Br J Surg 2012;99(7):964–72.

38. Agwunobi AO, Carlson GL, Anderson ID, et al. Mechanisms of intestinal failure in Crohn's disease. Dis Colon Rectum 2001;44(12):1834–7.

39. Shetty V, Teubner A, Morrison K, et al. Proximal loop jejunostomy is a useful adjunct in the management of multiple intestinal suture lines in the septic abdomen. Br J Surg 2006;93(10):1247–50.

40. Mulholland MW, Delaney JP. Proximal diverting jejunostomy for compromised small bowel. Surgery 1983;93(3):443–7.

41. de Vries Reilingh TS, Bodegom ME, van Goor H, et al. Autologous tissue repair of large abdominal wall defects. Br J Surg 2007;94(7):791–803.

42. Abdel-Malik R, Scott NA. Double near and far prolene suture closure: a technique for abdominal wall closure after laparostomy. Br J Surg 2001;88(1): 146–7.

43. Fischer JE. The importance of reconstruction of the abdominal wall after gastrointestinal fistula closure. Am J Surg 2009;197(1):131–2.

44. Wind J, van Koperen PJ, Slors JF, et al. Single-stage closure of enterocutaneous fistula and stomas in the presence of large abdominal wall defects using the components separation technique. Am J Surg 2009;197(1):24–9.

45. Greene MA, Mullins RJ, Malangoni MA, et al. Laparotomy wound closure with absorbable polyglycolic acid mesh. Surg Gynecol Obstet 1993;176(3): 213–8.

46. Ramirez OM, Ruas E, Dellon AL. "Components separation" method for closure of abdominal-wall defects: an anatomic and clinical study. Plast Reconstr Surg 1990;86(3):519–26.

47. Wangensteen OH. Repair of recurrent and difficult hernias and other large defects of the abdominal wall employing the iliotibial tract of fascia lata as a pedicled flap. Surg Gynecol Obstet 1934;59:766–80.

48. Depuydt K, Boeckx W, D'Hoore A. The pedicled tensor fasciae latae flap as a salvage procedure for an infected abdominal mesh. Plast Reconstr Surg 1998;102(1):187–90.

49. Kimata Y, Uchiyama K, Sekido M, et al. Anterolateral thigh flap for abdominal wall reconstruction. Plast Reconstr Surg 1999;103(4):1191–7.

50. Ninkovic M, Kronberger P, Harpf C, et al. Free innervated latissimus dorsi muscle flap for reconstruction of full-thickness abdominal wall defects. Plast Reconstr Surg 1998;101(4):971–8.

51. Sasaki K, Nozaki M, Nakazawa H, et al. Reconstruction of a large abdominal wall defect using combined free tensor fasciae latae musculocutaneous flap and anterolateral thigh flap. Plast Reconstr Surg 1998;102(6):2244–52.

52. Maxhimer JB, Hui-Chou HG, Rodriguez ED. Clinical applications of the pedicled anterolateral thigh flap in complex abdominal-pelvic reconstruction. Ann Plast Surg 2011;66:285–91.

53. Itani KM, Rosen MJ, Vargo D, et al. Prospective study of single-stage repair of contaminated hernias using a biologic porcine tissue matrix: the RICH study. Surgery 2012;152:498–505.
54. Blatnik J, Jin J, Rosen M. Abdominal hernia repair with bridging acellular dermal matrix–an expensive hernia sac. Am J Surg 2008;196(1):47–50.

Parastomal Hernia Repair

Nilay R. Shah, MD, MS[a], Randall O. Craft, MD[b],
Kristi L. Harold, MD[a],*

KEYWORDS

- Parastomal hernia • Sugarbaker technique • Keyhole technique • Laparoscopy
- Outcomes

KEY POINTS

- Parastomal hernia is an almost inevitable consequence of stoma formation. Most parastomal hernia appears within 2 years of stoma formation.
- Laparoscopic keyhole technique has higher rates of recurrence (34.6%) than laparoscopic Sugarbaker technique (11.6%).
- Overall, results of open and laparoscopic repair were similar in terms of morbidity and mortality. Length of stay is shorter with laparoscopic procedure.
- Prophylactic mesh placement during stoma formation lowers rates of parastomal herniation.

INTRODUCTION

Parastomal hernia (PSH) is the protrusion of abdominal contents next to a stoma through the abdominal wall defect created during ostomy formation. The incidence varies widely, ranging from 0% to 48%, largely dependent on the type of enterostomy created (**Table 1**).[1–3] The lack of a uniform definition of what constitutes a PSH and the inadequacy of physical examination in detecting early occurrences makes the true incidence difficult to quantify. Although laparoscopic and trephine stoma formation show a lower incidence of hernia formation, the studies published on these techniques are small series with short follow-up (none longer than 1 year). Several classification systems have been proposed but none are universally accepted (**Table 2**).[4–6] Seo and colleagues[7] proposed radiologic classification by computed tomography (CT) scan based on content of hernia sac (**Table 3**). However, the diagnosis can usually be made by history, physical examination, digital examination of stoma, and CT scan.

Funding Sources: None.
Conflict of Interest: None.
[a] Department of Surgery, Mayo Clinic Hospital, 5777 East Mayo Boulevard, MCSB SP 3-522 Gen Surg, Phoenix, AZ 85054, USA; [b] Plastic and Reconstructive Surgery, Division of Surgery, Banner MD Anderson Cancer Center, 2946 East Banner Gateway Drive, Gilbert, AZ 85234, USA
* Corresponding author.
E-mail address: Harold.Kristi@mayo.edu

Surg Clin N Am 93 (2013) 1185–1198
http://dx.doi.org/10.1016/j.suc.2013.06.011
0039-6109/13/$ – see front matter © 2013 Elsevier Inc. All rights reserved.

Table 1
Incidence of parastomal hernias after enterostomies

Type of Enterostomy	Incidence of Parastomal Hernias (%)
End colostomy	4–48
Loop colostomy	0–31
End ileostomy	1.8–28.3
Loop ileostomy	0–6
Laparoscopic stomal formation	0–6.7
Trephine stoma formation	6.7–12

Most hernias appear within 2 years of stoma formation.[2] Risk factors associated with formation of PSHs are advanced age, technical failure, increased intra-abdominal pressure, emphysema, obesity, malnutrition, steroid use, malignancy, and wound infection.[1,8–11] However, the exact cause for PSH formation remains unknown. There has been some speculation of the loss of tensile strength caused by a shift of the collagen ratio from mature type I collagen to immature type III collagen during healing.[8,10] Most PSHs are asymptomatic and are managed nonoperatively.[12] However, 11% to 70% require surgical intervention because of obstruction or incarceration, prolapse, giant hernia, pain, bleeding, appliance leakage, or discomfort from an ill-fitting appliance.[11,13]

PSH REPAIR
Open Repair

Various procedures have been used for PSH repair, including primary repair, stoma reversal, stoma relocation, and placement of prosthetic mesh. Primary fascial repair is technically simple, avoids an additional laparotomy incision, and has low morbidity but is associated with a reported 46% to 100% recurrence rate.[1,11] Stoma relocation requires an additional laparotomy, resulting in three potential hernia sites, and is

Table 2
Classification of parastomal hernias

	Rubin	Devlin	Gil and Szczepkowski
Type 1	Peritoneal hernia sac through dilated stomal canal	Interstitial hernia with hernia sac located between layers of abdominal muscles	Parastomal hernia without coexisting cicatricial hernia and without abdominal wall deformation
Type 2	Intrastomal hernia	Subcutaneous hernia	Parastomal hernia associated with cicatricial hernia without deformtion of abdominal wall
Type 3	Subcutaneous prolapse	Intrastomal hernia	Large, isolated parastomal hernia without coexisting cicatricial hernia with abdominal wall deformity
Type 4	Pseudohernia	Peristomal hernia with stomal prolapsed	Large parastomal hernias with coexisting cicatricial hernia with abdominal wall deformity

Type	Content of Hernia Sac
Table 3 Radiologic classification of parastomal hernia	
0	Peritoneum follows the wall of the bowel forming the stoma, with no formation of a sac
Ia	Bowel forming the colostomy with a sac <5 cm
Ib	Bowel forming the colostomy with a sac >5 cm
II	Sac containing omentum
III	Intestinal loop other than the bowel forming the stoma

associated with a recurrence rate of up to 24% to 86%.[5,6] Overall complication rates of 22.6% to 88% have been reported for primary fascial repair and stomal relocation.[5,11]

Prosthetic mesh repair of PSHs can be onlay, retromuscular, or intraperitoneal. In 1985, Sugarbaker was the first to describe the intraperitoneal mesh repair of a PSH.[14] His technique involved securing the mesh over the entire fascial defect circumferentially except laterally to create a mesh flap valve around the stoma (**Fig. 1**). This prevented herniation and contact with the stoma bud, theoretically reducing infection. In his published series of seven patients, there were no reported recurrences or complications after 4 to 7 years follow-up. In the Keyhole technique, a 2- to 3-cm "keyhole" cut-out is made to surround the ostomy while covering the entire hernia defect (**Fig. 2**).[15–18] However, there is a risk of obstructing the enterostomy if a smaller keyhole is made and a risk of recurrence if the hole is larger. In a review of reported series, overall morbidity was 22.2%. Recurrence rate was 9.4%.[19]

Laparoscopic Repair

The advent of laparoscopic surgery in ventral hernia repair has led to many benefits including less pain, shorter hospital stay, and faster recovery. Laparoscopic repair of PSH has the advantages of greater mesh overlap and transabdominal fixation while avoiding the creation of new hernia sites. Current described approaches for laparoscopic PSH repair include a modified Sugarbaker technique, a keyhole technique, and a "sandwich" technique, which incorporates elements of both.

Our clinical experience mirrors the current literature suggesting that the use of a solid piece of mesh versus a cut piece of mesh results in a lower hernia recurrence and a shorter operative time.

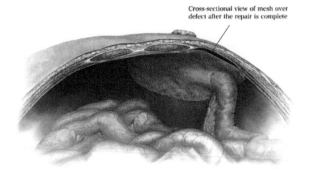

Cross-sectional view of mesh over defect after the repair is complete

Fig. 1. Sugarbaker repair. (*From* Huguet KL, Harol KL. Laparoscopic parastomal hernia repair. Oper Tech Gen Surg 2007;9(3):119; with permission.)

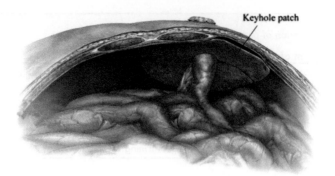

Fig. 2. Keyhole repair. (*From* Huguet KL, Harol KL. Laparoscopic parastomal hernia repair. Oper Tech Gen Surg 2007;9(3):121; with permission.)

Laparoscopic Technique

After induction of general anesthesia, the patient is placed in the supine position with both arms tucked at the sides (**Fig. 3**). A first-generation cephalosporin is given 1 hour before the incision. A Foley catheter is placed if needed and a monitor positioned on each side of the patient. The abdomen is prepared including the ostomy. An

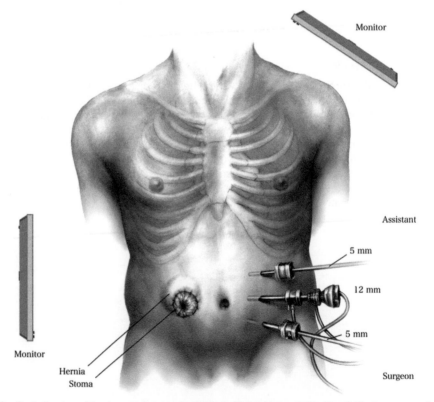

Fig. 3. Patient positioning and port placement. (*From* Huguet KL, Harol KL. Laparoscopic parastomal hernia repair. Oper Tech Gen Surg 2007;9(3):114; with permission.)

additional Foley balloon catheter is placed in the ostomy to assist with localization of the correct loop of intestine when dissecting adhesions (**Fig. 4**). An Ioban drape (3M Company, St. Paul, MN) is applied to the abdomen covering the stoma and the inserted Foley catheter. Access to the peritoneal cavity is gained using a Veress needle placed subcostally in the left upper quadrant at the midclavicular line. After adequate pneumoperitoneum (15 mm Hg of carbon dioxide), a 5-mm Optiview port is placed in the lateral position of the abdomen on the side opposite from the ostomy site. On the same side of the abdomen as the Optiview port, two additional 5-mm trocars are placed low and lateral in the abdomen. Lysis of any adhesions is performed using sharp dissection. At this stage, external manipulation of the Foley catheter placed in the stoma can greatly help in the identification of the loop of bowel ending in the ostomy. After adhesiolysis is complete, and the entire anterior abdominal wall is visualized with the stomal loop of bowel identified, spinal needles are used to measure the extent of the hernia defect. Any other coexisting ventral hernias are included in the measurement so that all defects are covered (**Figs. 5** and **6**). The defect is also measured and marked on the outside of the abdomen to later center the prosthesis. A sheet of ePTFE (Gore DUAL-MESH; W.L. Gore, Flagstaff, AZ) is trimmed to a size that allows for 5 cm of overlap beyond all fascial defects. Figures are drawn on the mesh as points of reference for orienting the mesh once placed intra-abdominally. A single Gore-Tex suture (CV-0) is placed at the edge of the mesh on three of the four sides. Two Gore-Tex sutures are placed on the fourth side to allow the mesh to encompass the stoma while allowing the bowel to exit through the created mesh flap-valve. A 5-mm port is placed in the lateral abdominal wall on the opposite side of the three working ports. A 12-mm port is placed in a position where it will later be covered by the mesh to prevent the possibility of trocar site hernia. The superior and inferior edges of the mesh are simultaneously rolled toward one another to facilitate unfurling once in the abdomen. A grasper is placed in the port ipsilateral to the ostomy, and the tip of the instrument brought out through the 12-mm port to grab the mesh and bring it into the abdomen (**Figs. 7** and **8**). The mesh is unrolled and oriented based on the markings. The open jaws of a laparoscopic atraumatic bowel grasper are used to measure a 5-cm overlap from the edge of the fascial defects (**Fig. 9**). This area is marked with a spinal needle, and the transfascial sutures are passed through these

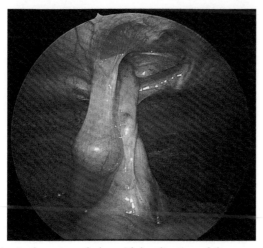

Fig. 4. Foley catheter in the ostomy helps with localization of the correct loop of intestine.

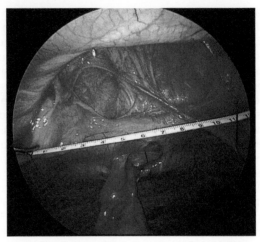

Fig. 5. Measurement of vertical defect size.

sites with a suture passer. It is important to orient sutures to avoid the stoma as it traverses the edge of the mesh; the mesh flap valve is created such that the stoma crosses the lateral or inferior edge. The mesh is then tacked circumferentially with spiral tacks except at the exit site of the stoma (**Fig. 10**). Additional 0-Gore-Tex transabdominal sutures are placed every 4 to 5 cm circumferentially around the mesh with a suture passer. The knots are tied in the subcutaneous tissues and the skin is released from the knot with a hemostat clamp. The 5- and 12-mm port sites are closed with a 4-0 monocryl suture. The stab incisions from the transabdominal sutures are closed with skin adhesive. **Figs. 11** and **12** show the final appearance of the repair.

Outcomes

Tables 4 and **5** show outcomes of open and laparoscopic repair of PSH. One multiinstitutional series consists of 25 consecutive patients who underwent laparoscopic

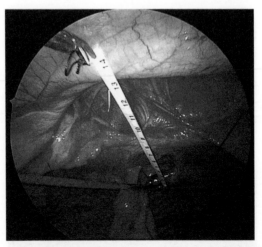

Fig. 6. Measurement of horizontal defect size. Ventral hernia defect size is incorporated with parastomal hernia defect.

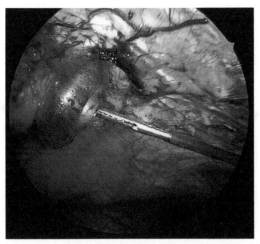

Fig. 7. A tip of grasper is passed through 12-mm port to grasp the mesh.

PSH repair with nonslit ePTFE mesh (Sugarbaker technique) followed for a median of 19 months (range, 2–38 months). Mean patient age was 60 years with a body mass index of 29 kg/m^2. Six of the patients had undergone previous mesh stoma repairs. The mean size of the hernia defect was 64 cm^2 with a mean mesh size of 365 cm^2. All procedures were successfully completed laparoscopically with no conversions to open surgery reported. Overall postoperative morbidity was 23% with a mean hospital length of stay of 3.3 days. One patient death was reported because of pulmonary complications, one patient had a trocar site infection, and one patient had a mesh infection requiring mesh removal. Of the 25 patients, one (4%) experienced a recurrence, similar to our own short-term outcomes.[35]

Hansson and colleagues[19] published a systematic review of surgical techniques for PSH repair. A total of 35 studies were included. The open and laparoscopic

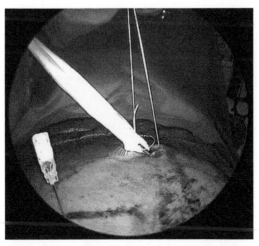

Fig. 8. Twelve-millimeter port is removed and mesh is brought into the abdominal cavity with help of the grasper.

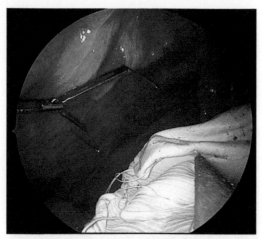

Fig. 9. Five-centimeter overlap from the edge of fascial defect is measured by open jaws of laparoscopic atraumatic bowel grasper.

techniques outcome was published in 23 and 12 studies, respectively. Pooled proportions of outcome were measured per surgical technique. A total of 106 repairs were done with primary fascial repair and had a highest number of recurrence (69.4%). Same pool of repairs had highest rate of wound infection (11.8%). The overall mesh infection rate of 2.4% was reported. Wound infection rate was even lower in mesh repair (4.1%) than in suture repair (11.7%). No wound or mesh infection was reported for pool of patients who underwent laparoscopic Sugarbaker and keyhole technique. Laparoscopic keyhole technique had higher rates of recurrence (34.6%) than laparoscopic Sugarbaker technique (11.6%). In contrast, open Sugarbaker technique had higher recurrence of 14.2% than open keyhole technique (7.2%). Laparoscopic sandwich technique had lowest rate of recurrence (2.1%). Overall, results of open and laparoscopic repair were similar in terms of morbidity and mortality. Only one study has

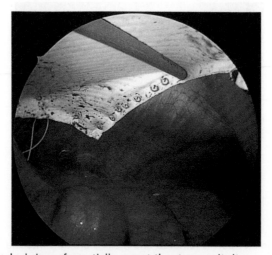

Fig. 10. Mesh is tacked circumferrentially except the stoma exit site.

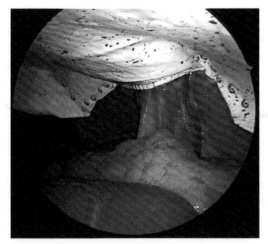

Fig. 11. Final appearance of the Sugarbaker repair.

compared open and laparoscopic repair retrospectively. Length of stay was significantly lower in laparoscopic group (3 days) compared with open group (5 days).

Choice of Mesh

Various meshes (polypropylene, ePTFE, biologic) have been used and none has proved to be the standard. There is no difference in complications that can be directly attributed to mesh choice.[19]

PSH PREVENTION

The ideal treatment of any hernia is to prevent its occurrence. In 1986, Bayer and coleagues[38] first described mesh insertion at the time of primary stoma formation. Since then, many observational studies have confirmed the safety and effectiveness

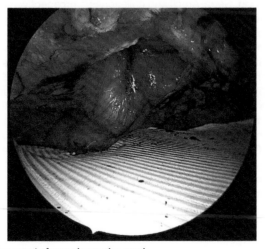

Fig. 12. View of the repair from above the mesh.

Table 4
Outcomes of different types of open parastomal hernia repair in studies with greater than or equal to 10 patients

Study	No. of Repairs	Recurrence (%)	Infection (%)	Erosion (%)	Follow-up (mo) (mean)
Open onlay mesh repair					
Ho & Fawcett,[20] 2004	15	6.7	0	—	(15)
Luning & Spillenaar-Bilgen,[21] 2009	16	19	6.2	0	6–110 (33)
de Ruiter & Bijnen,[22] 2005	46	15.9	6.6	—	12–156 (60)
Steele et al,[23] 2003	58	26	3.4	0	(36)
Geisler et al,[24] 2003	16	62.5	12.5	6.2	2–161 (39)
Subperitoneal mesh repair					
Longman & Thomson,[25] 2005	10	0	0	0	2–40 (30)
Guzman-Valdivia et al,[26] 2008	25	8	8	0	8–24 (12)
Egun et al,[27] 2002	10	0	20	0	22–69 (54)
Intraperitoneal mesh repair					
van Sprundel & Gerritsen van der Hoop,[15] 2005	15	13.3	0	0	5–52
Stelzner et al,[28] 2004	20	15	5	0	3–84 (42)
Hofstetter et al,[17] 1998	13	0	0	0	>96

Data from Refs.[15,17,20–28]

of prophylactic mesh insertion with low morbidity.[12,39,40] Three randomized controlled trials have been published. Janes and colleagues[41] conducted a randomized trial with 27 patients receiving a conventional stoma and an additional 27 patients had placement of a lightweight mesh in a sublay position at the time of ostomy creation. After 12 months of follow-up, PSH was present in 13 of 26 patients without mesh placement and in 1 of 21 in whom prophylactic mesh was placed. There was no incidence of wound infection, infection associated with the mesh, fistula formation, or pain during the observation period. Serra-Aracil and colleagues[42] prospectively evaluated the use of a lightweight mesh placed prophylactically at the time of end colostomy creation compared with standard ostomy formation alone. A total of 27 patients were randomized to each group and followed-up clinically and radiographically with abdominal CT by an independent clinician at 1 month and every 6 months after surgery. No mesh complications were reported. In the clinical follow-up (median, 29 months; range, 13–49), 11 (40.7%) of 27 hernias were recorded in the control group compared with 4 (14.8%) of 27 in the study group (P = .03). Abdominal CT identified 14 (44.4%) of 27 hernias in the control group compared with 6 (22.2%) of 27 in the study group (P = .08). Hammond and colleagues[43] prospectively evaluated the use of prophylactic Permacol mesh (Covidien, Mansfield, MA) placement in 20 patients. The median follow-up was only of 6.5 months, when 3 of 10 patients had PSH in the no-mesh group and no patients in the mesh group had PSH hernia. Recently, Shabbir and colleagues[3] did a systematic review with these three randomized controlled trials. A total of 128 patients (mesh 64, no mesh 64) were enrolled in these three studies. There was a statistically significant difference in the incidence of PSH in the mesh group (8 [12.5%] of 64) and in the no-mesh group (34 [53%] of 64). There was no difference in morbidity.

Table 5
Outcomes of different types of laparoscopic parastomal hernia repair in studies with greater than or equal to 10 patients

Study	Technique	No. of Repairs	Conversion (%)	Recurrence (%)	Infection (%)	Erosion (%)	Follow-up (mo) (median)
Mizrahi et al,[29] 2012	Keyhole	29	6.9	46.4	3.4	0	12–53 (30)
Wara & Andersen,[30] 2011	Keyhole	66	4	3	4.5	1.5	6–132 (36)
Hansson et al,[19] 2012	Keyhole	54	14.5	37	1.8	0	12–72 (36)
Pastor et al,[31] 2009	Keyhole/Sugarbaker	12	8.3	33.3	16.6	0	(13.9)[a]
Muysoms,[32] 2007	Keyhole/Sugarbaker	24	0	41.7	0	0	4–54 (21.2)[a]
Berger & Bientzle,[33] 2007	Sugarbaker/sandwich	66	1.5	12	4.5	0	3–72 (24)
Craft et al,[34] 2008	Keyhole/Sugarbaker	21	0	4.7	4.8	0	3–36 (14)[a]
Mancini et al,[35] 2007	Sugarbaker	25	0	4	4	0	2–38 (19)
LeBlanc et al,[36] 2005	Keyhole/Sugarbaker	12	0	8.3	0	0	3–39 (20)
McLemore et al,[37] 2007	Keyhole/Sugarbaker	19		10.5	2	—	20[a]

[a] Mean Follow-up.
Data from Refs.[19,29–37]

SUMMARY

PSH formation is an almost unavoidable complication of stoma formation. Various techniques have been described in the literature to repair these hernias. The laparoscopic Sugarbaker technique seems to be faster, technically feasible, and associated with a low rate of recurrence. It provides dependable mesh overlap, transabdominal mesh fixation, and it avoids creating new potential sites of hernia. However, long-term follow-up is necessary to assess the safety and efficacy of this approach. Prophylactic mesh placement should be considered during stoma creation to decrease the rate of parastomal herniation.

REFERENCES

1. Carne PW, Robertson GM, Frizelle FA. Parastomal hernia. Br J Surg 2003;90(7): 784–93.
2. Londono-Schimmer EE, Leong AP, Phillips RK. Life table analysis of stomal complications following colostomy. Dis Colon Rectum 1994;37(9):916–20.
3. Shabbir J, Chaudhary BN, Dawson R. A systematic review on the use of prophylactic mesh during primary stoma formation to prevent parastomal hernia formation. Colorectal Dis 2012;14(8):931–6.
4. Gil G, Owski MS. A new classification of parastomal hernias: from the experience at Bielanski Hospital in Warsaw. Pol Przegl Chir 2011;83(8):430–7.
5. Rubin MS, Bailey HR. Parastomal hernias. In: MacKeigan T, Cataldo P, editors. Intestinal stomas: principles, techniques and management. St Louis (MO): Quality Medical Publishing; 1993. p. 245–67.
6. Devlin HB. Peristomal hernia. In: Dudley HD, editor. Operative surgery volume I: alimentary tract and abdominal wall. 4th edition. London: Butterworths; 1983. p. 441–3.
7. Seo SH, Kim HJ, Oh SY, et al. Computed tomography classification for parastomal hernia. J Korean Surg Soc 2011;81(2):111–4.
8. Klinge U, Binnebosel M, Rosch R, et al. Hernia recurrence as a problem of biology and collagen. J Minim Access Surg 2006;2(3):151–4.
9. De Raet J, Delvaux G, Haentjens P, et al. Waist circumference is an independent risk factor for the development of parastomal hernia after permanent colostomy. Dis Colon Rectum 2008;51(12):1806–9.
10. Jansen PL, Mertens Pr P, Klinge U, et al. The biology of hernia formation. Surgery 2004;136(1):1–4.
11. Ripoche J, Basurko C, Fabbro-Perray P, et al. Parastomal hernia. A study of the French federation of ostomy patients. J Visc Surg 2011;148(6):e435–41.
12. Lopez-Cano M, Lozoya-Trujillo R, Quiroga S, et al. Use of a prosthetic mesh to prevent parastomal hernia during laparoscopic abdominoperineal resection: a randomized controlled trial. Hernia 2012;16(6):661–7.
13. Israelsson LA. Preventing and treating parastomal hernia. World J Surg 2005; 29(8):1086–9.
14. Sugarbaker PH. Peritoneal approach to prosthetic mesh repair of paraostomy hernias. Ann Surg 1985;201(3):344–6.
15. van Sprundel TC, Gerritsen van der Hoop A. Modified technique for parastomal hernia repair in patients with intractable stoma-care problems. Colorectal Dis 2005;7(5):445–9.
16. Morris-Stiff G, Hughes LE. The continuing challenge of parastomal hernia: failure of a novel polypropylene mesh repair. Ann R Coll Surg Engl 1998;80(3): 184–7.

17. Hofstetter WL, Vukasin P, Ortega AE, et al. New technique for mesh repair of paracolostomy hernias. Dis Colon Rectum 1998;41(8):1054–5.
18. Byers JM, Steinberg JB, Postier RG. Repair of parastomal hernias using polypropylene mesh. Arch Surg 1992;127(10):1246–7.
19. Hansson BM, Slater NJ, van der Velden AS, et al. Surgical techniques for parastomal hernia repair: a systematic review of the literature. Ann Surg 2012; 255(4):685–95.
20. Ho KM, Fawcett DP. Parastomal hernia repair using the lateral approach. BJU Int 2004;94(4):598–602.
21. Luning TH, Spillenaar-Bilgen EJ. Parastomal hernia: complications of extraperitoneal onlay mesh placement. Hernia 2009;13(5):487–90.
22. de Ruiter P, Bijnen AB. Ring-reinforced prosthesis for paracolostomy hernia. Dig Surg 2005;22(3):152–6.
23. Steele SR, Lee P, Martin MJ, et al. Is parastomal hernia repair with polypropylene mesh safe? Am J Surg 2003;185(5):436–40.
24. Geisler DJ, Reilly JC, Vaughan SG, et al. Safety and outcome of use of nonabsorbable mesh for repair of fascial defects in the presence of open bowel. Dis Colon Rectum 2003;46(8):1118–23.
25. Longman RJ, Thomson WH. Mesh repair of parastomal hernias: a safety modification. Colorectal Dis 2005;7(3):292–4.
26. Guzman-Valdivia G, Guerrero TS, Laurrabaquio HV. Parastomal hernia-repair using mesh and an open technique. World J Surg 2008;32(3):465–70.
27. Egun A, Hill J, MacLennan I, et al. Preperitoneal approach to parastomal hernia with coexistent large incisional hernia. Colorectal Dis 2002;4(2):132–4.
28. Stelzner S, Hellmich G, Ludwig K. Repair of paracolostomy hernias with a prosthetic mesh in the intraperitoneal onlay position: modified Sugarbaker technique. Dis Colon Rectum 2004;47(2):185–91.
29. Mizrahi H, Bhattacharya P, Parker MC. Laparoscopic slit mesh repair of parastomal hernia using a designated mesh: long-term results. Surg Endosc 2012;26(1): 267–70.
30. Wara P, Andersen LM. Long-term follow-up of laparoscopic repair of parastomal hernia using a bilayer mesh with a slit. Surg Endosc 2011;25(2):526–30.
31. Pastor DM, Pauli EM, Koltun WA, et al. Parastomal hernia repair: a single center experience. JSLS 2009;13(2):170–5.
32. Muysoms F. Laparoscopic repair of parastomal hernias with a modified Sugarbaker technique. Acta Chir Belg 2007;107(4):476–80.
33. Berger D, Bientzle M. Laparoscopic repair of parastomal hernias: a single surgeon's experience in 66 patients. Dis Colon Rectum 2007;50(10):1668–73.
34. Craft RO, Huguet KL, McLemore EC, et al. Laparoscopic parastomal hernia repair. Hernia 2008;12(2):137–40.
35. Mancini GJ, McClusky DA III, Khaitan L, et al. Laparoscopic parastomal hernia repair using a nonslit mesh technique. Surg Endosc 2007;21(9):1487–91.
36. LeBlanc KA, Bellanger DE, Whitaker JM, et al. Laparoscopic parastomal hernia repair. Hernia 2005;9(2):140–4.
37. McLemore EC, Harold KL, Efron JE, et al. Parastomal hernia: short-term outcome after laparoscopic and conventional repairs. Surg Innov 2007;14(3):199–204.
38. Bayer I, Kyzer S, Chaimoff C. A new approach to primary strengthening of colostomy with Marlex mesh to prevent paracolostomy hernia. Surg Gynecol Obstet 1986;163(6):579–80.
39. Janson AR, Janes A, Israelsson LA. Laparoscopic stoma formation with a prophylactic prosthetic mesh. Hernia 2010;14(5):495–8.

40. Hauters P, Cardin JL, Lepere M, et al. Prevention of parastomal hernia by intraperitoneal onlay mesh reinforcement at the time of stoma formation. Hernia 2012; 16(6):655–60.

41. Janes A, Cengiz Y, Israelsson LA. Randomized clinical trial of the use of a prosthetic mesh to prevent parastomal hernia. Br J Surg 2004;91(3):280–2.

42. Serra-Aracil X, Bombardo-Junca J, Moreno-Matias J, et al. Randomized, controlled, prospective trial of the use of a mesh to prevent parastomal hernia. Ann Surg 2009;249(4):583–7.

43. Hammond TM, Huang A, Prosser K, et al. Parastomal hernia prevention using a novel collagen implant: a randomised controlled phase 1 study. Hernia 2008; 12(5):475–81.

Soft Tissue Coverage in Abdominal Wall Reconstruction

Donald P. Baumann, MD, Charles E. Butler, MD*

KEYWORDS

- Abdominal wall reconstruction • Hernia • Surgical mesh
- Reconstructive surgical procedures • Surgical flaps

KEY POINTS

- Soft tissue reconstruction in the abdominal wall requires an algorithmic anatomic approach based on defect location.
- The decision to select a locoregional flap or a free flap is determined by defect surface area, local donor flap options, and availability of recipient vessels.
- Patient systemic comorbidities, locoregional wound conditions, and the possibility of early/late reoperation must be factored into flap selection.
- Reconstruction of complex abdominal wall defects that involve both musculofascial repair and soft tissue replacement highlight the importance of coordinated collaboration between general surgeons and plastic and reconstructive surgeons.

The need for soft tissue coverage in abdominal wall reconstruction suggests a loss of tissue beyond the availability of local tissue to be recruited to resurface the defect. Because most abdominal wall defects can be reconstructed with the redundant tissue usually found in the truncal area of most patients, these defects represent a more complex subset of abdominal wall reconstructions. Indications for flap coverage vary by cause of defect, defect type, and timeline for closure. Multiple clinical scenarios can lead to a loss of abdominal wall soft tissue requiring replacement including oncologic resection, traumatic injury, radiation-associated wounds, skin necrosis, superficial soft tissue infection, and septic evisceration. The amount of soft tissue loss and amount of coverage able to be performed with local skin advancement must be factored into the reconstructive plan. Abdominal wall defects requiring soft tissue coverage can be classified as partial-thickness defects, involving the skin and

Funding Sources: None.

Conflict of Interest: None.

Department of Plastic Surgery, Unit 1488, The University of Texas MD Anderson Cancer Center, 1400 Pressler, Houston, TX 77030, USA

* Corresponding author. Department of Plastic Surgery, Unit 1488, University of Texas MD Anderson Cancer Center, 1400 Pressler, FCT 19.500, Houston, TX 77030.

E-mail address: cbutler@mdanderson.org

Surg Clin N Am 93 (2013) 1199–1209

http://dx.doi.org/10.1016/j.suc.2013.06.005

0039-6109/13/$ – see front matter © 2013 Elsevier Inc. All rights reserved.

subcutaneous tissue only, or full-thickness composite defects, which involve loss of the abdominal wall musculofascia in addition to the overlying skin and subcutaneous tissue. The indications for soft tissue replacement in abdominal wall reconstruction also depend on the chronicity of the wound defect, with some defects benefiting from early soft tissue coverage and others being more appropriate for delayed flap coverage, whereas some defects might be better served with chronic wound care and healing by secondary intention.

In the past, abdominal wounds were treated with wound care and allowed to heal over time by secondary intention, or were reconstructed with a skin graft after the local wound environment was optimized. This approach resulted in a protracted course of care and significant morbidity. In time, the concept of delayed primary closure gained popularity, allowing certain patients with favorable wound characteristics to undergo closure after a short period of a few days instead of being committed to weeks or months of open wound care (**Fig. 1**).

Soft tissue flap reconstruction offers significant advantages compared with delayed primary or secondary healing wound closure. Flap reconstruction is performed in a single-stage procedure obviating chronic wound management. Flap reconstruction offers immediate and definitive wound closure mitigating the local milieu inflammatory response and local tissue injury. In reconstructions involving bioprosthetic mesh these two factors are critical in that, if the mesh is interposed between two well-vascularized tissue planes (posterior abdominal wall/peritoneal cavity and a soft tissue flap superficially), then bilaminar vascular ingrowth can be achieved, accelerating the period of bioprosthetic mesh revascularization and incorporation. In addition, a closed wound environment diminishes the proinflammatory state of an open wound, which limits the degree of enzymatic degradation of the bioprosthetic mesh during the incorporation phase.

Over the last 15 years, negative-pressure wound therapy (NPWT) has revolutionized the approach to wound care, particularly in the abdominal wall. NPWT allows preservation of the wound environment by managing fluid losses, decreasing bacterial contamination, and accelerating granulation tissue formation. In abdominal wall reconstruction this preserves the option for delayed closure by flap reconstruction or delayed primary closure.

Planning for flap reconstruction in the abdominal wall must factor defect type, defect location, availability of surrounding soft tissue, and, in certain cases, planned reoperation. Flap reconstructions can be classified by where the tissue is recruited and their blood supplies: local flaps, random or axial; regional flaps, pedicled; and free flaps, microanastomoses.

LOCAL FLAP OPTIONS

Local flaps involve recruiting tissue adjacent to the wound defect. Well-planned incisions are critical to preserve blood supply to the local flap and avoid wound healing complications at the donor site used to resurface the wound defect. There are various flap transposition designs available including advancement, rotation/advancement, interpolation, V-Y advancement, and bipedicled flaps. These flaps can be oriented in various dimensions, including vertical, oblique, and horizontal. These flaps are perfused through random or axial blood supplies, so understanding of the vascular anatomy in terms of abdominal wall angiosomes and perforator location is critical to designing robust local flaps.

It is also important to consider the impact of preexisting incisions in the abdominal wall when planning a flap design. A midline laparotomy may preclude harvesting a

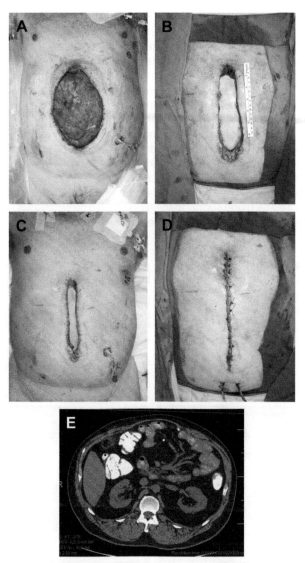

Fig. 1. Delayed primary fasciocutaneous flap closure. A 58-year-old man developed anastomotic leak after laparoscopic esophagectomy. The patient underwent multiple washouts and was treated as an open abdomen for 2 weeks (*A*). Abdominal wall closure with inlay bridging bioprosthetic mesh and bilateral component separation was performed and the patient underwent negative-pressure wound therapy (NPWT) for 2 weeks (*B*). Next he underwent skin debridement and advancement flap delayed primary closure (*C, D*). Two-year postoperative computed tomography follow-up (*E*). (*Courtesy of* D.P. Baumann, MD, Houston, TX. Copyright © 2009 Donald Baumann.)

local flap from the contralateral abdominal wall. However a midline defect bisected by a laparotomy scar can be divided in half and reconstructed by 2 local flaps, one from each hemiabdomen. Another key factor in performing a local flap reconstruction is limiting tension across the wound closure at both the defect site and the donor site. The flap perfusion, especially at the most distal part of the flap, can be compromised if the flap is placed on high tension either by pushing the limits of the flap design or by creating excessive biaxial tension across the flap when the donor site is closed. One strategy that can be used to mitigate excessive tension is to transpose the flap to cover the defect site and then skin graft the donor site.

For midline defects, a bipedicled flap is generally used for midline defects either unilaterally or bilaterally. The flap is oriented vertically with a minimum of a 3:1 length/width ratio and maintains a blood supply from both the superior and inferior aspects of the flap.[1] The flap is then directly transposed to resurface the defect and, by design, the donor site cannot be closed without an undue degree of tension. To offload the tension a skin graft is placed on the donor site, preserving blood supply to the distal flap to maximize wound healing. The keystone flap is one strategy to reconstruct large trunk defects (**Fig. 2**). The keystone flap enables 1-stage resurfacing of the both the defect and donor site. The flap is designed as a large 3:1 ellipse parallel to the long axis of the defect.[2] The blood supply to the flap is based on cutaneous perforators that shift toward the defect when the flap is advanced. Once the leading edge of the

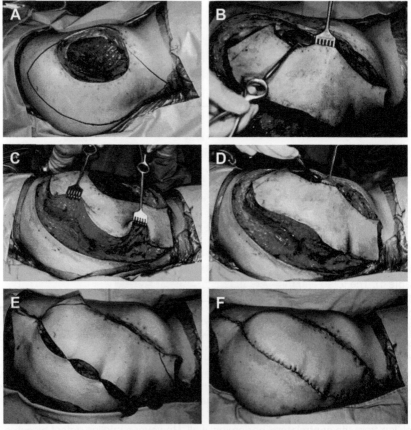

Fig. 2. Keystone flap. A 24-year-old woman with sarcoma of the upper lateral thigh. (*A*) The sarcoma has been removed and the resultant defect is marked for keystone island flap repair; note the large defect size. (*B–D*) The flap is freed and ready for inset without the need for undermining. (*E*) The redundant inner corners of the flap are marked and trimmed to prevent standing cutaneous deformity. (*F*) Final opposing V-Y primary closure.

keystone flap is inset the donor site is closed on itself from the poles of the long axis of the flap to the side of the flap remote from the defect. This flap succeeds because of the transposition tension from the advancement and closure being distributed over the long circumference of the flap skin island.

REGIONAL FLAP OPTIONS

In cases in which the defect size exceeds the availability of local soft tissue for coverage, the next option is to consider a regional flap. Regional flaps are pedicled flaps based on a dominant axial blood supply that can be delivered into the abdominal wall to support tissue perfusion in the flap's new location. Regional pedicled flaps are harvested from adjacent anatomic areas such as the chest, groin, thigh, or back. Pedicled flaps can be designed as either fasciocutaneous flaps, myocutaneous flaps, or muscle flaps resurfaced with a skin graft. When selecting a pedicled regional flap it is important to consider the donor morbidity incurred. In addition, not only must the flap's ability to reach the defect be considered but also how the transferred flap will tolerate the rotational and flexion/extension forces placed on it in the trunk. As an example, because the flap's pedicle vessels remain in their position of origin, the flap can traverse the groin or flank and have its blood flow compromised by compression or rotation in these areas (**Fig. 3**). Pedicled regional flap options for abdominal wall reconstruction include latissimus and serratus flaps for upper lateral defects and thigh-based flaps (anterolateral thigh [ALT], vastus lateralis/medialis, and tensor fascia lata [TFL]) for lower abdominal wall defects.

FREE TISSUE TRANSFER

Microsurgical free tissue transfer increases the capacity of the reconstructive surgeon to provide soft tissue coverage for abdominal wall defects that are not amenable to either local or regional flap coverage. Flaps of most sizes, volumes, dimensions, and compositions can be transferred from donor sites remote from the abdominal wall. Although more technically demanding, the evolution of microsurgical techniques enables successful free flap transfer in excess of 98% of cases.[3]

FLAP DONOR SITE OPTIONS

There are many free flap donor site options available for abdominal wall reconstruction (**Table 1**). The torso and thigh are the main areas of flap harvest for defects in the upper abdominal wall and epigastrium to the suprapubic region. Flaps can be harvested from these donor sites as either pedicled flaps or free flaps. The posterior chest wall donor site yields the latissimus dorsi and serratus anterior muscle flaps. These two flaps can be harvested as muscle flaps or myocutaneous flap designs. In addition, they can be harvested together as a chimeric flap to increase the tissue volume for flap transfer. These flaps can be transposed to the upper epigastrium or subcostal region as a pedicled flap. For defects beyond the reach of the thoracodorsal pedicle the flap can be converted to a free flap and transposed anywhere in the abdominal wall (**Fig. 4**).

In cases in which a large skin paddle is required for the abdominal wall defect, a free scapular or parascapular flap can be designed on the circumflex scapular branch of the subscapular arterial system. If a latissimus or serratus flap is harvested, the functional donor site impact must be considered as it relates to the weakened abdominal wall. In addition, in terms of logistical planning, the patient must undergo a position

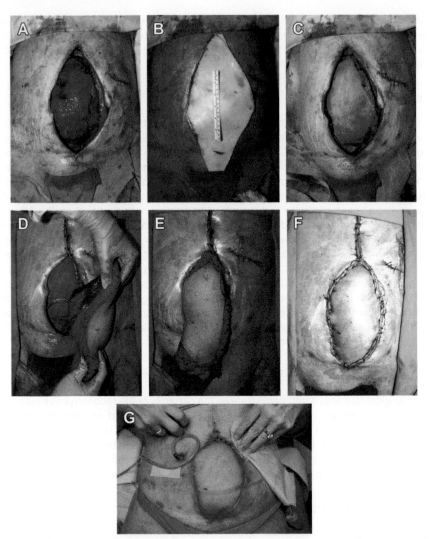

Fig. 3. Pedicled anterolateral thigh flap reconstruction of abdominal wall. A 45-year-old woman developed a pelvic abscess with fascial dehiscence after undergoing hysterectomy, oophorectomy, and abdominoperineal resection. She underwent multiple washouts and open-abdomen NPWT management (A). She then underwent exploration and reconstruction with inlay bridging bioprosthetic mesh (B, C). A left-sided anterolateral thigh flap was harvested and pedicled on the descending branch of the lateral femoral circumflex system up into the abdominal defect (D, E). The flap was then partially deepithelized and inset (F). The patient at 4-week follow-up (G). (*Courtesy of* D.P. Baumann, MD, Houston, TX. Copyright © 2011 Donald Baumann.)

change to facilitate flap dissection in the posterior chest wall, which adds complexity and additional time to the procedure.

The thigh represents the mainstay for flap donor sites. Both pedicled flaps for coverage of the infraumbilical abdominal wall and free flaps can be designed in several configurations: fasciocutaneous, myocutaneous, muscle, and chimeric flaps. The descending branch of the lateral circumflex femoral system provides blood supply

Table 1
Abdominal wall flap reconstruction algorithm

Location	Regional/Pedicled Flap	Free Flap
Epigastric region	Latissimus dorsi	Thigh-based flap
	Transposition flap (intramuscular perforators)	Latissimus dorsi
Periumbilical region	External oblique	Thigh-based flap
	Bipedicled fasciocutaneous	Latissimus dorsi
Hypogastric region	External oblique	Thigh-based flap
	Bipedicled fasciocutaneous	Latissimus dorsi
	Thigh-based flap	
	TFL	

to the vastus lateralis and rectus femoris muscles. The transverse branch of the lateral circumflex femoral system provides blood supply to the TFL muscle. These flaps can be harvested as muscle-only flaps or with overlying skin paddles. The anterolateral thigh flap is designed by including a skin paddle overlying the vastus lateralis muscle and can be designed as a myocutaneous or fasciocutaneous flap. The TFL flap can be designed to include the distal fascia of the iliotibial tract and a smaller proximal skin paddle if needed.[4] The anteromedial thigh flap can be designed on medial perforators from the descending branch of the lateral circumflex femoral system. The rectus femoris muscle is most commonly designed as a muscle flap; however, a skin island can be included over the central muscle when appropriately sized cutaneous perforators are present.

These thigh-based flaps can be designed in any combination as chimeric flaps (ie, ALT with anteromedial thigh (AMT) flaps, ALT with TFL, vastus lateralis with TFL). Taken to the extreme, the vastus lateralis, TFL, and the rectus femoris can be harvested with all overlying skin territory as a subtotal thigh flap for increased volume and skin coverage for massive abdominal wall defects (**Fig. 5**).[5]

RECIPIENT VESSELS

The success of any free tissue transfer relies on the availability of suitable recipient vessels providing arterial inflow and venous outflow to the free flap. There are several recipient vessels available for abdominal wall reconstruction with free flaps. The main vascular axis in the central abdominal wall is the internal mammary/superior epigastric/inferior epigastric system. The internal mammary and deep inferior epigastric vessels provide large-caliber recipient vessels of 2-mm to 3-mm diameter for microanastomosis. However, the vessels are present at the most cephalad and caudal limits of the abdominal wall. The main challenge for identifying recipient vessels is in the central aspect of the abdominal wall. In situ options include intramuscular components of the distal superior and inferior epigastric systems or the terminal intercostal branches. However, these vessels are smaller in caliber (1–2 mm) and present more technically challenging microanastomoses. In cases in which the internal mammary-epigastric axis is unavailable the thoracodorsal pedicle reach can be extended into the central abdomen by way of vein grafts.

Recipient vessel options exist beyond the abdominal wall itself. There are several options in the groin based on the superficial femoral system. The superficial inferior epigastric artery, the superficial circumflex iliac artery, and the deep circumflex iliac artery provide vessels of reasonable caliber for free flap transfer to the lower central and lateral abdominal wall. If primary anastomosis is not feasible then vein grafts or vein loops are required. Vein grafts are often harvested from the leg (greater or less

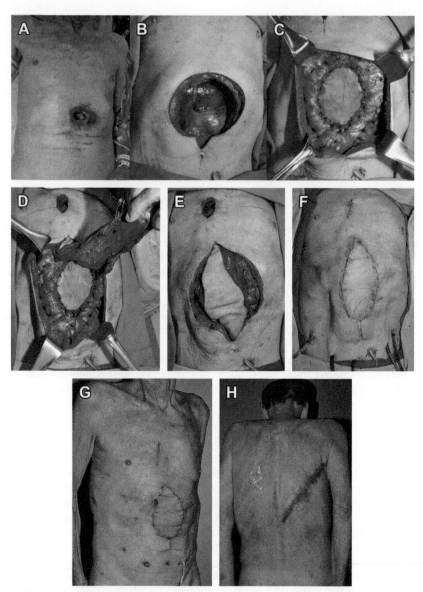

Fig. 4. Free latissimus myocutaneous flap reconstruction of epigastric defect. A 63-year-old patient with metastatic squamous cell carcinoma to abdomen and chest wall. Preoperative view of ulcerated erosive lesion into abdominal cavity. (*A*) Composite full-thickness resection of the abdominal wall including anterior reflection of diaphragm. Resultant thoracoabdominal composite defect. (*B*) Bioprosthetic mesh inlay bridging repair of the thoracoabdominal defect. (*C*) Free latissimus myocutaneous flap reconstruction of the epigastrium. Right internal mammary vessels used as recipient vessels. Pedicle tunneled under the lower chest wall skin flap (*D, E, F*). The patient at 3-week follow-up (*G, H*). (*Courtesy of* C.E. Butler, MD, Houston, TX. Copyright © 2011 Charles Butler.)

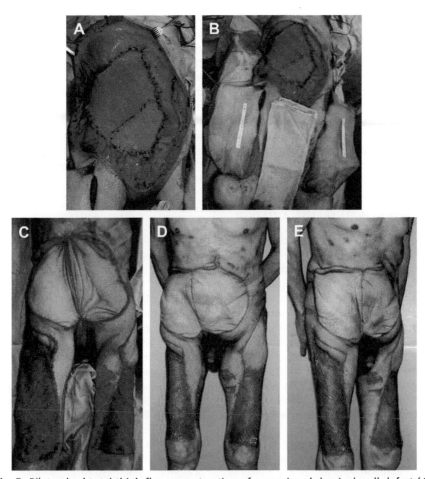

Fig. 5. Bilateral subtotal thigh flap reconstruction of a massive abdominal wall defect (*A*). Abdominal wall defect musculofascial reconstruction with bioprosthetic mesh (*B*). Flap harvest. Pedicled right subtotal thigh flap included the rectus femoris muscle and a skin paddle of 37 × 16 cm. Left subtotal thigh flap included the rectus femoris and tensor fasciae latae muscles and a skin paddle of 40 × 18 cm (*C*). Flap inset with donor site skin grafts (*D*). Postoperative view at 10 weeks (*E*). (*Courtesy of* C.E. Butler, MD, Houston, TX. Copyright © 2009 Charles Butler.)

saphenous vein) or arm (cephalic vein). In addition, in abdominal wall reconstructions with concurrent laparotomy intra-abdominal vessels can be used as recipients if there are no local options in the abdominal wall. The omental and gastroepiploic vessels can be easily mobilized to reach the undersurface of the abdominal wall. Care must be taken in insetting and supporting the flap pedicle so that there is no tension on the anastomoses when the visceral contents shift when the patient transitions from supine to sitting/standing. In addition, the morbidity of reentering the abdominal cavity must be considered if there is a vascular thrombosis. In addition, when bioprosthetic mesh is used for the musculofascial reconstruction as an adjunct to the fascia of the flap the pedicle traverses an aperture in the mesh, compromising the abdominal wall integrity and potentially leading to a hernia defect. For these reasons local recipient options should be explored before intra-abdominal vessels are selected.

Vein grafts and arterialized vein loops provide recipient vessels in the central abdominal wall. Vein grafts can be harvested from either the upper or lower extremity as a cephalic vein graft or saphenous vein graft. For central and lower abdominal defects an arterialized saphenous vein loop can be designed. The saphenous vein is dissected and transected distally and then anastomosed to the superficial femoral artery or a side branch. This technique allows delivery of the loop to the flap's recipient site where the loop is divided providing an arterialized afferent limb and a venous drainage efferent limb. This technique only requires 3 anastomoses instead of 4, as is the case with direct arterial and venous vein grafts. The main recipient vessel sites for vein grafts or arterialized vein loops are the thoracodorsal vessels; internal mammary vessels; branches of the superficial femoral system and the deep inferior epigastric vessels can be used to extend the reach of vein grafts to the central abdominal wall.

ABDOMINAL WALL TRANSPLANTATION

Abdominal wall transplantation represents the zenith of abdominal wall flap reconstruction. It is generally reserved for patients undergoing single-organ or multiorgan visceral transplants in which abdominal wall closure by autologous flaps is not technically feasible or presents significant donor morbidity. Abdominal wall closure after visceral organ transplantation is challenging in the setting of donor/recipient organ size mismatch and/or prior recipient abdominal surgery. Transplant patients can benefit from vascularized composite allotransplants as an additional strategy to expand the domain of the abdominal cavity to allow for either a graft/recipient size mismatch or inability for closure in the event of extreme intestinal edema. Although the risks of lifelong immunosuppression potentially outweigh the benefits of abdominal wall transplantation in healthy nontransplant patients, transplant patients are already bound to an immunosuppressive regimen and can benefit from the addition of allograft abdominal wall musculofascial tissue to reduce abdominal wall wound complication at the time of transplantation.

In the setting of transplant immunosuppression, the risk of an open abdominal wound, fascial dehiscence, septic evisceration, or fistula carries significant morbidity and potential mortality. When conventional abdominal wall closure techniques are insufficient, allotransplantation is performed. Extensive study of the vascular supply of the abdominal wall has allowed design of musculofasciocutaneous flaps based on the deep inferior epigastric (DIEP) system. These flaps can be transferred based on either the DIEP vessels through microsurgical techniques or the external iliac for a macrovascular anastomosis. Selvaggi and colleagues[6] describe a series of 15 abdominal wall transplants with 3 episodes of rejection salvage with modulating immunosuppression and 2 flap losses caused by vascular thrombosis.

Pediatric transplant patients present challenges in managing graft/recipient size mismatches and have the potential for needing advanced reconstructive options for abdominal wall closure. Given the microsurgical challenges associated with pediatric vessel caliber, alternative strategies for abdominal wall transplantation have been developed. Agarwal and colleagues[7] described a novel flap design for pediatric liver transplant patients.[8,9] They design a posterior rectus sheath fascioperitoneal flap based on the terminal branches of the hepatic artery via the falciform ligament, which enables transfer of the vascularized posterior sheath in continuity with the liver by means of the falciform ligament without the requirement for additional vascular anastomoses.

Abdominal wall transplantation is in its earliest stages. It has virtually eliminated the issue of donor site morbidity and future advances will likely focus on improved recipient site function. To this end, refining flap design even further to include dynamic neurotized flap transfers that can provide stable abdominal wall contour and preserved truncal core muscular stability will represent a new era in abdominal wall reconstruction.

REFERENCES

1. Smith PJ. The vascular basis of axial pattern flaps. Br J Plast Surg 1973;26(2): 150–7.
2. Khouri JS, Egeland BM, Daily SD, et al. The keystone island flap: use in large defects of the trunk and extremities in soft-tissue reconstruction. Plast Reconstr Surg 2011;127(3):1212–21.
3. Bui DT, Cordeiro PG, Hu QY, et al. Free flap reexploration: indications, treatment, and outcomes in 1193 free flaps. Plast Reconstr Surg 2007;119(7):2092–100.
4. Chalfoun CT, McConnell MP, Wirth GA, et al. Free tensor fasciae latae flap for abdominal wall reconstruction: overview and new innovation. J Reconstr Microsurg 2012;28(3):211–9.
5. Lin SJ, Butler CE. Subtotal thigh flap and bioprosthetic mesh reconstruction for large, composite abdominal wall defects. Plast Reconstr Surg 2010;125(4): 1146–56.
6. Selvaggi G, Levi DM, Cipriani R, et al. Abdominal wall transplantation: surgical and immunologic aspects. Transplant Proc 2009;41(2):521–2.
7. Agarwal S, Dorafshar AH, Harland RC, et al. Liver and vascularized posterior rectus sheath fascia composite tissue allotransplantation. Am J Transplant 2010;10(12):2712–6.
8. Lee JC, Olaitan OK, Lopez-Soler R, et al. Expanding the envelope: the posterior rectus sheath-liver vascular composite allotransplant. Plast Reconstr Surg 2013; 131(2):209e–18e.
9. Ravindra KV, Martin AE, Vikraman DS, et al. Use of vascularized posterior rectus sheath allograft in pediatric multivisceral transplantation–report of two cases. Am J Transplant 2012;12(8):2242–6.

Biology of Biological Meshes Used in Hernia Repair

Yuri W. Novitsky, MD

KEYWORDS

- Biological mesh • Hernia • Surgery • Abdominal wall • Grafts

KEY POINTS

- Ideally, use of biological grafts would be more advantageous in infected and contaminated fields, to incorporate and integrate into the ventral abdominal wall and ultimately to prevent recurrence. Although the use of biological meshes clearly has importance in ventral abdominal wall surgery, significant doubts about their indications and the implications of their use have arisen.
- Recent data have been disappointing on several fronts. Animal investigations have failed to demonstrate consistent evidence of biological mesh remodeling and replacement of biological grafts with collagen-like tissue. In addition, recent human experience has revealed that true remodeling of biologics occurs at the periphery of an implanted graft, if at all.
- Combining this evidence with disappointing clinical outcomes of biologics, particularly in the long term, has significantly cooled off enthusiasm about biological grafts. While investigations of biological grafts are still ongoing, the traditionally proposed notion of graft remodeling as an underlying principle of biological grafts is likely not representative of reality.
- It appears that the current design of biological constructs will have to undergo significant modifications to remain a part of the surgeon's armamentarium in the future.

INTRODUCTION

Throughout the United States and most of the world, hernia repair continues to be the most common surgical procedure performed by general surgeons.[1–3] Successful repair of most hernias requires the use of a prosthetic implant for reinforcement of the defect. Synthetic surgical meshes have been used for more than 50 years and are the most prevalent category of meshes used today. However, synthetic materials have been associated with a variety of complications related to foreign-body implantation. Some of the more serious adverse effects of synthetics include sensation of

Disclosures: Consultant/speaker bureau for Lifecell, CR Bard.
Department of Surgery, Case Comprehensive Hernia Center, University Hospitals Case Medical Center, Case Western Reserve University, 11100 Euclid Avenue, Cleveland, OH 44106, USA
E-mail address: yuri.novitsky@uhhospitals.org

Surg Clin N Am 93 (2013) 1211–1215
http://dx.doi.org/10.1016/j.suc.2013.06.014 surgical.theclinics.com
0039-6109/13/$ – see front matter © 2013 Elsevier Inc. All rights reserved.

the implant, limitation of movement, chronic pain, and, most concerning, prosthetic infection. In addition, synthetic meshes have traditionally been thought to be contra-indicated in infected or potentially contaminated fields.[4–8] Because of the need for prosthetic implants to resist infections and to support repairs in contaminated or potentially contaminated fields, biological meshes have been developed to take the place of nondegradable synthetic meshes. Clearly a biological matrix that would resist infection, while providing a durable reinforcement of a hernia repair, would be ideal for most, if not all, repairs. This article reviews the validity of assumptions that support the purported notion of the biological behavior of biological meshes.

BASIC CONCEPTS

One of the key factors in determining the success of the graft is its biocompatibility and the degree of evoked host tissue response. Implanted graft can become either in-corporated, resulting in neovascularization and deposition of collagen (remodeling) throughout the material; encapsulated, with deposition of fibrotic material at the periphery and around the graft; or resorbed/degraded, without any visible residual evidence of the mesh.

The purported function of biologics is to serve as a regenerative framework that sup-ports matrix remodeling and deposition of new collagen.[1–5] Factors that affect how a given mesh is reacted upon by the recipient include tissue sourcing, different methods of processing, decellularization, and sterilization used. Manufacturers use various pro-prietary methods and processing solvents that likely influence the innate biochemical and biomolecular structure of the collagen scaffold. Subsequently, these matrix alter-ations likely influence foreign-body recognition and antigen presentation. The resultant processing likely changes a variety of factors that are essential for matrix survival: immunogenic potential, biocompatibility, and foreign-body response to each implant.

COLLAGEN CROSS-LINKING

Of all the various processing techniques used by the manufacturers, collagen cross-linking appears to have the most profound impact on tissue responses to biological meshes. By using hexamethylenediisocyanate, carbodiimide, glutaraldehyde, or photo-oxidizing agents,[9,10] intentional cross-linking is used to prolong the life span of the mesh, using processing techniques that add to the 3-dimensional structure of the collagen to, essentially, mechanically strengthen the matrix and impede degrada-tion by collagenase. To help put this process in proper perspective, it is important to point out that "terminally" cross-linked animal dermis is leather. Even nonintentionally cross-linked products may undergo molecular structural changes, such as collagen cross-linking, from γ-irradiation during the sterilization process.[11] In addition, incom-plete removal of chemical cross-linking agents could result in cytotoxicity from resi-dues leaching from the mesh itself, which may induce prolonged toxic effects and heightened cellular responses.[9,10] Although clinical circumstances requiring long-term tissue reinforcement may provide some utility for a cross-linked graft, it is clear that such meshes display a significant immunologic disadvantage that likely translates into poor performance in a clinical setting, especially in the face of contamination.[12–15]

MESH INTEGRATION AND HOST REACTIONS

On implantation, rapid mesh integration remains an important and clearly desirable outcome. Unfortunately, this process is poorly understood and is often difficult to qualify and quantify. It appears that there is a cascade of events that follow initial mesh-host interaction. The author believes that acute inflammatory response takes place after mesh placement in the host. This event is a necessary one in wound healing and, obviously, is highly influential in the performance of biological mesh. The process of ingrowth begins with mononuclear cell (macrophages and mast cell) penetration into a mesh scaffold. Although meshes with diminished biocompatibility do not allow for such neocellularity, grafts that are positively recognized by a host will have host cells easily migrate from the periphery of the mesh inward. This step is often simultaneous with new proliferation of blood vessels within the graft. Once mononuclear cells populate the graft, the typical sequence of wound-healing events likely takes place. Mononuclear cells secrete cytokines and other signaling factors to attract fibroblasts. Once fibroblasts arrive, new collagen synthesis and deposition take place. Of importance, this process has to occur not only at the mesh/host interface but also within the graft itself; this would predispose a biological graft for ingrowth, incorporation, and deposition of new collagen within the mesh. Although this sequence is appealing, the author has not been unable to elucidate such a process in several animal models. Moreover, recent experience with mesh explants from humans has supported the notion that "remodeling" is not a typical event.

Inflammation appears to be a common component of host response to implanted biological prosthetics.[6,15–17] This reaction either may aid in the integration of the mesh via normal wound-healing mechanisms, or can induce a disproportionate inflammatory response. Such exaggerated reaction will likely result in excessive scarring, graft encapsulation, and/or degradation.[6,15,18] The balance between appropriate wound healing and detrimental sequelae is largely controlled by cytokines, growth factors, and other chemical signaling molecules produced by host macrophages at the site of the host/mesh interface. Orenstein and colleagues[15,19] were the first to evaluate the immunogenic potential of various human-derived and porcine-derived biological meshes in vitro. With regard to porcine meshes, non–cross-linked porcine dermis mesh and, to a lesser degree, porcine intestinal submucosa-derived mesh were associated with a markedly diminished cytokine production in comparison with the cross-linked porcine dermis materials. Although the exact clinical importance of the excessive macrophage activation in vitro is unclear, this early evidence of adverse effects of chemical cross-linking has subsequently been collaborated by several in vivo studies.[6,13,18,20] Most recently, Petter-Puchner and colleagues[12] reported a pronounced foreign-body response to intraperitoneal implantation of Collamend and Surgisis in rats. Both meshes were noted to be surrounded by a broad rim of foreign-body giant cells and granulomas. Consequently, the "biological" behavior of such grafts is somewhat limited.

BIOLOGICAL MESH REMODELING

The final and most important step in biological mesh placement is graft integration and remodeling with deposition of new collagen and regeneration of tissue. During this process, the implanted mesh is often resorbed by the host. Melman and colleagues[21] have suggested that when scaffold degradation is accompanied by cellular infiltration, extracellular matrix (ECM) deposition, and neovascularization, it can be viewed as remodeling. At times, however, when ECM deposition/neovascularization does not occur, mesh is likely replaced by a scar with a resultant detriment to a hernia repair. One of the other key factors that influence remodeling may be the rate of scaffold degradation.[21] Almost uniform failure of absorbable meshes may be due to a fairly rapid degradation of the graft without proper support for new ECM-component deposition. In fact, a gradual remodeling of an implanted tissue graft seems to be essential for abdominal wall repair because degradation or absorption of a scaffold not balanced with deposition of new collagen would predispose to mesh failure.[17] Deeken and colleagues[16] reported that non–cross-linked grafts showed more favorable remodeling characteristics. However, remodeling in their study was not associated with stronger reinforcement of native tissue repairs in the long term. As mentioned earlier, these paradoxic results may be a consequence of the animal model used. Another recent study revealed essential lack of matrix absorption and absence of remodeling of cross-linked graft after 6 months' implantation.[18] Of interest, most of the Collamend matrix samples were completely degraded by bacteria from associated wounds. The mesh samples that did not get infected were found to have no evidence of remodeling and poor or no integration.[18] While such mesh performance may at times result in an effective repair in the clean setting, this behavior of Collamend can hardly be viewed as "biological" reinforcement. Instead, given its lack of integration into the host and likely resultant fibrous encapsulation, cross-linked grafts often act as permanent foreign-body materials, similar to GoreTex–based synthetics. In fact, the author found in his mouse model that cross-linked grafts had no evidence of remodeling but a thick layer of fibrous encapsulation 3 months after implantation. It appears that the balance between ECM deposition and mesh degradation is critical for mesh remodeling and effective tissue reinforcement. Finally, although many investigators reported deposition of "new" matrix at the site of biological mesh implantations, a typical scar plate developed as a part of normal wound healing which likely to mimicked regeneration. Truly distinguishing regenerated collagen within degraded scaffold from fibrotic scar formation has contrived to be a tough challenge.

SUMMARY

Ideally, the use of biological grafts would be more advantageous in infected and contaminated fields, to incorporate and integrate into the ventral abdominal wall and ultimately to prevent recurrence. While biological meshes clearly have importance in ventral abdominal wall surgery, significant doubts about their indications and the implications of their use have arisen. Recent data have been disappointing on several fronts. Animal investigations have failed to demonstrate consistent evidence of biological mesh remodeling and replacement of biological grafts with collagen-like tissue. In addition, recent human experience has revealed that true remodeling of biologics occurs at the periphery of an implanted graft, if at all. Combining this evidence with disappointing clinical outcomes of biologics,[22] particularly in the long term, has significantly cooled off enthusiasm about biological grafts. While investigations of biological grafts are still ongoing, the traditionally proposed notion of graft remodeling as an underlying principle of biological grafts is likely not representative of reality. It appears that the current design of biological constructs will have to undergo significant modifications to remain a part of the surgeon's armamentarium in the future.

REFERENCES

1. Gaertner WB, Bonsack ME, Delaney JP. Experimental evaluation of four biologic prostheses for ventral hernia repair. J Gastrointest Surg 2007;11:1275–85.
2. Cornwell KG, Landsman A, James KS. Extracellular matrix biomaterials for soft tissue repair. Clin Podiatr Med Surg 2009;26:507–23.
3. Rosen MJ. Biologic mesh for abdominal wall reconstruction: a critical appraisal. Am Surg 2010;76:1–6.
4. Jansen PL, Mertens Pr P, Klinge U, et al. The biology of hernia formation. Surgery 2004;136:1–4.

5. Jin J, Rosen MJ, Blatnik J, et al. Use of acellular dermal matrix for complicated ventral hernia repair: does technique affect outcomes? J Am Coll Surg 2007; 205:654–60.
6. Sandor M, Xu H, Connor J, et al. Host response to implanted porcine-derived biologic materials in a primate model of abdominal wall repair. Tissue Eng Part A 2008;14:2021–31.
7. Marreco PR, da Luz Moreira P, Genari SC, et al. Effects of different sterilization methods on the morphology, mechanical properties, and cytotoxicity of chitosan membranes used as wound dressings. J Biomed Mater Res B Appl Biomater 2004;71:268–77.
8. Rueter A, Schleicher JB. Elimination of toxicity from polyvinyl trays after sterilization with ethylene oxide. Appl Microbiol 1969;18:1057–9.
9. Khor E. Methods for the treatment of collagenous tissues for bioprostheses. Biomaterials 1997;18:95–105.
10. Schmidt CE, Baier JM. Acellular vascular tissues: natural biomaterials for tissue repair and tissue engineering. Biomaterials 2000;21:2215–31.
11. Gouk SS, Lim TM, Teoh SH, et al. Alterations of human acellular tissue matrix by gamma irradiation: histology, biomechanical property, stability, in vitro cell repopulation, and remodeling. J Biomed Mater Res B Appl Biomater 2008;84:205–17.
12. Petter-Puchner AH, Fortelny RH, Silic K, et al. Biologic hernia implants in experimental intraperitoneal onlay mesh plasty repair: the impact of proprietary collagen processing methods and fibrin sealant application on tissue integration. Surg Endosc 2011;25:3245–52.
13. Butler CE, Burns NK, Campbell KT, et al. Comparison of cross-linked and non-cross-linked porcine acellular dermal matrices for ventral hernia repair. J Am Coll Surg 2010;211:368–76.
14. Pierce LM, Rao A, Baumann SS, et al. Long-term histologic response to synthetic and biologic graft materials Implanted in the vagina and abdomen of a rabbit model. Am J Obstet Gynecol 2009;200:546.e1–8.
15. Orenstein SB, Qiao Y, Klueh U, et al. Activation of human mononuclear cells by porcine biologic meshes in vitro. Hernia 2010;14:401–7.
16. Deeken CR, Melman L, Jenkins ED, et al. Histologic and biomechanical evaluation of crosslinked and non-crosslinked biologic meshes in a porcine model of ventral incisional hernia repair. J Am Coll Surg 2011;212:880–8.
17. Xu H, Wan H, Sandor M, et al. Host response to human acellular dermal matrix transplantation in a primate model of abdominal wall repair. Tissue Eng Part A 2008;14:2009–19.
18. de Castro Bras LE, Shurey S, Sibbons PD. Evaluation of crosslinked and non-crosslinked biologic prostheses for abdominal hernia repair. Hernia 2012;16: 77–89.
19. Orenstein SB, Qiao Y, Kaur M, et al. Human monocyte activation by biologic and biodegradable meshes in vitro. Surg Endosc 2010;24:805–11.
20. Burns NK, Jaffari MV, Rios CN, et al. Non-cross-linked porcine acellular dermal matrices for abdominal wall reconstruction. Plast Reconstr Surg 2010;125: 167–76.
21. Melman L, Jenkins ED, Hamilton NA, et al. Early biocompatibility of crosslinked and non-crosslinked biologic meshes in a porcine model of ventral hernia repair. Hernia 2011;15:157–64.
22. Rosen MJ, Krpata DM, Ermlich B, et al. A 5-Year clinical experience with single-staged repairs of infected and contaminated abdominal wall defects utilizing biologic mesh. Ann Surg 2013;257(6):991–6.

Clinical Outcomes of Biologic Mesh: Where Do We Stand?

Hobart W. Harris, MD, MPH

KEYWORDS

• Allograft • Xenograft • Prosthetics • Efficacy

KEY POINTS

- The cumulative data regarding biologic mesh use on ventral hernias under contaminated conditions do not support the claim that they are better than synthetic mesh used under the same conditions.
- Most of the available data pertain to the use of human acellular dermal matrix to repair complex ventral hernias, a product that both experts in the field and manufacturers now agree is inadequate for this clinical application.
- The highly promoted and frequently discussed practice of placing biologic mesh in contaminated surgical fields is being done outside of the products' original intended use and, in some instances, equates to off-label use of a medical device.
- Biologic mesh use, even in noncontaminated conditions, is questionable when the reported results are viewed in light of the high costs.

INTRODUCTION

Ventral hernias occur after 11% to 23% of laparotomy incisions. With 4 to 5 million laparotomies performed annually in the United States, there are an estimated 400,000 ventral hernia repairs each year, making it one of the most common procedures performed by general surgeons and adding more than $8 billion to US health care costs. A permanent prosthetic mesh repair during a clean case in which there is no bacterial contamination is the standard of care, yielding the best long-term results and reducing the hernia recurrence rate by 50%.[1] The management of ventral hernias in the setting of bacterial contamination remains, however, a major clinical challenge because placing a permanent synthetic prosthetic into a contaminated field is generally thought to result in an unacceptably high rate of complications, including surgical site infection, enterocutaneous fistula, and recurrent hernia formation. Therefore, until recently, the standard of care for repairing a complex ventral hernia (eg, one that involves a compromised surgical field in which gastrointestinal, biliary, and/or genitourinary procedures are performed or frank infection is present) was a 2-stage procedure. In the

Disclosures: The author has nothing to disclose.
Department of Surgery, UCSF, 513 Parnassus Avenue, Room S-301, Box 0104, San Francisco, CA 94143-0104, USA
E-mail address: Hobart.Harris@ucsfmedctr.org

first stage, the contaminated portion of the surgery is completed and the abdominal wall reconstructed using a temporary synthetic (absorbable) prosthetic. In the second stage, after approximately 6 to 12 months have elapsed and the wound contamination has been eliminated, the persistent ventral hernia is repaired using a permanent synthetic prosthetic. Although the 2-stage procedure is thought to reduce the risks of infection-related complications by avoiding placement of permanent prosthetic material into a contaminated wound, it unfortunately requires patients to undergo 2 separate operations, hospitalizations, and recovery periods, during which time they often cannot work and must endure a limited level of physical activity.

Several biomedical companies have recently introduced new biologic prosthetics (mesh) to address the clinical challenge of treating complex ventral hernias with a 1-stage repair. Because biologic mesh is derived from living tissue, these products are promoted as resisting infection and enabling wound healing in contaminated surgical fields. Currently, an intriguing variety of biologic meshes, derived from collagen-rich porcine, bovine, or human tissues, such as skin, intestinal submucosa, or pericardium, is available for the 1-stage repair of complex ventral hernias. These products are, however, expensive, and long-term outcome data are sparse. Furthermore, data are accumulating that question the overall clinical efficacy of such products, despite their intuitive appeal as more natural tissue replacements.

This article reviews currently available clinical data regarding the use of biologic mesh for the 1-stage repair of incisional hernias in the setting of wound contamination. Specifically, it attempts to answer the general question, "Should biologic mesh be used for incisional hernia repair?"

TYPES OF BIOLOGIC MESH

Biologic meshes derived from collagen-rich tissues of human (allograft) or animal (xenograft) origin were introduced into clinical practice in the 1990s.[2] Whereas synthetic prosthetics have been successfully used to reinforce the abdominal wall for more than a century, biologic meshes represent the newest effort to find the ideal material for hernia repair. In theory, biologic mesh provides a 3-D scaffold of extracellular matrix proteins that enables native cells to infiltrate and promotes neovascularization and the regeneration of healthy connective tissue that is resistant to infection. The biologic nature of the material is thought to provide an improved ability to reintegrate with surrounding tissues while reducing the risk of infection, erosion, extrusion, and rejection compared with the synthetic alternatives. Biologic meshes purportedly avoid some of the complications observed with the use of synthetic mesh, but, most importantly, biologic meshes can be deployed in the setting of wound contamination, a condition for which the use of synthetic mesh is generally discouraged.

More than a dozen different biologic meshes are currently available for abdominal wall reconstruction (**Table 1**). These products differ in their biologic source, processing to remove cellular components and reduce antigenicity, decontamination, size and thickness, amount of cross-linking, storage and handling characteristics, and costs. Although a detailed evaluation of these various differences is beyond the scope of this article, a brief discussion of cross-linking is warranted because it is frequently cited as a feature that has a critical impact on a prosthetic's clinical performance. Cross-links are covalent or ionic bonds that link one polymer chain to another, with a resultant increase in strength of the overall material. Cross-linking in the context of biologic mesh refers to bonds between extracellular matrix proteins, most commonly collagen fibers. Some degree of collagen cross-linking occurs naturally; yet, creating additional cross-links yields increased resistance to degradation by

Table 1
Summary of the commercially available biologic meshes

Biologic Source	Manufacturer	Notes
Human acellular dermis		
AlloDerm	LifeCell	Proprietary sterilization process
AlloMax	Davol/Bard	Sterilized via γ-irradiation
FlexHD	Ethicon	Hydrated dermis packaged in ethanol solution
Porcine acellular dermis		
CollaMend	Bard	Cross-linked collagen and elastin
Permacol	Covidien	Chemically cross-linked lysine/hydroxylysine residues
Strattice	LifeCell	Non–cross-linked, prehydrated matrix
XenMatrix	Davol/Bard	Proprietary dermal processing without cross-linking
Porcine intestinal submucosa		
FortaGen	Organogenesis	Low level of cross-linking
Surgisis	Cook	Multiple versions marketed since 2004
Bovine acellular dermis (fetal)		
SurgiMend	TEI Biosciences	Type III collagen-rich dermis in 1–4 mm thicknesses
Bovine pericardium		
Peri-Guard	Synovis	Gluteraldehyde cross-linking, NaOH sterilization
Tutopatch	Tutogen	Proprietary chemical and mechanical sterilization
Veritas	Synovis	Propylene oxide capped amine technology

either host or bacterial enzymes, thereby increasing mesh durability and reportedly decreasing hernia recurrence rates. Animal data indicate that although increased cross-linking is associated with a decreased rate of tissue degradation, it is also associated with decreased tissue integration.[3] Optimal tissue integration and mesh strength/durability define 2 ends of a spectrum. As the amount of cross-linking in a biologic mesh increases, so does the material's durability, but with the trade-off of decreased tissue integration. There is insufficient information to conclusively determine the effect of cross-linking on hernia recurrence rates, thereby rendering the clinical importance of this specific mesh characteristic unclear.

CLINICAL OUTCOMES

The overall clinical efficacy of biologic prosthetics for the repair of incisional hernias is unclear, despite their aggressive marketing, clinical popularity, and intuitive scientific appeal. A review of how these products reach the marketplace and the available clinical outcomes data is provided to help clinicians make as informed and prudent decisions as possible when considering the use of these intriguing biomaterials.

FDA Review of Biologic Meshes

The Food and Drug Administration (FDA) is responsible for protecting and promoting public health through the regulation and safety of food, tobacco, dietary supplements, drugs, vaccines, biopharmaceuticals, radiation emitting devices, veterinary products, and medical devices. Although clinicians are not expected to be experts in federal regulatory processes, the substantial difference between FDA clearance versus approval is important. Biologic meshes can be allografts or xenografts, with each class having a different regulatory pathway. Biologic xenografts are considered intermediate risk (class 2) medical devices that frequently obtain the agency's clearance via the

510(k) pathway. This regulatory requirement determines that a product either has the same intended use and characteristics of a product already on the market or the same use but with different characteristics that are substantively equivalent to what already exists in the marketplace. For most such products, clinical trials are not necessary to satisfy these requirements. Alternatively, to obtain FDA approval, a product must provide clinical trial evidence of safety and efficacy, which is routine and familiar for the introduction of a new drug. In contrast, a new medical device can be marketed once it obtains FDA clearance, which is generally a matter of safety alone. The FDA classifies allografts (eg, AlloDerm) as human tissue for transplantation, resulting in a different regulatory pathway than that for xenografts, one that requires neither FDA clearance nor approval. Consequently, surgeons are effectively using biologic meshes for abdominal wall reconstruction that are safe but clinically unproved. In addition, whereas the FDA cleared biologic meshes for the "intended for use as a soft tissue patch to reinforce soft tissue where weakness exists and for the surgical repair of damaged or ruptured soft tissue membranes,"[4] that clearance does not include the use of these biomaterials to repair hernias in contaminated fields. Understandably, in the absence of robust, high-quality clinical trial data and potentially vague regulatory restrictions, 2 of the most commonly asked questions regarding biologic meshes are, "Which one should I use?" and "How well do they work?"

Literature and Systemic Reviews

Despite the number of different biologic meshes available for incisional hernia repair, most published reports involve the use of 4 specific products: AlloDerm (non–cross-linked human dermis), Permacol (cross-linked porcine dermis), Strattice (non–cross-linked porcine dermis), and Surgisis (non–cross-linked porcine intestine). Consequently, the data analyzed by recent clinical and systematic reviews examining the use of biologic mesh for incisional hernia repair reflect the performance of these prosthetics.[5–10] A summary of the available clinical data represents an analysis of more than 60 published studies, involving more than 1700 surgical repairs and an overall mortality rate of less than 4% (**Table 2**). Several observations deserve attention when considering this analysis.

- Poor quality primary data

First and foremost, the general quality of the available data is poor, thereby significantly limiting the ability to draw definitive conclusions, let alone derive strong treatment recommendations. The studies included in the analyses are either case series or

Table 2
Summary of clinical outcomes for incisional hernia repair using biologic mesh

Biologic Source	Repairs (N)	Wound Complications (%)	Hernia Recurrences (%)	Mean Follow-up (mo)	Contaminated Wounds (%)
Human acellular dermis	1232	48	22	14	<20
Porcine acellular dermis	298	51	16	10	<30
Cross-linked	133				
Non–cross-linked	165				
Porcine intestinal submucosa	135	83	8	15	<35
Other	36	—	—	—	—
Summary	1701	51	20	13	<23

case reports, all of which are considered a low level of evidence.[7,11–14] This concern is further compounded these data reported inconsistently, with different inclusion and exclusion criteria, outcome variables, and follow-up periods. These inconsistencies make it difficult to legitimately compare studies and render most conclusions unsupported or premature. For example, important variables, such as surgical technique or level of wound contamination, are not reported with sufficient detail to appropriately stratify the outcome data, thereby forfeiting the opportunity to accurately combine or compare data between studies. Ultimately, the shortcomings of poor-quality primary data cannot be overcome, no matter how rigorous and robust the analytic methods, and must not be forgotten when attempting to use this information to guide clinical decision making. These serious concerns notwithstanding, the data analysis yields several interesting and provocative observations.

- Allografts (human acellular dermal matrix) dominate the hernia repair literature

A majority of available data pertain to a biomaterial that is experiencing decreasing clinical popularity. As highlighted in **Fig. 1**, more than 70% of procedures reported in the literature detailing the use of biologic mesh for incisional hernia repair involve the use of human acellular dermal matrix. Beyond the statistical impact on the data from such numerical dominance by a single product (AlloDerm), the use of human dermal allografts for incisional hernia repair has been seriously questioned. Many surgeons, including experts in hernia repair, have become disillusioned with human allografts for incisional hernia repair because of high wound complication and hernia recurrence rates.[15–18] In the author's experience, the industry seems to be moving away from promoting human allografts for incisional hernia repair in favor of biologic meshes that are more readily available and display more consistent and predictable physical properties and characteristics.

- High rate of wound complications

All types of biologic mesh are associated with a significant rate of wound complications, ranging from 50% to 80%. Approximately half of the wound complications are

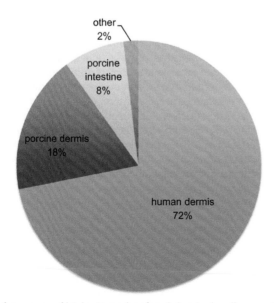

Fig. 1. Estimated frequency of biologic meshes for abdominal wall reconstruction by source.

infections, but biologic meshes are also associated with seromas, hematomas, fistulas, skin necrosis, and mesh disintegration, independent of source, processing, or degree of cross-linking.[6,7] Many of the published articles on biologic mesh for hernia repair comment that synthetic mesh is contraindicated in contaminated conditions and go on to highlight how biologic mesh can address this difficult situation. The complication rates with the use of biologic mesh are, however, comparable to those of synthetic mesh, bringing into question the fundamental indication for the biologic class of prosthetic.[9,10]

- High rate of hernia recurrences at 1-year follow up

Recurrence rates of 15% to 25% are frequently reported after repair of an incisional hernia. Consequently, an estimated cumulative recurrence rate of 20% after incisional hernia repair using a biologic mesh seems to fall within that range, until considering when in a patients' follow-up period the recurrence rate is measured. The best available data suggest that the incidence of recurrent incisional hernias increases with time.[19] Therefore, patient follow-up periods must be comparable if accurately comparing recurrence rates as a function of prosthetic material. Accordingly, recurrence rates at approximately 1 year of follow-up are reasonably estimated to be 5% for synthetic mesh versus 20% for biologic mesh.[20] These relative estimates should be evaluated in light of the lack of high-quality data regarding incisional hernia repair (previously discussed). Still, it can reasonably be concluded that there is insufficient information to support a reduced hernia recurrence rate for biologic meshes versus the synthetic alternatives. Furthermore, solid data indicate that using biologic mesh to bridge a fascial defect is associated with failure rates of 38% to 88% at 1 year.[15,16,21]

- Greater experience in noncontaminated wounds

Published reviews on biologic mesh use for ventral hernia repair under contaminated conditions all conclude by supporting the continued use of these meshes for that indication. The ability to use a natural, tissue-derived biomaterial that develops neovascularity and thus can resist infection is the central indication that separates biologic versus synthetic prosthetics. But, a closer look at the primary data contained in these reviews indicates that such positive conclusions are unwarranted, for several reasons. Beyond the primary concerns of poor quality clinical data, only 6 studies used the standardized Centers for Disease Control and Prevention wound classification system of clean, clean-contaminated, contaminated, and dirty[22–28]; the remainder either did not define what was meant by "contamination," listed a few scenarios that the investigators considered "unclean," or used another classification system that combined contaminated wounds with wounds at high-risk for contamination.[7] Unfortunately, the arbitrary designation of contamination, or not using a standard classification system for such an important definition, leaves open the possibility for provider bias in what is considered a contaminated field and, thus, can affect how the data are interpreted. In addition, well under 25% of incisional hernia repairs using a biologic prosthetic were performed clearly contaminated conditions. It is, therefore, not surprising that there is no consensus among surgeons regarding how or when biologic meshes should be used during abdominal wall reconstruction.[29]

Cost Analyses

Cost is an important but underevaluated issue of concern regarding the use of biologic meshes, which can be 10 to 20 times more expensive than synthetic meshes. Of the 5 recent review articles, 3 either included charts illustrating examples of what these prostheses cost[5,10] or briefly discussed how cost should be an important deciding factor when choosing which mesh to use.[10,30] But, only 1 of the 5 articles actually stated that biologic meshes are more expensive than synthetics. Of the 25 primary articles used by the clinical review articles, 9 mention cost in their discussion sections and all conclude that biologic mesh materials are substantially more expensive than other prosthetics available. A recent cost analysis demonstrated that the use of biologic mesh more than doubled the direct cost of ventral hernia repair using synthetic mesh, converting a marginally profitable procedure into a significant financial loss.[31] A vast majority of the reviews and primary articles having not paid special attention to cost does not lessen its importance. Specific cost data are not always obtainable because of hospital-manufacturer contracts, but it is undeniable that on average, the price for biologic mesh material is significantly more than for standard mesh.[31] Considering the economic strains that the health care field is currently experiencing, along with the cumulative weakness of the available data on biologic meshes, a rigorous and prospective cost analysis should be undertaken if they are to remain in use. Accordingly, 2 FDA-supported randomized controlled trials are currently underway to compare the use of biologic versus synthetic prosthetics for repair of complex ventral hernias in the setting of wound contamination. Study outcome variables include hernia recurrence and relative costs of treatment.

SUMMARY

Analysis of the current data highlights several important issues that surgeons should consider when evaluating the use of biologic mesh for incisional hernia repair:

- The cumulative data regarding biologic mesh use on ventral hernias under contaminated conditions do not support the claim that they are better than synthetic mesh used under the same conditions.
- The highly promoted and frequently discussed practice of placing biologic mesh in contaminated surgical fields is being done outside of the products' original intended use and, in some instances, equates to off-label use of a medical device.
- Biologic mesh use, even in noncontaminated conditions, is questionable when the reported results are viewed in light of the high costs.

After evaluation of the available clinical data, including significant wound complications, a noteworthy failure rate at 1 year, and high product costs, it is difficult to support the continued use of biologic meshes in incisional hernia repair outside of well-designed and rigorously conducted clinical trials. Alternatively, a strong and reasonable argument can be made for creating an industry-sponsored, publicly available registry of biologic prosthetic use for ventral hernia repairs. This straightforward mandate, if properly constructed and implemented, would significantly expand knowledge regarding how these intriguing biomaterials are used and their overall clinical efficacy.[7,9]

REFERENCES

1. Luijendijk RW, Hop WC, van den Tol MP, et al. A comparison of suture repair with mesh repair for incisional hernia. N Engl J Med 2000;343(6):392–8.
2. Smart NJ, Marshall M, Daniels IR. Biological meshes: a review of their use in abdominal wall hernia repairs. Surgeon 2012;10(3):159–71.
3. Liang HC, Chang Y, Hsu CK, et al. Effects of crosslinking degree of an acellular biological tissue on its tissue regeneration pattern. Biomaterials 2004;25(17): 3541–52.

4. 510(k) Premarket notification K070560. Available at: http://www.accessdata.fda. gov/cdrh_docs/pdf7/K070560.pdf.
5. Bachman S, Ramshaw B. Prosthetic material in ventral hernia repair: how do I choose? Surg Clin North Am 2008;88(1):101–12, ix.
6. Beale EW, Hoxworth RE, Livingston EH, et al. The role of biologic mesh in abdominal wall reconstruction: a systematic review of the current literature. Am J Surg 2012;204(4):510–7.
7. Bellows CF, Smith A, Malsbury J, et al. Repair of incisional hernias with biological prosthesis: a systematic review of current evidence. Am J Surg 2013;205(1):85–101.
8. Gray SH, Hawn MT, Itani KM. Surgical progress in inguinal and ventral incisional hernia repair. Surg Clin North Am 2008;88(1):17–26, vii.
9. Primus FE, Harris HW. A critical review of biologic mesh use in ventral hernia repairs under contaminated conditions. Hernia 2013;17(1):21–30.
10. Shankaran V, Weber DJ, Reed RL 2nd, et al. A review of available prosthetics for ventral hernia repair. Ann Surg 2011;253(1):16–26.
11. Petrisor B, Bhandari M. The hierarchy of evidence: levels and grades of recommendation. Indian J Orthop 2007;41(1):11–5.
12. Rosenberg W, Donald A. Evidence based medicine: an approach to clinical problem-solving. BMJ 1995;310(6987):1122–6.
13. Sackett DL, Rosenberg WM, Gray JA, et al. Evidence based medicine: what it is and what it isn't. BMJ 1996;312(7023):71–2.
14. The Oxford 2011 levels of evidence. Available at: http://www.cebm.net/index. aspx?o=5653.
15. Blatnik J, Jin J, Rosen M. Abdominal hernia repair with bridging acellular dermal matrix—an expensive hernia sac. Am J Surg 2008;196(1):47–50.
16. Candage R, Jones K, Luchette FA, et al. Use of human acellular dermal matrix for hernia repair: friend or foe? Surgery 2008;144(4):703–9 [discussion: 709–11].
17. Janis JE, Nahabedian MY. Acellular dermal matrices in surgery. Plast Reconstr Surg 2012;130(5 Suppl 2):7S–8S.
18. Patel KM, Bhanot P. Complications of acellular dermal matrices in abdominal wall reconstruction. Plast Reconstr Surg 2012;130(5 Suppl 2):216S–24S.
19. Flum DR, Horvath K, Koepsell T. Have outcomes of incisional hernia repair improved with time? A population-based analysis. Ann Surg 2003;237(1):129–35.
20. Sanders DL, Kingsnorth AN. The modern management of incisional hernias. BMJ 2012;344:e2843.
21. Itani KM, Rosen M, Vargo D, et al. Prospective study of single-stage repair of contaminated hernias using a biologic porcine tissue matrix: the RICH Study. Surgery 2012;152(3):498–505.
22. Bellows CF, Albo D, Berger DH, et al. Abdominal wall repair using human acellular dermis. Am J Surg 2007;194(2):192–8.
23. Diaz JJ Jr, Conquest AM, Ferzoco SJ, et al. Multi-institutional experience using human acellular dermal matrix for ventral hernia repair in a compromised surgical field. Arch Surg 2009;144(3):209–15.
24. Diaz JJ Jr, Guy J, Berkes MB, et al. Acellular dermal allograft for ventral hernia repair in the compromised surgical field. Am Surg 2006;72(12):1181–7 [discussion: 1187–8].
25. Helton WS, Fisichella PM, Berger R, et al. Short-term outcomes with small intestinal submucosa for ventral abdominal hernia. Arch Surg 2005;140(6):549–60 [discussion: 560–2].
26. Kim H, Bruen K, Vargo D. Acellular dermal matrix in the management of high-risk abdominal wall defects. Am J Surg 2006;192(6):705–9.

27. Parker DM, Armstrong PJ, Frizzi JD, et al. Porcine dermal collagen (Permacol) for abdominal wall reconstruction. Curr Surg 2006;63(4):255–8.
28. Patton JH Jr, Berry S, Kralovich KA. Use of human acellular dermal matrix in complex and contaminated abdominal wall reconstructions. Am J Surg 2007;193(3): 360–3 [discussion: 363].
29. Harth KC, Krpata DM, Chawla A, et al. Biologic mesh use practice patterns in abdominal wall reconstruction: a lack of consensus among surgeons. Hernia 2013;17(1):13–20.
30. Ventral Hernia Working Group, Breuing K, Butler CE, et al. Incisional ventral hernias: review of the literature and recommendations regarding the grading and technique of repair. Surgery 2010;148(3):544–58.
31. Reynolds D, Davenport DL, Korosec RL, et al. Financial implications of ventral hernia repair: a hospital cost analysis. J Gastrointest Surg 2013;17(1):159–67.

Safety of Prosthetic Mesh Hernia Repair in Contaminated Fields

Alfredo M. Carbonell, DO*, William S. Cobb, MD

KEYWORDS

- Prosthetic • Synthetic • Biological • Mesh • Hernia • Repair

KEY POINTS

- Several investigators have shown the acceptably low morbidity associated with the use of heavyweight polypropylene mesh in clean-contaminated and contaminated fields.
- The development of lightweight polypropylene mesh constructs has provided surgeons with a less dense mesh containing significantly decreased surface area and wide pores. These newer meshes may act more favorably in contaminated fields.
- The surgical dictum that permanent synthetic mesh is contraindicated in clean-contaminated and contaminated fields is unfounded, as an overwhelming amount of literature currently supports the use of prosthetic mesh in contaminated fields in a myriad of clinical scenarios, from the trauma open abdomen, to fascial dehiscence, incisional and parastomal hernia prophylaxis, emergent strangulated hernias, and elective procedures with breaching of the gastrointestinal tract.

INTRODUCTION

The management of a hernia or loss of abdominal wall substance in the presence of contamination has changed considerably. Historically, this has ranged from simple skin closure, to primary suture repair, myofascial release, laparostomy technique with eventual skin graft, synthetic mesh, absorbable mesh, and most recently biological mesh. For years, surgical dictum has posited that permanent synthetic mesh is contraindicated in the repair of a hernia in a contaminated field. The origin of this belief likely arose from the scattered reports of mesh extrusion through the skin, enteric fistula complications, and chronic draining sinuses that occurred when heavyweight polypropylene mesh was being used for the closure of the infected open abdomen with loss of abdominal wall substance. At the time, the mesh was allowed to granulate through and later epithelialize or undergo a skin graft. Despite these reports, several investigators have shown the acceptably low morbidity associated with the use of

Disclosures: The authors have nothing to disclose.
Division of Minimal Access and Bariatric Surgery, Department of Surgery, Hernia Center, Greenville Health System, University of South Carolina School of Medicine – Greenville, 701 Grove Road, Greenville, SC 29605, USA
* Corresponding author.
E-mail address: acarbonell@ghs.org

Surg Clin N Am 93 (2013) 1227–1239
http://dx.doi.org/10.1016/j.suc.2013.06.012
0039-6109/13/$ – see front matter © 2013 Elsevier Inc. All rights reserved.

surgical.theclinics.com

heavyweight polypropylene mesh in clean-contaminated and contaminated fields. Recently, the development of lightweight polypropylene mesh constructs has provided surgeons with a less dense mesh, containing significantly decreased surface area and wide pores. The experience with using these more modern mesh constructs in contaminated fields has grown considerably. This article reviews the use of prosthetic mesh in contaminated fields from its first description to the present and in many clinical scenarios. The time has now come to critically reevaluate the unfounded fear of using permanent mesh in contaminated fields.

EARLY EXPERIENCE

Polypropylene mesh was developed in the 1950s by Dr Francis Usher for the purposes of reinforcement during inguinal and incisional hernia repairs.[1] Citing the growing experience with polypropylene mesh, and the fact that despite infection, the mesh rarely required removal, Schmitt and Grinnan[2] reported the seminal series of polypropylene mesh for bridging large, contaminated abdominal wall defects caused by military blast injuries during the Vietnam war. They reported their outcomes in 3 patients in whom the mesh was placed as a sublay with the skin left open. After daily wet to dry dressing changes to the wound, the mesh became granulated, and when the granulation bed was adequate, a split-thickness skin graft was placed. The investigators identified multifilament braided sutures, such as silk and polyester, as well as crumpled or folded-over mesh, as the cause of all of their local wound complications. As a result, they stressed the importance of using monofilament suture for mesh fixation, and gave painstaking detail to how the mesh is placed to ensure that it lies flat without any buckling.

This war-time practice spread to the civilian trauma arena, in which Mathes and Stone[3] first reported their management of 11 trauma victims with contaminated loss of abdominal wall substance, in which polypropylene mesh was used as a bridged closure of the devastated abdominal wall and, subsequently, allowed to granulate. The granulation bed was either covered with a skin graft or an adjacent skin flap was mobilized for coverage. In follow-up, these investigators noted that only 3 (27%) patients required partial mesh excision because of infection. Similarly, Gilsdorf and Shea[4] published their outcomes in 6 patients with septic fascial wound dehiscence in which polypropylene mesh was placed as a sublay with full-thickness, transabdominal, braided, polyester suture fixation. No patients developed fistulas, and in only 1 patient did "any of the mesh extrude and then not as an infected foreign body but as an irritating protrusion", which again indicates the importance of ensuring that the mesh is placed flat and in a taut position. Boyd[5] subsequently reported his success in 8 patients with infected abdominal wall loss from infection and electrical injury managed with polypropylene mesh bridging. He described placing the mesh in a sublay position, using polypropylene suture placed through the folded edge of the mesh with the free edge on top. The sutures are placed perpendicular to the wound edge, taking smaller bites through the mesh than through the abdominal wall, so as to prevent the mesh from gathering up. Despite several other similar case reports, the existing experience at the time failed to mention any of the significant long-term outcomes of these techniques.

It was not until Voyles and colleagues[6] published their 5-year experience with polypropylene mesh in heavily contaminated emergency abdominal wall reconstructions that surgeons began to understand more about the sequelae of synthetic mesh in these scenarios. They operated on 31 patients, 25 with necrotizing fascial tissue infections (often with accompanying intra-abdominal sepsis), 3 shotgun blasts, and

3 patients with massive bowel distention precluding fascial closure. All patients had severe wound contamination at the time of surgery, classified as dirty wounds. All mesh was placed in the sublay position with omentum interposed below, and the mesh fixated with either interrupted or running sutures. There were 7 early deaths, leaving 24 patients who were followed until death or complete wound stabilization. Six patients had their mesh removed and the fascia closed primarily. Six patients had the mesh left in situ and allowed to granulate and epithelialize. Of these patients, 1 developed enteric fistula and 5 a mesh extrusion. Nine other patients had a split-thickness skin graft placed over the mesh/granulation bed with 3 developing fistulae, and all 9, a mesh extrusion. The technique was changed in the last 3 patients, in whom the mesh/granulation bed was covered with mobilization of an adjacent flap of skin and fat. These 3 wounds healed without fistula or extrusion.

Adding to the literature, Stone and colleagues[7] published a 20-year experience with acute full-thickness losses of the abdominal wall. Over this period, 124 patients underwent polypropylene mesh bridge closure of large abdominal wall defects in severely contaminated scenarios. There was a 30% wound morbidity and only a 5% incidence of enteric fistula. Reporting for the first time in the literature, these investigators found differences between the mesh types used. Marlex (Bard Davol, Cranston, RI) had twice the incidence of postoperative wound sepsis, 6 times as many associated bowel fistulas, and less than one-third as many successful skin graft takes for cover. On the other hand, Prolene (Ethicon, Bridgewater, NJ) was retained permanently once skin closure had been obtained in one-third of the patients in whom that had been planned, whereas Marlex required removal in almost all in whom it had been inserted. In addition, ease of removal, subjectively, was significantly better with the more pliable and smooth Prolene. The astute clinical observations of Stone and colleagues in this immense series highlighted the difficulty in managing these patients with devastated abdominal walls. Considering the clinical scenarios, the available mesh constructs, and the techniques of the time, they had respectable clinical outcomes.

The existing data regarding the use of polypropylene mesh in contaminated fields through the mid-1980s was essentially limited to placing heavyweight, dense polypropylene mesh in severely contaminated wounds with little control of bacterial burden, on an emergent and semiemergent basis. In addition, the mesh was used as a bridge with exposed viscera below, and a massive skin wound, which was left open. Either the mesh underwent planned removal or was left in situ to granulate, with a planned subsequent skin graft, or was allowed to epithelialize. Most of the mesh extrusions occurred in patients in whom the mesh/granulation bed was allowed to epithelialize or in those who underwent split-thickness skin grafting. The take-home points were that the mesh should either be removed, and the abdominal wall reconstructed, or a thick pedicled flap of skin and fat be mobilized for mesh coverage.

MIDTERM EXPERIENCE

It seemed that polypropylene mesh closure of dirty wounds was generally well accepted. In 1986, Dayton and colleagues[8] reported their 8-patient case series using an absorbable, woven, polyglycolic acid mesh, Dexon (Covidien, Mansfield, MA), for the reconstruction of contaminated abdominal wall defects. Although this was an innovative and novel concept at the time, using an absorbable mesh, the discussion section of the article made a damaging argument against polypropylene mesh in contaminated fields. The investigators mention that review of the current, polypropylene mesh series of the time showed that 50% to 90% of patients required removal of the mesh at some time in the postoperative period. This, we believe, was a misinterpretation of the literature at the time. The polypropylene mesh bridge was a temporizing measure for some patients, in that many patients had planned mesh removal with primary fascial closure once the abdominal wall sepsis had cleared. Of those in whom the mesh was left in situ, it was understood that skin grafting or epithelialization was associated with mesh extrusion, so those techniques were abandoned in favor of flap closure. Thus, to say that 90% of the mesh was removed is not completely accurate, because it implies removal as a result of complications. Nevertheless, the seed of doubt was planted.

Detailed wound management was elucidated by Fansler and colleagues[9] when they discussed their outcomes in 26 critically ill patients undergoing polypropylene mesh closure of a contaminated abdominal wall. These investigators reported no fistulas in patients in whom the mesh was either excised or left in situ and covered by a flap. When a skin graft was placed, they had a 50% rate of enteric fistula, and when allowed to epithelialize, a 40% rate. In a series of 70 patients, Brandt and colleagues[10] showed that when omentum was placed between the bowel and the mesh, a fistula could be completely avoided versus a rate of 26% when there was no omentum interposed. In addition, complications of mesh extrusion and hernia occurred less often when flap coverage of the mesh was used as opposed to skin graft or epithelialization (5% vs 52%, $P<.01$). These data were strikingly similar to what Stone[7] and Voyles[6] had described 10 years earlier. We thus continue to see the importance of well-vascularized coverage of the mesh-granulation bed as the most important predictor of wound healing and the sole factor that helps avoid fistula formation. The repeated dressing changes abrading the bowel granulation through the mesh or the chronic exposure to the air with desiccation likely explains the increased risk of fistula formation when the mesh/granulation bed is not protected.

PROSTHETIC HERNIA REPAIR IN ELECTIVE CONTAMINATED SETTINGS

Although many surgeons were using polypropylene mesh in an effort to bridge the abdominal wall of patients with devastating dirty wounds and open abdomens at the time, perhaps it was believed that these were worst-case scenarios, and despite some potential mesh morbidity, the benefits of mesh use outweighed the risks. However, the same argument did not hold true for elective surgery. For example, when presented with a patient with midline incisional and parastomal hernia after a Hartmann procedure who was undergoing restoration of intestinal continuity, surgeons were unwilling to use synthetic mesh for the fear of potential mesh complications. Although mesh extrusion, draining sinuses, and enterocutaneous fistulae were understood potential complications when using mesh in dirty wounds, there had never been any evidence to suggest that mesh was contraindicated in clean-contaminated or contaminated fields during elective surgery. In the case mentioned earlier, most surgeons would restore intestinal continuity and perform a primary suture repair of the parastomal and incisional hernia defects. The landmark Dutch trial showing the superiority of mesh repair over primary suture repair for incisional hernia was not published until 2000 and the long-term results were not published until 2004.[11,12] Essentially, surgeons were still preferentially performing suture repair of even large incisional hernias. Add to this the fear of potential mesh infection in contaminated fields, and it is no coincidence that it took decades to see any change in clinical practice.

The first description in the American literature of using mesh in elective clean-contaminated and contaminated cases was published by McLanahan and colleagues,[13] who reported a 106-patient case series of retromuscular incisional hernia repairs, 9 of whom had hernias repaired in clean-contaminated and contaminated fields. The wound morbidity for the entire series was 18%, and no patients required mesh removal in long-term follow-up. Despite some favorable results in this small series, the concept never gained traction in the United States, and surgeons still perpetuated the fear of using mesh in potentially contaminated fields.

Despite the reluctance of most surgeons in the United States to use mesh in potentially contaminated fields, European surgeons, on the other hand, saw things differently. Vix and colleagues[14] from France reported on 47 cases of open retromuscular incisional hernia repairs with braided polyester mesh in a "potentially septic" field (clean-contaminated and contaminated wounds), compared with an equal case-matched control of incisional hernia repair in clean wounds. These investigators found no statistical difference in abdominal wall infection, intestinal fistula, or mesh infection between the 2 groups. One prosthesis was removed in the contaminated group at the time of reoperation for an anastomotic leak, and thus was not a mesh-related complication. Subsequently, in 2000, Birolini and colleagues[15] published their series of 20 patients undergoing elective colorectal surgery and concomitant hernia repair. The case mix comprised restoration of intestinal continuity after enterostoma (75%) and colectomy with primary anastomosis (25%). The hernia repairs were performed by primary midline fascial reapproximation with a running absorbable suture, accompanied by subcutaneous dissection and anterior rectus sheath relaxing incisions if needed. Different from the retromuscular repair popularized in France, Birolini and colleagues,[15] from Brazil, used polypropylene mesh placed as an onlay and sutured to the abdominal wall using absorbable sutures. With 2-year follow-up in all patients, these investigators reported 1 superficial skin infection, 1 deep wound infection, and 1 patient with a draining sinus, which healed after partial excision of a small area of unincorporated mesh.

Despite American surgical dictum stating the contrary, Kelly and Behrman,[16] in 2002, reported their experience with 24 cases of preperitoneal inguinal, retromuscular incisional, and intraperitoneal parastomal hernia repairs with polypropylene mesh in clean-contaminated and contaminated fields. They had an 18% wound morbidity rate and no mesh removals after an average of 6 months to 3 years follow-up. Similarly, Geisler and colleagues[17] published 30 patients undergoing elective colorectal surgery and incisional or parastomal hernia repair with polypropylene mesh placed as an onlay or sublay. The series reported a 7% wound morbidity, with only 1 mesh removal because of bowel erosion after keyhole parastomal hernia repair.

Over the next several years, other investigators continued to share their successful experience with synthetic mesh in contaminated fields.[18–23]

A unique report was published by Scholtes and colleagues.[24] This was an insightful look at their 8-year experience managing 114 patients with fascial dehiscence and open abdomen classified as either contaminated or dirty. Composite monofilament polyester mesh, composite multifilament polyester mesh, and a composite polyvinylidine fluoride-polypropylene was used in the intraperitoneal position in 51 patients, and no mesh was used in 63 patients. The only difference was a lower incidence of incisional hernia formation, long-term, when mesh was used. Wound complications were not reported, but the enteric fistula rate was 10% to 17%, although this was unrelated to mesh use.

EMERGENT PROSTHETIC REPAIR OF ACUTELY STRANGULATED HERNIAS

One recurring question that arises during the American certifying examination for surgeons is how to handle the acutely strangulated inguinal or incisional hernia requiring bowel resection. Despite evidence to the contrary, the safe answer remains to address the nonviable bowel and repair the hernia primarily with suture, avoiding the use of a prosthetic. In this section, the current data showing the safety of prosthetic repair in these scenarios are reviewed.

Nieuwenhuizen and colleagues,[25] reported the outcomes of inguinal and ventral hernias operated on for acute incarceration and strangulation, in which 99 had mesh placed and 103 underwent primary suture repair. These investigators found wound infection rates of 7% with mesh and 18% without mesh, and multivariate analysis pointed to bowel resection as a significant risk factor for wound infection. Despite the higher rate of wound infection in patients with bowel resection, no mesh was ever removed. In 60 cases of acutely incarcerated incisional hernias with bowel obstruction repaired with onlay polypropylene mesh, Zafar and colleagues[26] noted a 38% wound complication rate when a bowel resection was performed versus 28% without bowel resection. Despite slightly higher infections with bowel resection, no mesh required removal, even in 5 patients who developed deep infections. On the other hand, Abd-Ellatif and colleagues[27] used polypropylene mesh onlay repair for incisional hernias, Lichtenstein repairs for inguinal hernias, and open anterior preperitoneal repairs for femoral hernias in a large group of patients presenting with emergent hernia strangulation. Their group experienced a low rate of wound infections between the patients with and without bowel resection (3% vs 5%, $P = .6$).

The theme remains the same throughout other series of strangulated inguinal hernias repaired with polypropylene mesh and also requiring bowel resection. Although the wound complication rate may be increased with bowel resection, the mesh never required removal.[28,29] Bessa and Abdel-Razek[30] analyzed the combined results of prosthetic mesh repair in cases of strangulated inguinal and incisional hernias available in the literature. Combined analysis of 572 patients revealed that bowel resection was required in 14.7% of cases, with a wound infection rate of 4%, seroma rate of 3.8%, and mesh infection in 1 patient (0.2%). Thus, the data support the safety of prosthetic mesh for the repair of hernias that present strangulated, requiring bowel resection.

PROSTHETIC INCISIONAL HERNIA PROPHYLAXIS

Incisional hernias are not uncommon after laparotomy and many well-known risk factors for incisional hernia have been shown. Interesting work has been carried out in the area of attempting to prevent hernias from forming by placing mesh at the index laparotomy. Investigators have looked at obese patients undergoing open bariatric surgery in an attempt to see whether hernia prophylaxis is safe and effective in this clean-contaminated surgery. In the only randomized controlled trial of mesh versus suture closure in this bariatric population, Strzelczyk and colleagues[31] placed polypropylene mesh in the retromuscular position in patients undergoing roux-en-Y gastric bypass. These investigators found a significant reduction in incisional hernia (0% vs 21%) and no difference in wound morbidity with the prophylactic placement of mesh. Similarly, Curro and colleagues,[32] in a group of patients undergoing biliopancreatic diversion, reported reduced rates of incisional hernia with prophylactic mesh placed retromuscularly (4% vs 32%, $P = .009$), and 1 surgical site infection (SSI) in each group, with no mesh infections. Despite being a clean-contaminated case with entry into the gastrointestinal tract, the use of mesh at the time of open bariatric surgery seems to be safe.

PROSTHETIC PARASTOMAL HERNIA PROPHYLAXIS

Parastomal hernia is a well-recognized consequence of stoma creation. Although various techniques exist for repair, one of the latest concepts has been prevention of parastomal hernia by placing mesh at the index stoma creation. Stoma creation is at minimum a clean-contaminated field, and placing mesh around the bowel has the potential implication of mesh/bowel erosion. The first report of parastomal hernia prevention was a retrospective study of 36 patients who had heavyweight polypropylene mesh that was placed as an onlay on the anterior rectus sheath. The bowel was subsequently brought up through a central 20-mm cut in the mesh and the ostomy matured. Although no mean follow-up period was stated, some patients were reported to have been followed for 48 months, with only 1 patient suffering ostomy stenosis, and a second, a suture granuloma. There were no infectious complications, mesh removals, or erosions.[33] It was 10 years until the next prospective trials using prophylactic placement of mesh in an onlay,[34] sublay,[35] and intraperitoneal[36] position. In long-term follow-up, parastomal hernia rates were reported of 8.3%, 9.5%, and 0%, respectively. There were no infections or stenoses, but 1 patient in the sublay study developed early stoma necrosis, requiring stoma revision; however, the mesh was left undisturbed.[35]

Two randomized controlled trials examined the use of lightweight polypropylene mesh in the sublay position versus no mesh. Jänes and colleagues[37] reported a dramatic reduction in parastomal hernia rate with mesh (12.3% vs 81%) with no infections, necrosis, or stenosis, whereas Serra-Aracil and colleagues[38] reported a parastomal hernia rate of 22% with mesh versus 44% without. These investigators reported 1 infection in each group, 1 necrosis in each group, and 1 stenosis in the mesh group. Even more impressive was a consecutive series of prophylactic mesh placement in 73 patients presented by Jänes and colleagues,[39] in which 55 of the cases were contaminated, with a 5% wound infection rate, and 18 were dirty cases, with a 16% infection rate. Despite the series including patients undergoing a Hartmann procedure with fecal and purulent peritonitis, no mesh-related complications were reported and it was thus concluded that "in routine surgery a stoma can be created with a prophylactic mesh in most patients and does not increase the rate of complications. A prophylactic mesh can be used in severely contaminated wounds."

RETROSPECTIVE DATABASE OUTCOMES

Despite multiple series showing the safety and efficacy of using synthetic mesh in clean-contaminated and contaminated fields, there have been 2 retrospective database studies which have severely impaired the progress of this clinical practice, in the United States in particular.

Xourafas and colleagues[40] performed a 15-year retrospective review of incisional hernia repairs in clean-contaminated and contaminated fields performed with mesh in 51 and without mesh in 126 patients. These investigators reported a significantly higher wound infection rate (22% vs 5%, $P = .001$), other complication rate (24% vs 8%, $P = .009$), and reoperation rate (27% vs 10%, $P = .004$) with mesh versus without. In addition, they found no difference in recurrence (22% vs 24%, $P = .85$). Thus, the investigators recommended "caution in using mesh when performing a ventral hernia repair with a simultaneous bowel resection because of the significantly higher risk of complications and reoperations." It is difficult to draw any real conclusions from this study, because of its retrospective nature, in that the choice of using mesh or not was clearly variable and cases were performed by 23 surgeons over a 15-year period. There was also a significant difference in mesh use versus not, based on defect size. The investigators categorized the defects into 2 groups: 1 to 3 cm and greater than 3 cm. The largest and most difficult hernia defects received mesh, and thus, this may account for the increased infectious complications with mesh. One could argue there was little or no standardization in mesh choice or surgical technique. The mesh data point included both permanent synthetic mesh of different varieties grouped with absorbable and biologic meshes. These are mesh types that we now know all act differently from an infectious as well as hernia recurrence standpoint. The investigators then draw the conclusion that the infectious risks being higher with mesh and the recurrence rate being no different shows no advantage to using mesh, when the recurrence rate in the no-mesh group is 24%. This figure is lower than the known 63% rate of hernia recurrence with suture alone in the iconic Dutch randomized controlled trial comparing mesh with suture repair of hernias.[12] Despite the negative connotation that mesh received in this study for the higher associated infectious risk, there were only 7 mesh removals because of deep infection, and it is not known which type, where they had been placed, or the circumstances surrounding their removal.

A second, misleading study used the National Surgical Quality Improvement Program database to look at 33,832 patients who underwent mesh repair of incisional hernias from 2005 to 2010. The study also analyzed a concurrent group of patients with nonmesh hernia repair. Clean mesh repairs totaled 29,931, clean-contaminated mesh repairs, 3879, and contaminated mesh repairs, 22. Compared with ventral hernia repairs with mesh in a clean field, procedures performed in a clean-contaminated and contaminated field had a 2.53 and 3.84 times higher odds of developing a superficial SSI, respectively. The use of mesh in a clean-contaminated field also showed a higher odds ratio of having at least 1 postoperative complication than in repairs without mesh (3.56 vs 2.52). The effect of mesh on postoperative complications in contaminated fields could not be definitively assessed because of a small sample population in the mesh group ($P = .875$). The investigators concluded that there is significant risk associated with mesh use in a field with any level of contamination, and "thus discourage the use of mesh in ventral hernia repairs in clean-contaminated and contaminated fields." This conclusion is incriminating to the use of mesh in any level of contamination, and it will take years to undo the damage that this study has done to the known safety in using prosthetics in contaminated fields. The principal study flaw is that it fails to identify which types of mesh were used to repair these hernias. It is unlikely that most of the mesh used during the study period was prosthetic, because it has been common practice to use biological mesh in contaminated scenarios in the United States since before 2005, which is when the study began its data query. It has been well shown that biological mesh incisional hernia repair in clean-contaminated and contaminated fields is associated with wound complication rates of 41.7% to 66%.[41,42] Thus, the infectious complications may be overinflated because of the mesh type, but is impossible to tell, because the mesh implant procedure code contained within the database does not differentiate between prosthetic, biological, or absorbable mesh. In addition, the main study finding was the increased rate of SSI as the level of contamination in the wound increased. Of course, this finding stands to reason. It is not an effect of the mesh but rather a function of the bacterial burden of the wound. When the data are analyzed closer, there seems to be little difference in SSI between the mesh and nonmesh groups for every level of contamination: superficial SSI, clean 2.7 versus 3.0%; clean contaminated 6.6% versus 5.0%; contaminated 9.1% versus 10%, respectively. The deep SSI rates were: clean, 1.0% versus 1.0%; clean-contaminated, 3.0 versus 2.3; and contaminated, 4.5% versus 5.1%, respectively. The study analyzed a large group of patients undergoing hernia repair in different wound classes. The only conclusion that can be drawn from the study is that wound infections increase as the level of contamination increases.

THE MODERN ERA AND LIGHTWEIGHT MESH

The advent of lightweight polypropylene mesh, which contains wide pores and less dense fibers, has revolutionized hernia repair. Not only has it been associated with less postoperative pain, increased patient satisfaction, and improved abdominal wall physiology and compliance, it is likely the most ideal mesh to resist infection.[43–51]

The ideal mesh to resist infection should contain the least surface area possible for bacterial adherence. Multifilament and laminar mesh constructs have increased surface area for bacterial attachment, and are not preferable for contaminated field use. Blatnik and colleagues[51] tested the rate of bacterial clearance of several mesh constructs in a live rat model. Monofilament, unprotected polypropylene and polyester mesh cleared a larger proportion of methicillin-resistant *Staphylococcus aureus* compared with other multifilament mesh constructs and composite meshes with an antiadhesive barrier. As the level of contamination increased, there was a proportional decrease in bacterial clearance.

The concept that decreased mesh surface area is beneficial also applies to large mesh pore size. As pore size increases, so does the area for increased cellular response and tissue ingrowth. A fast and close incorporation of the mesh by the host tissue decreases the chance for bacteria to adhere on the biomaterial surface and thus decreases infection rates.[52] Díaz-Godoy and colleagues[50] compared different polypropylene meshes of medium (0.8 mm), large (1.5 mm), and very large (3.6 mm) pore width. In a rabbit appendiceal puncture-aspiration model, the retromuscular space was developed for mesh placement, and the abdominal cavity, mesh, and subcutaneous tissue were inoculated with the fecal aspirate. None of the rabbits that received very-large-pore mesh developed an SSI, compared with a 30% and 33% rate of infection in the medium-pore and large-pore mesh groups, respectively.

These animal data fully support what surgeons are seeing clinically with the use of lightweight polypropylene mesh, particularly in contaminated fields. Despite gross purulent contamination and mesh-wound exposure to the atmosphere, lightweight, wide-pore mesh granulates over quickly and heals in the most compromised situations. Berrevoet and colleagues[53] published their results with the management of 63 patients who developed deep SSIs involving mesh located retromuscularly in 54 patients and intraperitoneally in 9. Affected mesh types were wide-pore polypropylene mesh (n = 60) and multifilament polyester mesh (n = 3). All patients were treated with negative-pressure wound therapy, and the mean time to complete wound closure was 19 days for umbilical wounds, 34 days for midline incisional wounds, and 62 days for wounds with mesh located intraperitoneally. All 3 infected multifilament polyester meshes required complete or partial removal for complete wound healing, whereas every polypropylene mesh was salvaged complete. Others have found similar results.[54] This finding again emphasizes the importance of decreased surface area for decreased bacterial attachment and rapid and increased tissue incorporation.

We are publishing the largest series in the literature describing our experience with the retromuscular placement of lightweight, wide-pore polypropylene mesh in clean-contaminated and contaminated field hernia repair. A total of 100 patients with a mean body mass index of 32 ± 9.3 kg/m^2 met inclusion criteria. There were 42 clean-contaminated and 58 contaminated cases. The incidence of surgical site occurrence including seroma, wound breakdown, and SSI was 26.2% in clean-contaminated cases and 34% in contaminated cases. The 30-day SSI rate was 7.1% for clean-contaminated and 19.0% for contaminated cases. There were a total of 7 recurrences, with a mean follow-up of 10.8 ± 9.9 months (range, 1–63). Mesh removal was required in 4 patients: 2 because of early anastomotic leaks, 1 because of stomal disruption and retraction in a morbidly obese patient, and 1 from a long-term enterocutaneous fistula in a patient who had undergone an open, retromuscular parastomal hernia repair.[55] This study represents the largest review of the clinical outcomes for synthetic mesh use in a contaminated setting. Although perhaps not yet considered standard of care in the United States, we have shown favorable infection, recurrence, and mesh removal rates associated with the use of synthetic mesh in contaminated ventral hernia repair, compared with similar cases in which biological meshes were used.[41,42] We believe that the importance of the retromuscular space cannot be overstated. This well-vascularized space helps protect the mesh if there is a wound complication involving the skin or subcutaneous tissue. Although the recommendations regarding the use of biological mesh and synthetic mesh in contaminated fields are evolving, our results challenge the status quo, further corroborating the necessity for a large-scale prospective randomized trial with the goal of providing reasonable practice guidelines. To that end, we are also participating in a prospective randomized controlled trial comparing biological versus synthetic mesh in repair of ventral hernias in contaminated fields (NCT01746316).

One of the scenarios missing from the literature is whether or not an infected prosthesis can be removed from a patient and a subsequent prosthesis placed. We have begun this practice in selected cases in which the tissue bed is favorable for new mesh implant. If we believe that we are compromising the repair to place the new prosthesis, we perform the operation in 2 stages. This rationale does not need to apply only to cases of infected prosthesis removals but rather should be used selectively when it is in the patient's best interest. Each scenario should be tailored to the patient's desires and expected outcomes. By addressing the contaminated scenario first, and deferring the hernia repair until a second operation, the surgeon can subsequently perform a hernia repair in a clean field with an ideal outcome.

SUMMARY

No other area of hernia repair has sparked so much debate and encouraged the zeal that prosthetic use is contraindicated in contamination. However, we have compiled an overwhelming amount of literature from around the world that supports the use of prosthetic mesh in contaminated fields in a myriad of clinical scenarios from the trauma open abdomen, to fascial dehiscence, incisional and parastomal hernia prophylaxis, emergent strangulated hernias, and elective procedures with breaching of the gastrointestinal tract. We believe that the time has come to put to rest the notion that prosthetics should not be used in contaminated fields.

REFERENCES

1. Usher FC, Ochsner J, Tuttle LL. Use of Marlex mesh in the repair of incisional hernias. Am Surg 1958;24:969–74.
2. Schmitt HJ, Grinnan GL. Use of Marlex mesh in infected abdominal war wound. Am J Surg 1967;113:825–8.
3. Mathes SJ, Stone HH. Acute traumatic losses of abdominal wall substance. J Trauma 1975;15:386–91.
4. Gilsdorf RB, Shea MM. Repair of massive septic abdominal wall defects with Marlex mesh. Am J Surg 1975;130:634–8.
5. Boyd WC. Use of Marlex mesh in acute loss of the abdominal wall due to infection. Surg Gynecol Obstet 1977;144:251–2.

6. Voyles CR, Richardson JD, Bland KI, et al. Emergency abdominal wall reconstruction with polypropylene mesh: short-term benefits versus long-term complications. Ann Surg 1981;194:219–23.
7. Stone HH, Fabian TC, Turkleson ML, et al. Management of acute full-thickness losses of the abdominal wall. Ann Surg 1981;193:612–8.
8. Dayton MT, Buchele BA, Shirazi SS, et al. Use of an absorbable mesh to repair contaminated abdominal-wall defects. Arch Surg 1986;121(8):954–60.
9. Fansler RF, Taheri P, Cullinane C, et al. Polypropylene mesh closure of the complicated abdominal wound. Am J Surg 1995;170:15–8.
10. Brandt CP, McHenry CR, Jacobs DG, et al. Polypropylene mesh closure after emergency laparotomy: morbidity and outcome. Surgery 1995;118:736–40 [discussion: 740–1].
11. Luijendijk RW, Hop WC, van den Tol MP, et al. A comparison of suture repair with mesh repair for incisional hernia. N Engl J Med 2000;343:392–8.
12. Burger JWA, Luijendijk RW, Hop WCJ, et al. Long-term follow-up of a randomized controlled trial of suture versus mesh repair of incisional hernia. Ann Surg 2004;240:578–83 [discussion: 583–5].
13. McLanahan D, King LT, Weems C, et al. Retrorectus prosthetic mesh repair of midline abdominal hernia. Am J Surg 1997;173:445–9.
14. Vix J, Meyer C, Rohr S, et al. The treatment of incisional and abdominal hernia with a prosthesis in potentially infected tissues–a case series of 47 cases. Hernia 1997;1:157–61.
15. Birolini C, Utiyama EM, Rodrigues AJ, et al. Elective colonic operation and prosthetic repair of incisional hernia: does contamination contraindicate abdominal wall prosthesis use? J Am Coll Surg 2000;191:366–72.
16. Kelly ME, Behrman SW. The safety and efficacy of prosthetic hernia repair in clean-contaminated and contaminated wounds. Am Surg 2002;68:524–8 [discussion: 528–9].
17. Geisler DJ, Reilly JC, Vaughan SG, et al. Safety and outcome of use of nonabsorbable mesh for repair of fascial defects in the presence of open bowel. Dis Colon Rectum 2003;46:1118–23.
18. Campanelli G, Nicolosi FM, Pettinari D, et al. Prosthetic repair, intestinal resection, and potentially contaminated areas: safe and feasible? Hernia 2004;8:190–2.
19. Stringer RA, Salameh JR. Mesh herniorrhaphy during elective colorectal surgery. Hernia 2005;9:26–8.
20. Antonopoulos IM, Nahas WC, Mazzucchi E, et al. Is polypropylene mesh safe and effective for repairing infected incisional hernia in renal transplant recipients? Urology 2005;66:874–7.
21. Machairas A, Liakakos T, Patapis P, et al. Prosthetic repair of incisional hernia combined with elective bowel operation. Surgeon 2008;6:274–7.
22. El-Gazzaz GH, Farag SH, El-Sayd MA, et al. The use of synthetic mesh in patients undergoing ventral hernia repair during colorectal resection: risk of infection and recurrence. Asian J Surg 2012;35:149–53.
23. Souza JM, Dumanian GA. Routine use of bioprosthetic mesh is not necessary: a retrospective review of 100 consecutive cases of intra-abdominal midweight polypropylene mesh for ventral hernia repair. Surgery 2013;153:393–9.
24. Scholtes M, Kurmann A, Seiler CA, et al. Intraperitoneal mesh implantation for fascial dehiscence and open abdomen. World J Surg 2012;36:1557–61.
25. Nieuwenhuizen J, van Ramshorst GH, Brinke Ten JG, et al. The use of mesh in acute hernia: frequency and outcome in 99 cases. Hernia 2011. http://dx.doi.org/10.1007/s10029-010-0779-4.

26. Zafar H, Zaidi M, Qadir I, et al. Emergency incisional hernia repair: a difficult problem waiting for a solution. Ann Surg Innov Res 2012;6:1.
27. Abd Ellatif ME, Negm A, Elmorsy G, et al. Feasibility of mesh repair for strangulated abdominal wall hernias. Int J Surg 2012;10:153–6.
28. Topcu O, Kurt A, Soylu S, et al. Polypropylene mesh repair of incarcerated and strangulated hernias: a prospective clinical study. Surg Today 2012. http://dx. doi.org/10.1007/s00595-012-0397-0.
29. Sawayama H, Kanemitsu K, Okuma T, et al. Safety of polypropylene mesh for incarcerated groin and obturator hernias: a retrospective study of 110 patients. Hernia 2013. http://dx.doi.org/10.1007/s10029-013-1058-y.
30. Bessa SS, Abdel-Razek AH. Results of prosthetic mesh repair in the emergency management of the acutely incarcerated and/or strangulated ventral hernias: a seven years study. Hernia 2013;17:59–65.
31. Strzelczyk JM, Szymański D, Nowicki ME, et al. Randomized clinical trial of postoperative hernia prophylaxis in open bariatric surgery. Br J Surg 2006;93:1347–50.
32. Currò G, Centorrino T, Musolino C, et al. Incisional hernia prophylaxis in morbidly obese patients undergoing biliopancreatic diversion. Obes Surg 2011;21:1559–63.
33. Bayer I, Kyzer S, Chaimoff C. A new approach to primary strengthening of colostomy with Marlex mesh to prevent paracolostomy hernia. Surg Gynecol Obstet 1986;163:579–80.
34. Gögenur I, Mortensen J, Harvald T, et al. Prevention of parastomal hernia by placement of a polypropylene mesh at the primary operation. Dis Colon Rectum 2006;49:1131–5.
35. Vijayasekar C, Marimuthu K, Jadhav V, et al. Parastomal hernia: is prevention better than cure? Use of preperitoneal polypropylene mesh at the time of stoma formation. Tech Coloproctol 2008;12:309–13.
36. Berger D. Prevention of parastomal hernias by prophylactic use of a specially designed intraperitoneal onlay mesh (Dynamesh IPST). Hernia 2008;12:243–6.
37. Jänes A, Cengiz Y, Israelsson LA. Preventing parastomal hernia with a prosthetic mesh: a 5-year follow-up of a randomized study. World J Surg 2009;33:118–21 [discussion: 122–3].
38. Serra-Aracil X, Bombardo-Junca J, Moreno-Matias J, et al. Randomized, controlled, prospective trial of the use of a mesh to prevent parastomal hernia. Ann Surg 2009;249:583–7.
39. Jänes A, Cengiz Y, Israelsson LA. Experiences with a prophylactic mesh in 93 consecutive ostomies. World J Surg 2010;34:1637–40.
40. Xourafas D, Lipsitz SR, Negro P, et al. Impact of mesh use on morbidity following ventral hernia repair with a simultaneous bowel resection. Arch Surg 2010;145:739–44.
41. Rosen MJ, Krpata DM, Ermlich B, et al. 5-Year clinical experience with single-staged repairs of infected and contaminated abdominal wall defects utilizing biologic mesh. Ann Surg 2013;257:991–6.
42. Itani KMF, Rosen M, Vargo D, et al. Prospective study of single-stage repair of contaminated hernias using a biologic porcine tissue matrix: the RICH Study. Surgery 2012;152:498–505.
43. Cobb WS, Kercher KW, Heniford BT. The argument for lightweight polypropylene mesh in hernia repair. Surg Innov 2005;12:63–9.
44. Cobb WS, Burns JM, Peindl RD, et al. Textile analysis of heavy weight, mid-weight, and light weight polypropylene mesh in a porcine ventral hernia model. J Surg Res 2006;136:1–7.

45. Welty G, Klinge U, Klosterhalfen B, et al. Functional impairment and complaints following incisional hernia repair with different polypropylene meshes. Hernia 2001;5:142–7.
46. Weyhe D, Belyaev O, Müller C, et al. Improving outcomes in hernia repair by the use of light meshes–a comparison of different implant constructions based on a critical appraisal of the literature. World J Surg 2007;31:234–44.
47. Conze J, Kingsnorth AN, Flament JB, et al. Randomized clinical trial comparing lightweight composite mesh with polyester or polypropylene mesh for incisional hernia repair. Br J Surg 2005;92:1488–93.
48. O'Dwyer PJ, Kingsnorth AN, Molloy RG, et al. Randomized clinical trial assessing impact of a lightweight or heavyweight mesh on chronic pain after inguinal hernia repair. Br J Surg 2005;92:166–70.
49. Post S, Weiss B, Willer M, et al. Randomized clinical trial of lightweight composite mesh for Lichtenstein inguinal hernia repair. Br J Surg 2004;91:44–8.
50. Díaz-Godoy A, García-Ureña MÁ, López-Monclús J, et al. Searching for the best polypropylene mesh to be used in bowel contamination. Hernia 2011;15:173–9.
51. Blatnik JA, Krpata DM, Jacobs MR, et al. In vivo analysis of the morphologic characteristics of synthetic mesh to resist MRSA adherence. J Gastrointest Surg 2012;16:2139–44.
52. Merritt K, Shafer JW, Brown SA. Implant site infection rates with porous and dense materials. J Biomed Mater Res 1979;13:101–8.
53. Berrevoet F, Vanlander A, Sainz-Barriga M, et al. Infected large pore meshes may be salvaged by topical negative pressure therapy. Hernia 2013;17:67–73.
54. Meagher H, Clarke Moloney M, Grace PA. Conservative management of mesh-site infection in hernia repair surgery: a case series. Hernia 2013. http://dx.doi.org/10.1007/s10029-013-1069-8.
55. Carbonell AM, Criss CN, Cobb WS, et al. Outcomes of synthetic mesh in contaminated ventral hernia repairs. J Am Coll Surg, in press. http://dx.doi.org/10.1016/j.jamcollsurg.2013.04.039.

Economics of Abdominal Wall Reconstruction

Curtis Bower, MD, J. Scott Roth, MD*

KEYWORDS

- Abdominal wall reconstruction • Hernia • Cost • Economics

KEY POINTS

- More than 348,000 ventral hernia repairs are performed in the United States each year, accounting for at least $3.2 billion in health care.
- Mesh incisional herniorrhaphy is cost-effective compared with suture-based repairs, considering overall societal costs.
- Laparoscopic and open ventral hernia repairs have similar costs.
- The role for prophylactic mesh placement has not been clearly defined but may be beneficial in selected patient populations.
- The use of biological materials in ventral hernia repair is associated with significant financial losses for hospitals during the sentinel admission.

INTRODUCTION

Abdominal wall hernia repairs represent one of the most commonly performed surgical procedures. The volume of ventral hernia repairs escalates annually while recurrence rates have remained unchanged. At the same time, the incidence of new ventral hernias occurring following laparotomy remains as high as 20%, resulting in newly created hernias yearly. As a result of increased life expectancy, increases in the United States population, and the frequency of abdominal operations, the overall costs of ventral hernia repairs can be expected to continue to increase. Overall societal costs include the costs to employers, third-party payers, patients, and hospitals. The costs become even more staggering considering the lost productivity as a result of extended absences from employment related to the treatment of hernias and subsequent complications.

Funding Sources: Dr Bower, none to report; Dr Roth, CR Bard, Ethicon EndoSurgery, Covidien.
Conflict of Interest: Dr Bower, none to report; Dr Roth, Consultant for CR Bard; Board member of the Musculoskeletal Transplant Foundation; on the speaker bureau for Ethicon.
Section of Gastrointestinal & Minimally Invasive Surgery, Division of General Surgery, A. B. Chandler Medical Center, University of Kentucky, 800 Rose Street, UKMC - C224, Lexington, KY 40536-0298, USA
* Corresponding author.
E-mail address: s.roth@uky.edu

Significant research has been performed in the areas of hernia outcomes addressing questions of technique, biomaterials, and outcomes. However, studies evaluating the costs of hernia repairs, both direct and indirect, are lacking. In the changing economic environment, the delivery of health care must not only be of high quality but must also be cost-efficient. A thorough appreciation of costs and revenues is essential to the delivery of efficient health care.

SCOPE OF THE PROBLEM

Estimating the incidence of ventral and incisional hernias performed annually is a significant challenge, even before estimating the associated costs. Some investigators have estimated the number of hernias based on the annual number of laparotomies performed (in itself a difficult number to pinpoint) multiplied by published rates of incisional hernia formation.[1] Certainly this is one way to approximate the numbers and show significance; however, from a health policy standpoint, the error involved in such estimations is staggering, resulting in either underestimation or overestimation.

In 2003, Rutkow[2] attempted to quantify the numbers of hernia repairs in the United States and estimated the costs of hernia repair (including groin hernias) to be approximately $2.5 billion annually by compiling estimates of the numbers of procedures performed using the 1996 National Hospital Discharge Survey (NHDS) and the National Survey of Ambulatory Surgery (NSAS). Although this represents one of the best attempts to quantify hernia costs, there are significant limitations to this report, including the omission of hernia repairs performed in Veterans Administration (VA) hospitals, the necessity of estimating population growth, and a sampling error of approximately 10%. Based on these assumptions there were 105,000 incisional hernias, 175,000 umbilical hernias, and 80,000 ventral hernias performed annually at that time. During the same year, Flume and colleagues[1] estimated there were 153,000 incisional hernias being created each year, of which approximately one-third would require repair. This wide discrepancy highlights the challenge of accurately estimating the incidence of ventral hernias, which directly affects our ability to appreciate the overall societal costs of this condition.

In 2012, an inquiry into the number of ventral hernias was performed. Poulose and colleagues[3] evaluated data obtained from the 2001-2006 Nationwide Inpatient Sample (NIS) and the 2006 NSAS, and evaluated all abdominal wall hernias excluding inguinofemoral hernias. Owing to the lack of availability of cost data, cost estimation was performed using cost-to-charge ratios. In this report, the annual incidence of abdominal wall hernias was 348,000. To give some perspective, there were 16,662 general surgeons in the United States in 2005. Dividing the number of hernias by the number of general surgeons results in 21 ventral hernia repairs per surgeon per year.[4] From the NIS data, there were 126,548 abdominal ventral hernia repairs in 2001 and 154,278 in 2006: a 22% increase. The annual cost estimate for both inpatient and outpatient ventral hernia repairs was $3.2 billion. Based on these calculations, the authors conclude that each 1% reduction in hernia recurrence would result in a saving of at least $32 million in procedural costs. This figure is likely an underestimation, as this analysis excludes both physician fees and other societal costs, including those related to absence from work. In addition, this study also excluded procedures performed in the VA system, and therefore underestimates the total number of procedures performed.

Estimating the cost of delivering health care is a significant challenge not only in estimating the annual incidence of an individual procedure but also as it relates to the complexity of the health care system. Overall, health care costs include both direct and indirect costs to facilities as well as professional fees. Although direct costs are more obvious (including items such as supplies, equipment, and personnel), indirect costs (including overhead, facility fees, and unreimbursed personnel) represent real costs incurred by hospitals, which must be accounted for. Indirect costs may vary significantly between facilities based on infrastructure and resources. Similarly, direct costs may vary between facilities based on purchasing contracts, resulting in further variability in costs.

Hospital reimbursement for any individual procedure is most commonly based on a prospective payment system using diagnosis-related groups (DRG).[5] In 2013, hospitals receive payments based on a patient's DRG, which is calculated by using a "grouper," which accounts for the patient's age, gender, diagnosis(es), procedures performed, and discharge status. Payments for individual DRGs are based on complications occurring during the hospital stay, with varying payments for patient care based on the presence or absence of complications and comorbidities (CC) or major complications and comorbidities (MCC).

Hernia DRG codes include 353.0 (hernia procedures except inguinal and femoral with MCC), 354.0 (hernia procedures except inguinal and femoral with CC), and 355.0 (hernia procedures except inguinal and femoral without CC and MCC). Hospital reimbursement may vary significantly for an individual hernia repair based on the patient's hospital course according to CCs and MCCs defined by the Center for Medicare and Medicaid Services (CMS).

Reimbursement varies further between facilities based on the case-mix index (CMI). The CMI reflects the average weight of a health care facility's DRG. The higher a facility's CMI, the greater the number of high cost services the facility performs. The more high-cost services that are performed, the more money per patient the facility receives.

Accordingly, this complex system of hospital reimbursement results in significant variability in cost between facilities, based on both patient outcomes and the complexity of care provided at an individual facility. Considering these factors, a tertiary care referral center is more likely than a smaller medical facility to receive higher reimbursement for an individual procedure. However, this added reimbursement may help to defray the added costs associated with delivery of care with a higher degree of medical acuity to patients.

Aside from costs attributable to the medical facility, additional costs of medical care are incurred through professional fees (physician reimbursement). These fees result in separate charges to patients or third-party payers based on current procedural terminology (CPT) codes. Each CPT code describes a unique medical procedure and service. Hernia CPT codes include unique codes for both laparoscopic and open ventral hernia procedures. Payments are provided for professional services based on the respective CPT code documented and charged. Medicare provides payments for services based on relative value units (RVUs) assigned to each CPT code that includes RVUs for physician work, practice expenses, and malpractice expenses **(Table 1)**. Geographic practice cost indices (GPCI) are used as a multiplier to the RVUs to determine the total RVU value for a CPT. GPCIs effectively alter the RVU value for any given CPT code to accurately reflect the cost of providing care in varying regions throughout the United States. The total RVU value for a procedure is multiplied by a conversion factor to determine the physician payment for a CPT code **(Box 1)**. For 2013, the conversion factor was valued at $34.0230.[6]

The future of health care reimbursement in the United States is evolving because of the unsustainable rising overall costs of health care. In an effort to constrain costs, many models for reimbursement are developing and undergoing evaluation. Current

Table 1
Current procedural terminology codes, relative value units, and reimbursement

Procedure	CPT Code	wRVU	mpRVU	peRVU	2012 National Reimbursement (US$)
Initial incisional hernia—reducible	49560	11.92	2.48	7.35	731.47
Initial incisional hernia—incarcerated	49561	15.38	3.24	8.82	922.76
Recurrent incisional hernia—reducible	49565	12.37	2.60	7.72	762.44
Recurrent incisional hernia—incarcerated	49566	15.53	3.29	8.93	933.31
Implantation mesh	49568	4.88	1.03	1.97	266.51
Laparoscopic umbilical hernia—reducible	49652	11.92	7.54	0.83	683.82
Laparoscopic umbilical hernia—incarcerated	49653	14.94	9.34	1.07	854.00
Laparoscopic initial incisional hernia—reducible	49654	13.76	8.30	0.97	776.74
Laparoscopic initial incisional hernia—incarcerated	49655	16.84	10.12	1.19	948.29
Laparoscopic recurrent incisional hernia—reducible	49656	15.08	8.85	1.08	839.71
Laparoscopic recurrent incisional hernia—incarcerated	49657	22.11	12.23	1.57	1205.95

Abbreviations: CPT, current procedural terminology; mpRVU, malpractice RVU; peRVU, practice expense RVU; RVU, relative value units; wRVU, work RVU.

health care payment models reimburse hospitals and physicians based on the volume of care provided rather than the quality of care. Quality metrics are evolving whereby payment may be at least partially reimbursed based on defined patient outcomes (pay for performance). Accountable care organizations (ACO) represent a model of health care in which groups of providers are accountable for quality, cost, and overall care of a cohort of patients. These groups of providers (hospitals, physicians, postacute facilities) will provide health care to large cohorts of patients at a fixed cost in an effort to encourage the practice of cost-effective medicine.[7] In this model of health care, ACOs will hope to reduce unnecessary medical spending. ACOs will then share in the savings or losses associated with the delivery of care to this cohort of patients. It is unclear as to how this model might be implemented in the delivery of surgical care.

Box 1
Formula to calculate physician payment

Payment = [(RVU work × GPCI work) + (RVU practice expense × GPCI practice expense) + (RVU Malpractice × GPCI Malpractice)] × conversion factor

Bundled payment programs provide a single payment to both hospitals and physicians for providing care on the basis of expected costs for defined clinical episodes of care. This strategy for providing reimbursement attempts to reduce costs and unnecessary testing by providing a single lump-sum payment for an episode of care such as a hernia repair. As a result, extraneous procedures and testing will reduce overall profit to a facility. Both facilities and providers are likely to be motivated to reduce costs in providing care so as to maximize revenue. The Patient Protection and Affordable Care Act called for pilot programs evaluating bundled payments to begin in 2013, with subsequent expansion of the program in 2016.[8]

Undoubtedly the reimbursement system for health care in the United States is being closely scrutinized. It will be imperative for physicians to work with hospitals and other health care facilities to eliminate waste and improve efficiencies as the health care reimbursement model in the United States evolves. In light of the frequency of ventral hernia repairs and the tremendous variability within hernia care, hernia repair might serve as an excellent model to evaluate new strategies for reimbursement for surgical procedures.

COST-EFFECTIVENESS OF MESH FOR HERNIA REPAIR

Despite compelling evidence that mesh placement will result in lower recurrence rates, there is still a significant number of repairs being performed without mesh.[9] Rather than looking at this issue from the perspective of recurrence rate, another way to examine it is to look at the costs involved. Does a mesh repair reduce recurrence rates enough to offset the increased costs involved (longer time in the operating room, increased cost of materials, and complications)? In a study by Israelsson and colleagues[10] evaluating hernia repairs between 1991 and 2000, the hospital and societal costs of mesh and nonmesh hernia repairs were evaluated. A cost analysis of suture repair in comparison with mesh repair was performed. Not surprisingly, mesh repairs were more expensive from an operating room and anesthetic standpoint (longer cases). However, the mesh patients left the hospital sooner and returned to work earlier, resulting in an overall lower cost for mesh patients. In their follow-up, none of the mesh patients had a recurrence, whereas approximately 40% of primary-closure patients developed recurrences. Although this study does not look at the costs of the recurrences, recurrent hernias would clearly lead to increased costs should the patients undergo re-repair. The study is fairly limited because it is a small cohort of patients and the costs are calculated based on the Swedish system of providing social security to citizens while they are out of work, making it difficult to apply the results globally. In this study, the duration of follow-up was 30 months for the mesh group and 67 months for the nonmesh group, skewing the recurrence rate. Nevertheless, the study strongly suggests the cost-effectiveness of mesh-based hernia repairs from the standpoint of returning to work following the initial procedure.

A more recent study from 2009 by Finan and colleagues[11] also compared costs between open hernia repairs with and without mesh. This study hypothesized that the increased costs of materials, operating room time, and potential complications from mesh (infection, fistula, and so forth) would be offset by the reduced recurrence rates. Their cost analysis attempted to define the cost of preventing a recurrence. Decision analysis is a complex mathematical model with multiple variables entered to predict certain outcomes. The model relies on predicting outcomes based on published rates of many different factors, including recurrence rates and complication rates. In this study, the incremental cost to prevent 1 recurrence was $1878. This number is heavily influenced by the cost of materials and supplies (particularly mesh) and also accounts for the costs of mesh complications and recurrences, and includes the costs associated with any additional care required. This study does not take into account the societal costs of lost productivity from patients being out of work, and therefore likely underestimates the costs of complications and recurrences. In a subanalysis, small hernias, defined as smaller than 10 cm^2, were always less expensive than suture repairs when repaired with mesh, with no incremental cost to prevent a recurrence. This finding was due in large part to the difference in recurrence rates between mesh and suture repairs in small hernias (9.1% vs 46%). Based on this analysis, there is a definite cost associated with mesh placement, even when taking into account the reduced recurrence rates, except in the group of small hernias.

In considering the true cost of the use of mesh in preventing recurrences, it is imperative in determining cost-effectiveness to consider lost wages, decreased work productivity, and disability payments as well as hospital costs. A better understanding of the complex relationships influencing the economic impact of mesh utilization is needed.

ECONOMIC IMPACT OF LAPAROSCOPIC HERNIA REPAIR

Much has been published comparing laparoscopic with open repair of ventral hernias and citing the many benefits of laparoscopic ventral hernias, although not in a randomized controlled fashion. From a cost perspective, laparoscopic ventral hernia repairs have several advantages, including typically shorter hospital stays and quicker return to work. However, the barrier meshes used tend to be more expensive than uncoated polypropylene and polyester meshes, and the equipment costs associated with laparoscopy are also more than for open surgery.

A single institution analysis of 884 consecutive incisional hernia repairs was performed by Earle and colleagues[12] whereby laparoscopic repair was carried out in 53% and open procedures in 47%. The study evaluated hospital costs for the procedure and also included any hospital encounters in the 30-day postoperative period. This study did not evaluate the costs associated with recurrent hernias. The length of stay for laparoscopic repair was significantly shorter (1 ± 0.2 vs 2 ± 0.6 days) but had higher operating room supply costs and longer procedural times. There was no significant difference between the two groups in 30-day hospital follow-up encounters. The final analysis demonstrated the laparoscopic repair to be less costly than the open repair ($6725 vs $7445), although it was not statistically significant. By comparing hospital costs alone up to 30 days postoperatively, there was no difference in cost. The decreased length of stay offset the increased operating room costs associated with supplies and increased operative time. It stands to reason that if laparoscopic repairs result in a reduced recurrence of hernia and the complication rates are no higher, the long-term costs will be less. However, not all hernias are amenable or ideally suited to laparoscopic repair. Patients with wide defects may have noticeable bulges postoperatively and may not be satisfied with the cosmetic results, despite a successful hernia repair.[13] Based on the available literature, the laparoscopic repair remains an excellent choice, and in appropriately selected patients may be a less costly repair than open ventral hernia.

HERNIA PROPHYLAXIS

While the incidence of incisional hernia following laparotomy is reported to be as high as 20%, certain populations may be at greater risk for hernia formation.[14] In certain high-risk populations, it may be cost-effective to use techniques to minimize the risk of developing an incisional hernia. At present, the use of mesh as prophylaxis against incisional hernia formation is not often performed, although several ongoing studies are evaluating the clinical benefit of prophylactic mesh in reducing the incidence of incisional hernia formation with this strategy.[15] Although mesh placement may reduce the incidence of hernia formation in high-risk populations, there is no current method for reimbursing hospitals and physicians for the added costs associated with these procedures. In addition, costs associated with potential complications from mesh placement would need to be considered in any financial analysis. Until methods for identifying patients with the highest risk for hernia are available, routine hernia prophylaxis cannot be supported by clinical or economic models.

Parastomal hernia prophylaxis is one area in which a clear benefit has been demonstrated.[14,16,17] Reported incidence of parastomal hernia has been reported to be as high as 48%.[18,19] Reported figures for parastomal hernias that require subsequent intervention range from 18% to 30%.[14,19,20] In a study by Figel and colleagues,[21] biological mesh was used prophylactically at the time of end-stoma creation. In this study with a median clinical follow-up of 38 months (range 24–53 months), there were no parastomal hernias. Biological mesh was placed as either a Sugarbaker technique or a keyhole around the stoma. A cost analysis was performed to determine if the cost of the biological mesh would offset a reduction in the need for subsequent parastomal hernia repairs. By 2 different calculations it was determined that if the cost of the mesh remained the same ($5900), the reoperative rate for parastomal hernia would need to be higher than 39% to be cost-effective. Alternatively, the mesh would need to cost less than $2267. Financially it seems reasonable to consider prophylactic mesh placement in this subset of patients who are having a permanent stoma placed, as the risk of parastomal hernia does not appear to taper off even after many years. However, several other investigators have demonstrated good success with parastomal hernia prophylaxis using synthetic mesh.[16,17] The utilization of prophylactic synthetic mesh at the time of stoma creation may be significantly more cost-effective in light of the reduced cost of synthetic meshes relative to biological mesh materials.

ECONOMIC IMPACT OF COMPONENT SEPARATION PROCEDURES (OPEN AND ENDOSCOPIC)

Abdominal wall reconstruction is not infrequently performed for patients with complex and complicated ventral and incisional hernias. Numerous techniques exist for abdominal wall reconstruction following the initial description by Ramirez and colleagues[22] of the separation of components technique for hernia repair. Since its initial description, there have been numerous other descriptions of techniques for abdominal wall reconstruction. Many of these techniques have evolved in an attempt to reduce the associated morbidity of raising large skin flaps and dividing the periumbilical perforating vessels to the abdominal wall skin. These perforator-preserving component separations have been widely adopted in an attempt to reduce the wound morbidity associated with the component separation technique.[23,24]

Although a cost saving can be inferred from a reduction of postoperative morbidity, there is little evidence evaluating the cost differences. A recent innovation in the separation of components armamentarium is the endoscopic release of the external oblique, whereby the space between the external and internal oblique is dissected using a pneumatic balloon dissector, and an endoscope and cautery are used to then divide the external oblique.[25] This technique obviates large skin flaps that are associated with frequent postoperative wound complications.[26] Although a reduction in patient morbidity has been demonstrated, the increased costs associated may potentially offset the economic benefits of the reduced morbidity.[24]

In a retrospective study evaluating 54 patients, 59% of whom underwent an endoscopic approach and 41% an open approach, the cost-effectiveness of the two operations was analyzed.[27] Overall 6-month costs were reduced in the endoscopic group when total costs including mesh were considered, with the overall cost of the endoscopic group $12,528 compared with $20,326 ($P = .05$) for the open group. However, differences in the preoperative characteristics of the patient groups resulted in a greater utilization of biological mesh materials in the open group. An economic analysis including 6-month costs exclusive of mesh demonstrated no difference in costs between the two operations. In this study, wound morbidity was not significantly reduced in the endoscopic group, although other investigators have demonstrated significant reductions in wound morbidity with the endoscopic approach.[24] The modest increases in costs associated with the minimally invasive equipment required for component separation is likely to be offset by the reduction in costs associated with reduced morbidity. In the study by Rosen and colleagues,[25] the 2 largest impacts on expense were the cost of biological mesh and postoperative encounters related to wound complications. Further prospective trials will help further define the role of endoscopic component release and other perforator-preserving component-separation procedures.

Alternative techniques for abdominal wall reconstruction include posterior component separation, whereby the transversus abdominis muscle is released through the posterior rectus sheath.[23] These techniques preclude skin flaps as well, and do not require any specialized equipment. No cost data are available for posterior component separation procedures, so it is difficult to determine the financial implication of these operations.

HOSPITAL COSTS OF ABDOMINAL WALL HERNIA REPAIRS

As previously discussed, hospital reimbursement for abdominal wall hernias in 2013 is prospectively determined through DRG-based payments. As a result, hospitals must be aware of the costs of delivering care for each population of patients. As ventral hernia repairs represent one of the more frequently performed general surgical procedures, an understanding of the financial implications of these operations is essential.

A cost-effectiveness study of hernia repairs by Ibañez and colleagues[28] evaluated primary abdominal wall hernias including inguinofemoral, umbilical, epigastric, and Spigelian, and found that hernia surgery consumes 1.12% of their hospital budget. In their extensive cost analysis of 400 patients, they evaluated direct costs of the hospital, lost income, and travel expenses. In this study, the anesthetic choice was a major contributor to costs, with cases performed under local anesthesia having the lowest overall costs.[28] While feasible in many circumstances, local anesthesia may not be possible in many large and complicated ventral hernias. Although it is imperative for physicians and hospitals to provide optimal medical care, the costs of operating room supplies can actually be more than the DRG payment, which remunerates facilities for the entire hospitalization associated with the hernia repair. As a result, physicians and hospitals are motivated to contain costs through management of supplies as well as encouraging timely hospital discharges.

In a 2012 study, the costs, profits, and losses of providing hernia care at a tertiary care hospital were examined, evaluating open ventral hernia repairs over a 3-year period.[29] This study analyzed costs associated with operating room supplies, total direct costs, indirect costs, and hospital reimbursement. Review of the records identified 415 patients who underwent open ventral or incisional hernia repair as either a primary (hernia repair alone) or secondary procedure (concomitant to other abdominal operation). Although hospital payments were greater for those who underwent hernia repair as a secondary procedure, the overall hospital costs were greater than in those who underwent ventral hernia repair as a primary procedure, resulting in greater financial losses with secondary hernia repairs. An analysis of primary inpatient hernia repairs evaluated the costs of hernia repairs using 1 of 3 techniques: no mesh, synthetic mesh, or biological mesh. The synthetic mesh repairs garnered a modest $60 net profit, whereas primary repairs without mesh resulted in overall financial losses of $500. Even more staggering were the financial losses associated with the use of biological mesh materials, with financial losses of $8370. Operating room supply costs accounted for the majority of the costs associated with the losses in the biological mesh group. In this retrospective study, there are clear differences in the patient populations between those undergoing synthetic and biological mesh repairs.[29]

Biological mesh materials are most commonly used in hernia repairs with a non-clean wound classification, whereas synthetic meshes are most commonly used in the setting of a clean wound. Accordingly, it may not be appropriate to use synthetic meshes in the group of patients in which biological mesh is used. The adjunct of biological mesh to abdominal wall reconstruction has been shown to reduce hernia recurrence rates when compared with repairs without reinforcement.[30] As a result, the decision to implant a biological mesh may be in the best long-term interest of a patient while at the same time resulting in significant financial losses for tertiary care hospitals. In a study by Reynolds and colleagues,[29] there was also an increased incidence of hospital readmissions among the patients who underwent a hernia repair with biological mesh, again representing a more complex group of patients with greater risks for complications. As this study did not evaluate costs beyond the sentinel hospitalization, it is unclear whether the frequent hospital readmissions increased hospital losses or resulted in long-term profitability in this patient group.

Although net revenue for inpatient ventral hernia repairs overall resulted in losses, the contribution margin, defined as revenue minus direct costs, was positive in the synthetic and no-mesh patient groups. The biological mesh group demonstrated a negative contribution margin of $4560. This staggering loss is largely driven by the significant cost of these biological materials. As a result of the financial disincentive to providing care to this challenging group of patients, strategies for providing adequate hospital reimbursement for this group is needed. This financial analysis represented a 3-year average at a tertiary care facility. The applicability of this study to community hospitals is unclear. However, the study highlights the financial burden of providing care to complex patient groups that are not adequately reimbursed by the DRG system. As financial models for hospital and physician payments continue to evolve, it will be essential to ensure that health care systems are not unduly burdened by costs exceeding reimbursements.

BIOLOGICAL MESH

The introduction of biological mesh materials has dramatically changed the methods by which hernia care is provided, particularly for contaminated and infected hernia cases. Previous to 1999, surgical options for the repair of infected hernias were limited.[31] Apart from primary fascial closure, with or without a component separation procedure, options were limited to absorbable mesh, serial mesh excision, placement of a synthetic mesh, or a planned ventral hernia. Although the advent of biological mesh has increased surgical options in challenging cases, the costs associated with these materials is not insignificant. The clinical superiority of allografts over xeno-grafts or cross-linked grafts over non–cross-linked grafts remains an area of tremen-dous controversy (mainly due to a lack of clinical data), but there is no question that they are all very expensive.

Beyond the simple comparison of the nominal cost of uncoated polypropylene with the expense of acellular dermal matrices (as high as $30/cm^2), there have been several cost analyses that show definite increased costs associated with this type of mesh. As previously discussed, Reynolds and colleagues[29] noted that their inpatient ventral hernia repairs with synthetic mesh had a positive $3110 at the contribution margin, whereas the biological mesh patients had a negative $4560. Further analysis of operating room costs found the hernia mesh to be significantly more expensive in the biological group than in the synthetic group ($10,230 vs $1830), and this, presum-ably, was the largest contributor to the differences between the groups.

Poulose and colleagues[3] also noted during the time period from 2001 to 2006 that inpatient ventral hernia repair procedural costs steadily increased. It was also noted that during this period, biological meshes were becoming more available and more widely used. Although the cost of biological mesh was not clearly shown to be the rationale for rising costs, it certainly is another possible indicator of the financial impact of biological meshes.

In the cost comparison between open and endoscopic component release, two cost contributors were identified: wound morbidity and the use of biological grafts. The two groups had an approximately $7000 difference in their operating room costs, and the largest contributor to this difference was biological mesh.[27]

Given these findings, there is no doubt that the financial impact of biological mesh is significant and cannot be dismissed. On the other hand, there are definitely patients who benefit from the use of these meshes. A lack of meaningful data limits surgeons' ability to make evidence-based decisions. One of the primary advantages of a biolog-ical mesh over a synthetic material in a contaminated or infected setting is the reduc-tion in the risk of mesh infection that requires mesh removal. In the presence of infection, biological mesh materials often liquefy and deteriorate without the need for operative debridement. The use of synthetic mesh in a contaminated field may result in the development of prosthetic infection, which might potentially require mesh removal. Although the cost of a mesh infection is ill-defined, the costs associ-ated with infected implants have been reported to be as high as $50,000.[32]

Biological mesh materials have also been widely used in patients thought to be at high risk for abdominal wall infections.[33] Patients with multiple comorbid conditions have been shown to be at increased risk for abdominal infections.[34] Houck and col-leagues[35] demonstrated that patients with ventral hernia and prior abdominal wall in-fections have a 3-fold increased incidence of postoperative wound complications relative to patients without a prior history of wound complications.[35] Although patients with multiple comorbid conditions may have a higher likelihood of postoperative wound complications, only a small percentage of wound complications will result in the need for mesh explants. In a study of high-risk hernia patients by Krpata and colleagues,[34] only 3 of 88 patients required mesh explantation. Although the risk of mesh explant in this group is only 3%, the added costs and burdens associated with mesh removal for both the patient and the surgeon may support its use in selected high-risk situations. Comparative prospective trials evaluating not only clinical but also economic out-comes are necessary to help determine strategies that are efficacious and efficient.

As the role of biological meshes in hernia care is evaluated, it is imperative that these issues are studied from a health policy perspective. The burden of providing care should not rest on the shoulders of the tertiary care facilities. Third-party payers must appreciate the nuances of hernia surgery and the need to appropriately compensate facilities for providing care to their customers.

SUMMARY

Abdominal wall hernia repairs are common procedures performed with significant heterogeneity. The costs associated with providing care to hernia patients are significant, and the cost of materials is often the single greatest expense. This cost can be offset somewhat or even completely in some cases by reducing recurrences and readmissions, a shorter length of stay in hospital, and fewer complications. Further studies are needed to specifically examine biological meshes and their role in the complex hernia patient. From a health policy standpoint, research in hernia repair needs to look beyond the clinical outcomes of recurrence and infections. As a society, we need to appreciate the financial implications of hernia care and develop care pathways that are cost efficient.

REFERENCES

1. Flum DR, Horvath K, Koepsell T. Have outcomes of incisional hernia repair improved with time? A population-based analysis. Ann Surg 2003;237: 129–35.
2. Rutkow IM. Demographic and socioeconomic aspects of hernia repair in the United States in 2003. Surg Clin North Am 2003;83:1045–51, v–vi.
3. Poulose BK, Shelton J, Phillips S, et al. Epidemiology and cost of ventral hernia repair: making the case for hernia research. Hernia 2012;16:179–83.
4. Lynge DC, Larson EH, Thompson MJ, et al. A longitudinal analysis of the general surgery workforce in the United States, 1981-2005. Arch Surg 2008;143:345–50 [discussion: 351].
5. Mayes R. The origins, development, and passage of Medicare's revolutionary prospective payment system. J Hist Med Allied Sci 2007;62:21–55.
6. Centers for Medicare & Medicaid Services. Physician Fee Schedule. Available at: http://www.cms.gov/Medicare/Medicare-Fee-for-Service-Payment/Physician FeeSched/index.html?redirect=/physicianfeesched/. Accessed January 30, 2013.
7. Song Z, Lee TH. The era of delivery system reform begins. JAMA 2013;309:35–6.
8. Berwick DM. Making good on ACOs' promise—the final rule for the Medicare shared savings program. N Engl J Med 2011;365:1753–6.
9. Luijendijk RW, Hop WC, van den Tol MP, et al. A comparison of suture repair with mesh repair for incisional hernia. N Engl J Med 2000;343:392–8.
10. Israelsson LA, Jönsson L, Wimo A. Cost analysis of incisional hernia repair by suture or mesh. Hernia 2003;7(3):114–7.
11. Finan KR, Kilgore ML, Hawn MT. Open suture versus mesh repair of primary incisional hernias: a cost-utility analysis. Hernia 2009;13:173–82.
12. Earle D, Seymour N, Fellinger E, et al. Laparoscopic versus open incisional hernia repair: a single-institution analysis of hospital resource utilization for 884 consecutive cases. Surg Endosc 2006;20:71–5.
13. Tse GH, Stutchfield BM, Duckworth AD, et al. Pseudo-recurrence following laparoscopic ventral and incisional hernia repair. Hernia 2010;14:583–7.
14. Jänes A, Cengiz Y, Israelsson LA. Preventing parastomal hernia with a prosthetic mesh: a 5-year follow-up of a randomized study. World J Surg 2009;33:118–21 [discussion: 122–3].

15. Prevention of Incisional Hernia by Mesh Augmentation After Midline Laparotomy for Aortic Aneurysm Treatment (PRIMAAT). Available at: http://clinicaltrials.gov/ct2/show/NCT00757133. Accessed January 30, 2013.

16. Ventham NT, Brady RR, Stewart RG, et al. Prophylactic mesh placement of permanent stomas at index operation for colorectal cancer. Ann R Coll Surg Engl 2012;94:569–73.

17. Serra-Aracil X, Bombardo-Junca J, Moreno-Matias J, et al. Randomized, controlled, prospective trial of the use of a mesh to prevent parastomal hernia. Ann Surg 2009;249:583–7.

18. Londono-Schimmer EE, Leong AP, Phillips RK. Life table analysis of stomal complications following colostomy. Dis Colon Rectum 1994;37:916–20.

19. Carne PW, Robertson GM, Frizelle FA. Parastomal hernia. Br J Surg 2003;90:784–93.

20. Rieger N, Moore J, Hewett P, et al. Parastomal hernia repair. Colorectal Dis 2004;6:203–5.

21. Figel NA, Rostas JW, Ellis CN. Outcomes using a bioprosthetic mesh at the time of permanent stoma creation in preventing a parastomal hernia: a value analysis. Am J Surg 2012;203:323–6 [discussion: 326].

22. Ramirez OM, Ruas E, Dellon AL. "Component separation" method for closure of abdominal-wall defects: an anatomic and clinical study. Plast Reconstr Surg 1990;86:519–26.

23. Novitsky YW, Elliott HL, Orenstein SB, et al. Transversus abdominis muscle release: a novel approach to posterior component separation during complex abdominal wall reconstruction. Am J Surg 2012;204:709–16.

24. Giurgius M, Bendure L, Davenport DL, et al. The endoscopic component separation technique for hernia repair results in reduced morbidity compared to the open component separation technique. Hernia 2012;16:47–51.

25. Rosen MJ, Jin J, McGee MF, et al. Laparoscopic component separation in the single-stage treatment of infected abdominal wall prosthetic removal. Hernia 2007;11:435–40.

26. de Vries Reilingh TS, van Goor H, Charbon JA, et al. Repair of giant midline abdominal wall hernias: "components separation technique" versus prosthetic repair: interim analysis of a randomized controlled trial. World J Surg 2007;31:756–63.

27. Harth KC, Rose J, Delaney CP, et al. Open versus endoscopic component separation: a cost comparison. Surg Endosc 2011;25:2865–70.

28. Ibañez Rde M, Al Saied SA, Vallejo JA, et al. Cost-effectiveness of primary abdominal wall hernia repair in a 364-bed provincial hospital of Spain. Hernia 2011;15:377–85.

29. Reynolds D, Davenport DL, Korosec RL, et al. Financial implications of ventral hernia repair: a hospital cost analysis. J Gastrointest Surg 2013;17:159–67.

30. Espinosa-de-los-Monteros A, de la Torre JI, Marrero I, et al. Utilization of human cadaveric acellular dermis for abdominal hernia reconstruction. Ann Plast Surg 2007;58:264–7.

31. Rosen MJ. Biologic mesh for abdominal wall reconstruction: a critical appraisal. Am Surg 2010;76:1–6.

32. Darouiche RO. Treatment of infections associated with surgical implants. N Engl J Med 2004;350:1422–9.

33. Kanters AE, Krpata DM, Blatnik JA, et al. Modified hernia grading scale to stratify surgical site occurrence after open ventral hernia repairs. J Am Coll Surg 2012;215:787–93.

34. Krpata DM, Blatnik JA, Novitsky YW, et al. Evaluation of high-risk, comorbid patients undergoing open ventral hernia repair with synthetic mesh. Surgery 2013;153:120–5.
35. Houck JP, Rypins EB, Sarfeh IJ, et al. Repair of incisional hernia. Surg Gynecol Obstet 1989;169:397–9.

Pediatric Abdominal Wall Defects

Katherine B. Kelly, MD, Todd A. Ponsky, MD*

KEYWORDS

- Pediatric hernia • Umbilical hernia • Inguinal hernia • Gastroschisis • Omphalocele

KEY POINTS

- Indirect inguinal hernias occur in 4% of infants, and are more common in males and on the right side. Risk of incarceration is around 15%. Today pediatric inguinal hernias are frequently repaired laparoscopically or with laparoscopic guidance. These newer techniques have recurrence rates that are approaching the recurrence rate of open repair (1%). In neonates, hernias should be repaired before discharge from the hospital.
- Umbilical hernias occur in 10% to 30% of children. The fascial defect will continue to close over the first several years of the child's life. Other forms of abdominal wall hernias (femoral, epigastric, Spigelian) occur less frequently.
- Gastroschisis occurs in 3 of every 10,000 births. There is no overlying sac in gastroschisis, and the condition is not typically associated with congenital defects. A fibrous peel coats the bowel and makes manual reduction more difficult. Repeated trips to the operating room and silos can be used to achieve closure over time.
- Omphalocele occurs in 2 of every 10,000 births. This condition is more typically associated with congenital defects such as Beckwith-Wiedemann syndrome, pentalogy of Cantrell, bladder/cloacal extrophy, and Down syndrome. Bridging mesh can be used to close larger defects.

INTRODUCTION

Abdominal wall defects, in the form of hernias (inguinal, epigastric, umbilical, and so forth), gastroschisis, and omphalocele, make up a significant portion of a pediatric surgeon's operative practice. This article presents an overview of these pediatric conditions.

INGUINAL HERNIAS

Inguinal hernia repair is the most frequently performed pediatric surgical operation.

Epidemiology

The overall incidence of pediatric inguinal hernia is approximately 4%.[1] Inguinal defects are 10 times more common in males than in females.[2] Prematurity is also

Disclosures: None.
Division of Pediatric Surgery, Pediatric Surgery Center, Akron Children's Hospital, One Perkins Square, Akron, OH 44308, USA
* Corresponding author.
E-mail address: TPonsky@chmca.org

Surg Clin N Am 93 (2013) 1255–1267
http://dx.doi.org/10.1016/j.suc.2013.06.016
0039-6109/13/$ – see front matter © 2013 Elsevier Inc. All rights reserved.

associated with an increased incidence of inguinal hernia. Thirty percent of infants weighing less than 1 kg have inguinal hernias.[3]

Right-sided hernias predominate, accounting for 60% to 75% of inguinal hernias. This predominance is attributed to the later descent of the right testicle in males.[1] Bilateral hernias occur in 15% to 20% of cases. Female sex, prematurity, and left-sided inguinal hernias are risk factors for bilateral defects.[4]

Embryology and Anatomy

In the third month of gestation the processus vaginalis develops from the peritoneal lining. In the seventh to ninth month, the testes pass through the processus as it elongates along the course of the gubernaculum. The testes end up in the scrotum and the processus typically obliterates. A congenital inguinal hernia results when the proximal processus vaginalis fails to obliterate, allowing fat, bowel, or other organs to enter the processus and the surrounding inguinal canal.[5]

In females, the canal of Nuck corresponds to the processus vaginalis. This pouch communicates with the labia majora and typically closes in the seventh month of gestation.[1]

Clinical Presentation and Examination

Most inguinal hernias are recognized as intermittent bulging in the groin, scrotum, or labia. Such bulging is exacerbated by the increased intra-abdominal pressures seen when an infant cries or strains to have a bowel movement. Often a hernia is not seen on physical examination in the office despite the parent's description of a groin bulge that comes and goes. Many surgeons operate on this history alone. A recent and novel study suggests that parents take digital pictures of the bulge to document its presence.[6]

Examination of a hernia begins by identifying the testes within the scrotum. If no testis is found in the scrotum, the bulge may be an undescended testicle. The external ring, lateral to the pubis, is then palpated with a single finger. The spermatic cord and associated structures can be felt by rolling one's finger over them. Thickening of the cord structures or the "silk glove sign" signals the presence of a hernia sac. This clinical sign has a reported sensitivity of 91% and specificity of 97.3%.[7] Often, no bulge is initially seen. It is then helpful to induce increased intra-abdominal pressure by asking the child to perform a Valsalva maneuver or by making him/her laugh or cry.

Risk of Incarceration

Incarcerated inguinal hernias occur in 5% to 15% of pediatric hernia presentations. The rate of incarcerated hernia is up to 30% in infants.[8,9] Incarcerated hernias can typically be reduced with taxis.

Bowel entrapment typically occurs at the internal ring.[1]

Any inguinal hernia that cannot be reduced should be promptly taken to the operating room. The process of intestinal strangulation and infarction can develop in as little as 2 hours.[1]

Diagnostic Imaging

Although rarely used in the United States, Groin ultrasonography can be used to augment the physical examination for inguinal hernias. The finding of a hypoechoic structure measuring greater than 6 mm in the mid-inguinal canal is consistent with the presence of a hernia.[10] In one study, in-office ultrasonography increased the diagnostic accuracy from 84% to 97.9%.[11]

Timing of Surgery

When discussing the timing of an operation it is helpful to divide cases of inguinal hernia into 3 age groups: preterm infant, infant, and child.

Preterm infants have a higher incidence of inguinal hernia (25%–30%) and higher rates of incarceration (up to 31%).[4,12] Therefore, there is an impetus to repair these hernias before the infant is discharged from the neonatal intensive care unit. However, there are no data to suggest that surgery before discharge is better than waiting.[13–15] Indeed, preterm infants have an increased risk of postoperative apnea and/or bradycardia.[1] Furthermore, recent pediatric anesthesiology literature highlights the relationship between early exposure to anesthesia and long-term effects on neurodevelopment.[16] Therefore, the surgeon and parents must weigh the risk of incarceration against the risk of anesthesia.

Term infants can have their inguinal hernias repaired electively. Nevertheless, some argue for expedient surgery because of the higher rate of incarceration seen in infants. Typically children of up to 60 weeks postconceptual age are monitored overnight.[1]

Older children have a low rate of incarceration and can therefore be repaired electively.

Patent Processus or Hernia?

The presence of a patent processus vaginalis is necessary, but not sufficient, for the diagnosis of an indirect inguinal hernia. At 2 years of age, 20% of male children are thought to have a patent processus. However, the incidence of clinically appreciated hernias is far less. In recent studies on adults with indirect hernias, a contralateral patent processus has been found in 12% to 14% of patients. Of these, only 12% to 14% develop a contralateral hernia. However, patients with a contralateral patent processus are more likely than their counterparts with no patent processus vaginalis to develop a contralateral hernia.[17,18]

Assessing the Contralateral Groin for a Hernia

In the 1950s, it became standard practice to perform bilateral groin dissections in children with a unilateral hernia after work by Rothenberg and Barnett.[19] However, today most pediatric surgeons believe that bilateral groin exploration is not warranted. Although the rate of a patent contralateral processus vaginalis is 60% to 80% in infants and 40% in older children, the majority never become clinical hernias. Approximately 20% of children presenting with a unilateral hernia develop a clinically apparent hernia on the contralateral side.[1]

Furthermore, open groin dissection is not risk free. Testicular atrophy and injury to the vas deferens may contribute to higher rates of infertility among men who had their hernias repaired as a child.

Laparoscopy allows for visualization of bilateral groins and makes easy the diagnosis of a contralateral hernia or patent processus. Such procedures can be conducted through the hernia sac (ie, "the laparoscopic look") or through the umbilicus with the optional use of additional ports.

Open Repair

Czerny published the first report of high ligation of a hernia sac in 1887, and this repair continues to be the mainstay of pediatric inguinal hernia repair.[2] There is usually no weakness of the inguinal floor in these cases, as most are congenital indirect inguinal hernias. Therefore, no reinforcement of the tissues is needed and high ligation of the sac is adequate.

The pubic tubercle and anterior superior iliac spine are identified externally. The external ring lies just inferior and lateral to the pubic tubercle. Next, the skin is incised in the inguinal crease just superior and lateral to the pubic tubercle. In young children, the external and internal rings overlap. As the child grows, the internal ring moves laterally.

The incision continues through the dermis, Camper fascia, and Scarpa fascia. The inferior epigastric vein is avoided when incising the fascia of Scarpa. The external oblique muscle is identified and the inguinal ligament is cleared. The external oblique muscle is then incised, and the undersides of the cut edges are cleared with blunt dissection. This allows for visualization of the inguinal canal, which contains the spermatic cord and the associated hernia sac. Under the spermatic cord is the floor of the inguinal canal, the transversalis fascia. Also within the canal are the iliofemoral and ilioinguinal nerves. The cremasteric muscle fibers are also seen here, and these are spread to reveal the hernia sac. The sac is next dissected away from the cord structures (vas deferens and testicular vessels). The sac is divided and opened. Ovaries, fallopian tubes, or uterus may be found in the hernia. The proximal portion of the sac is dissected free up to the internal ring. It is then twisted on itself and ligated with a stick tie, usually using an absorbable suture.

The incision is then closed in layers and the skin is approximated with sutures.

Recurrences and complications

Open repair has a recurrence rate of approximately 1%, and therefore has been considered the gold standard of pediatric hernia repair. The largest case series of open repairs consists or more than 6300 patients and reports a recurrence rate of 1.2%.[20]

Additional complications of open inguinal hernia repair include testicular ischemia and atrophy, iatrogenic cryptorchidism, and injury to the vas deferens. The rate of testicular ischemia is higher in cases of incarcerated inguinal hernias.[21–23] However, this ischemia is caused by compression from the hernia, not the repair itself. In their series of 6361 repairs, Ein and colleagues[20] report a 0.3% rate of testicular atrophy. The rate among other studies ranges from 2% to 13%.[24]

Iatrogenic cryptorchidism is believed to occur when the testis slips out of the scrotum during dissection of the hernia sac. The testis then becomes bound up in scar tissue, resulting in an undescended testicle. This injury occurs in 0.8% to 2.8% of boys undergoing inguinal hernia repair.[25]

Finally, direct injury to the vas deferens occurs in 0.13% to 0.53% of repairs.[26,27] The rate of wound infection is low, at 1.2%.[20]

Laparoscopic Repair

Laparoscopic repair of pediatric inguinal hernias is becoming more common among pediatric surgeons. The procedure was first described in females in 1997, and subsequently in males 2 years later.[28,29] The greatest benefit to laparoscopic repair is the ability to look for defects bilaterally as well as to identify and repair hernias in the femoral or direct positions. Moreover, some argue that laparoscopic repair may be less traumatic to the spermatic cord and may also be a safer approach to very large or incarcerated hernias.

In general there are 2 approaches, intracorporeal ligation and laparoscopic assisted percutaneous ligation. Within these 2 classes of repair there are numerous techniques that have been proposed, only a few of which are mentioned here.

Intracorporeal repair

The largest published series of intracorporeal hernia repairs is attributable to Schier. His original technique was to primarily close the peritoneum with interrupted sutures, lateral to the cord structures.[30] Schier then modified his technique to a Z-suture at the internal ring.[31] His series of 712 inguinal hernias repaired with a Z-stitch reported a recurrence rate of 2.6%.[32]

Riquelme and colleagues[33] argue for an intracorporeal dissection and resection of the hernia sac with no ligation. This study of 71 patients argues that the scarring that occurs from sac dissection is all that is needed to close the defect. The investigators report a 0% recurrence rate with a follow-up period of 5 months to 4 years.

Extracorporeal (percutaneous) ligation

One of the earlier extracorporeal techniques is the SEAL technique (Subcutaneous Endoscopically Assisted Ligation).[34] In brief, a 5-mm 30° laparoscope is placed through the umbilical port. A stitch is placed extracorporeally in the groin, and the needle is guided in the preperitoneal plane around the internal ring under laparoscopic visualization. The spermatic cord travels in this preperitoneal plane and the suture is brought into the peritoneal cavity to "skip" over the spermatic cord near the 6 o'clock position. The suture is then directed back into the preperitoneal plane. The needle is backed out of the skin though the same stab incision and the suture is tied down, thus closing the internal ring.

There is concern among pediatric surgeons that "skipping" over the spermatic cord results in a weak repair. One approach to achieving a circumferential stitch while protecting the cord structures is hydrodissection. Injecting the preperitoneal space with water or local anesthetic lifts the peritoneum from the cord structures and creates a plane through which the suture is advanced. The authors have found that this technique has often led to pain attributable to the gathering up of extra anterior tissue.

The authors' current technique is a modification of that described by Patkowski and colleagues.[35] A 3-mm trocar is placed through the umbilicus and a 3-mm 70° scope inserted. Next, a 3-mm stab incision is made in the left lower quadrant, through which a 3-mm Maryland dissector is inserted. Based on the authors' published experience with rabbits, the anterior portion of the internal ring is then cauterized with the Maryland dissector. Next, the preperitoneal space is injected with Marcaine to hydrodissect the peritoneum from the cord structures. An 18-gauge needle, threaded with looped Prolene, is then inserted into the groin at the 12-o'clock position over the internal ring and is passed laterally between the peritoneum and cord structures to the medial side of the cord; the looped Prolene is then pushed through the needle. The needle is removed. A second needle with a looped Prolene thread is guided to the same 12-o'clock position but travels medially to meet the other looped Prolene, and is pushed through the original looped Prolene. The original Prolene is then pulled upon, and acts as a snare to pull the second Prolene around the internal ring and through the skin. A 2-0 Ethibond is then threaded through the Prolene loop. The Prolene is pulled back through its tract while the Ethibond, now looped, trails along. This maneuver brings the Ethibond loop around the internal ring. The looped end is then cut and the Ethibond is tied down to doubly ligate the internal ring. The knot rests within the subcutaneous tissue.

Open or Laparoscopic Repair?

Proponents of laparoscopic repairs argue that this approach involves no handling of the spermatic cord, which may result in a decreased risk of cord injury; they also argue that laparoscopic repair poses no risk of injury to the inguinal floor. Many believe that laparoscopic repair of hernias is less painful and has better cosmesis.

The numerous techniques used for laparoscopic repair makes it difficult to compare recurrence rates. Reported rates for early recurrence range from 1% to 4%.[32,36–38]

However, as surgeons have become more practiced at laparoscopic repair of inguinal hernia, several case series have reported recurrence rates close to the gold standard of open repair.[38,39]

In 2011, Yang and colleagues[40] published a meta-analysis of studies comparing laparoscopic and open repairs, and concluded that laparoscopic repair has a lower rate of metachronic hernia and shorter operative times for bilateral hernia. Laparoscopic and open repairs were similar with regard to operative times for unilateral hernias, recurrence, length of stay in hospital, and complications.

Nevertheless, larger randomized studies must be performed to directly address the superiority of one operative approach over another.

Direct Inguinal Hernias

Congenital direct inguinal hernias are unusual, but can occur. Direct defects are found in up to 5% of cases.[41]

Repair can be approached laparoscopically or through an open incision, and usually consists of primary closure of the defect. Mesh is avoided in the repair of hernias in adolescents.

Inguinal Hernias in Adolescents

There is debate regarding how best to address the inguinal hernia in an adolescent patient. Essentially the question is whether high ligation of the sac is a sufficient repair. Some propose that a Lichtenstein repair with mesh is the more appropriate repair for these children approaching adulthood.

In the Lichtenstein repair, the patient is positioned and prepped as if one were going to perform a high ligation of the hernia sac. A transverse groin incision is made to expose the external oblique muscle, and this is then incised transversely through the external ring. A space is then created below the external oblique from the anterior iliac spine to the Cooper ligament using blunt dissection. The inferior edge of the external oblique is also dissected free to expose the shelving edge of the inguinal ligament. The hernia sac and cord structures are then lifted out of the inguinal canal. The hernia sac is dissected from the associated cord structures. Care is taken to isolate the vas deferens, spermatic vessels, and genital branch of the genitofemoral nerve. The freed hernia sac is then reduced into the abdomen through the internal ring. A piece of polypropylene mesh is sutured to the Cooper ligament, and sewn to the shelving edge of the inguinal ligament inferiorly and the aponeurosis of the internal oblique superiorly. A slit in the mesh accommodates the cord structures. The tails of the mesh are then overlapped laterally and placed below the external oblique. A stitch can be placed through the 2 tails to create a ring around the cord structures. The external oblique is then closed over the mesh, which reconstructs the external ring. Care is taken at the end of the operation to ensure that the testicle is pulled down into the scrotum.

Alternatively, an adolescent inguinal hernia may be repaired laparoscopically through a TEP (totally extraperitoneal) and TAPP (transabdominal preperitoneal) repair, as performed in the adult population. The details regarding these procedures are beyond the scope of this article.

Proponents of high ligation point to the fact that adolescent hernias are congenital in nature and are very rarely due to acquired weakness in the inguinal floor. There is also concern regarding the impact of mesh on a patient's future fertility.[42–44] Those who support an adult-type repair are typically adult general surgeons who argue that adolescents are essentially adults and that the mesh repair will have a lower recurrence rate. There is little evidence to support this, however. With scant evidence to guide one's practice, the decision to perform high ligation versus mesh repair depends on the patient's age, size, and findings at groin exploration. The surgeon's clinical judgment continues to hold sway as regards surgical repair of adolescent inguinal hernia.

FEMORAL HERNIAS

The incidence of femoral hernias in children is rare, making up less than 1% of childhood groin hernias.[41] Often they are misdiagnosed as inguinal hernias and are repaired as such. These children re-present with early recurrences, and only then is it recognized that the defect is actually a femoral hernia.[45,46]

The open approaches to repairing these hernias include the classic McVay repair. However, laparoscopic approaches are becoming more common. The laparoscopic approach also affords the surgeon the opportunity to visualize and identify the femoral hernia.[45]

UMBILICAL HERNIAS

All neonates have a small umbilical defect at birth through which the umbilical vessels pass. Typically the umbilical ring closes in the early days to weeks of infancy. However, in 10% to 30% of children the defect fails to close and is apparent on physical examination. The incidence of umbilical hernia is associated with race, birth weight, and certain syndromes.[47]

African American infants are 6 to 10 times more likely than Caucasian infants to have an umbilical hernia.[48]

Likewise, infants born weighing less than 1200 g are nearly 4 times more likely to have an umbilical defect than their counterparts weighing greater than 2500 g. Children with Beckwith-Wiedemann and Down syndrome also have an increased risk of umbilical hernia.[49]

The vast majority of umbilical hernias present in early infancy will close spontaneously by the second or third year of life. Some believe that the likelihood of a defect closing depends on the size of the defect and the age of the child. Pediatric surgeons will wait to close a defect until the child is at least 3 to 5 years old. In a retrospective study of 489 children at the Mayo Clinic, the mean age of repair was 3.9 years and the mean size of the defect was 1.3 cm.[50]

The authors are currently conducting a study looking at the correlation between the size of an umbilical hernia and the likelihood that it will close spontaneously.

Incarceration of the pediatric umbilical hernia is considered uncommon. However, several studies report the cause for repair to be incarceration in up to 5% of cases. Strangulation occurs in less than 1% of cases.[50]

Repair of an umbilical hernia is typically done through a curved infraumbilical incision. The umbilical stalk is divided, and the hernia sac is removed and reduced. The fascial defect is the closed with interrupted transverse sutures. The umbilicus is tacked to the fascia and the skin is closed. Rates of reported recurrence are low (2%).

A minority of umbilical hernias are proboscoid umbilical hernias. The size of the fascial defect is similar to that in typical umbilical hernias, but there is a large amount of redundant overlying skin. Some support umbilicoplasty to achieve an aesthetic repair.[51]

Further study into the genetic mechanisms associated with the normal programmed umbilical closure may reveal additional novel approaches to the repair of these hernias.

EPIGASTRIC HERNIAS

During the final stages of abdominal wall formation, the rectus muscles are expected to approximate at the linea alba. If this fails to occur in the upper midline, an epigastric hernia is the result. Epigastric hernias are relatively common in children, with an incidence of up to 5%, half of which are symptomatic.

According to Coats and colleagues,[52] these hernias present as an epigastric bulge. Often they are painless. However, some children experience epigastric pain with increased activity. The bulge is reducible more than half of the time.

The epigastric hernia defect is usually small (0.7 cm) and can be closed primarily.[52] It is essential to mark the location of the hernia before the patient is paralyzed so that the precise site of the hernia can be located once the bulge reduces.

LUMBAR HERNIAS

The largest reported series of congenital lumbar hernias is 18 patients from India.[53,54] The etiology of these defects is unclear, but has been associated with anoxia during the third to fifth week of embryogenesis. Defects are more common in the superior lumbar triangle.[55]

In the series of Sharma and colleagues,[53] the median age of presentation was 3 months and the median defect size was 6 cm. Lumbocostovertebral syndrome was seen in 22% of the patients. A primary tissue repair was performed in most cases. However, 2 defects were greater than 10 cm and were repaired with polypropylene mesh.

SPIGELIAN HERNIAS

Spigelian hernias occur rarely in children. There are 34 case reports in the literature.[56]

These hernias can be bilateral and they occur equally on both sides of the abdomen. The diagnosis is typically made during a physical examination when a defect is detected lateral to the rectus below the level of the umbilicus. The size of the hernia defects are most commonly 1 to 3 cm.

Repair is a primary tissue repair. Losanoff and colleagues[56] make the point that in cases of suspected appendicitis with a normal appendix, a Spigelian hernia should be looked for on the anterior abdominal wall.

CONGENITAL ABDOMINAL WALL DEFECTS
Gastroschisis and Omphalocele

Gastroschisis and omphalocele (exomphalos) present unique challenges to the pediatric surgeon. Gastroschisis occurs in 3 of every 10,000 births, and omphalocele has an incidence of about 2 per 10,000 births.[57–59]

The etiology of these 2 entities is a matter of ongoing research. Gastroschisis is theorized to be less affected by genetics and more dependent on environmental factors such as ischemic insults. Therefore, there is an association between gastroschisis and intestinal atresias. By contrast, omphalocele is typically thought of as a being caused by genetic factors.[60,61]

Gastroschisis is characterized by protruding small bowel and other intra-abdominal organs without an overlying sac. The abdominal wall defect is typically smaller than 4 cm and to the right of the umbilicus. Exposure of the viscera to amniotic fluid and a compromised blood supply results in bowel that is edematous, thick, shortened, and covered in fibrinous exudate. The thickening of the bowel and the fibrous peel on the bowel makes manual reduction more difficult and can lead to prolonged ileus.

Omphalocele is characterized by bowel and viscera covered by a membrane that herniates through a defect, larger than 4 cm, at the umbilicus. The viscera are functionally normal as the membrane protects them from the environment. Omphalocele is associated with anomalies such as Beckwith-Wiedemann syndrome, pentalogy of Cantrell, bladder/cloacal extrophy, and Down syndrome.

Gastroschisis and omphalocele may be suspected if the prenatal maternal serum α-fetoprotein is elevated. Fetal ultrasonography can detect these defects in 75% to 80% of these defects. If omphalocele is identified, amniocentesis and/or chorionic villous sampling are recommended for karyotype analysis.

Postnatal care

Neonates with gastroschisis or omphalocele typically have a nasogastric tube placed for decompression. The herniated viscera is handled delicately and covered with moist gauze. These infants have large evaporative and third-space fluid losses. Judicious intravenous fluid resuscitation is needed to correct or avoid hypovolemia. For gastroschisis, prophylactic intravenous antibiotics are administered.

Surgical intervention

Omphalocele Emergent operation is not necessary for intact omphaloceles, and operative delay allows time to work the neonate up for concurrent abnormalities. Small or medium-sized defects should be closed primarily if possible. The omphalocele sac is excised. Next, the umbilical vessels are ligated. Skin flaps are created to develop fascial edges for closure. The viscera are reduced and the fascia is closed transversely. A purse-string suture can be placed in the overlying skin to create an umbilicus.

In some cases primary closure cannot be achieved at the first operation. Options for closure in these infants include the Gross technique, the Schuster technique, sequential sac ligation, tissue expanders, and nonoperative escharotic therapy.

The Gross technique uses synthetic or biological mesh to bridge the fascial defect. The resultant hernia is repaired at a later time.

Schuster proposed the use of a silastic silo to reduce the viscera over time. The silo is attached to the skin with nonabsorbable suture and is hung above the abdomen to use gravity to help reduce the viscera. The silo is tightened each day as the viscera reduce. Once all of the viscera have been reduced, the silo is removed and the fascia and skin are closed.

If the omphalocele membrane is thick and free from the viscera, it can be used as a silo. As the viscera reduce, the sac is sequentially twisted and ligated.

Tissue expanders can be used to slowly stretch the abdominal wall to increase the abdominal domain. The viscera can then be completely reduced and the fascia closed.

Nonoperative escharotic therapy can be used in giant omphaloceles in neonates who are poor surgical candidates. A topical escharotic such as silvadene is applied to the omphalocele membrane itself. With time, granulation tissue and epithelial tissue grow over the membrane. The resultant hernia is then repaired at a later time.

Gastroschisis Gastroschisis or ruptured omphalocele requires immediate operation to cover the viscera and prevent desiccation of the tissues. Attempts are initially made at primarily closing the defect. If this is not possible, a silo can be used to provide a protected and moist environment while waiting for the viscera to reduce.

It is necessary to run the bowel in cases of gastroschisis, owing to the intestinal atresias associated with this defect.

The authors' preferred approach to gastroschisis is to attempt primary, sutureless closure at the bedside as described by Sandler and colleagues.[62] The infant is intubated and sedated, and the bowel is reduced. The umbilical-cord remnant is used to cover the abdominal wall defect, and this is covered with gauze and a clear, plastic, adhesive covering. The dressing is changed every 4 days until the wound has completely epithelialized. There is a small incidence of resulting umbilical hernia, but most of these will close over time. This technique is safe, easy, and cosmetically superior.

Outcomes Long-term outcomes in cases of omphalocele depend on the prognoses associated with any concurrent chromosomal or structural abnormalities. Mortality rates of up to 30% have been reported.

Gastroschisis outcome depends on the extent of the exteriorized bowel and associated atresias. Prolonged ileus and delay in enteral feeding is common in these patients.[63]

REFERENCES

1. Glick PL, Boulanger S. Inguinal hernias and hydroceles. In: Grosfeld JL, O'Neill J, Coran A, et al, editors. Pediatric surgery. Philadelphia: Elsevier; 2006. p. 1172–92.
2. Lloyd D. Inguinal and femoral hernia. In: Ziegler M, Azizkhan R, Weber T, editors. Operative pediatric surgery. New York: McGraw-Hill; 2003. p. 543–54.
3. Kurkchubasche A, Tracy T. Unique features of groin hernia repair in infants and children. In: Fitzgibbons R, Greenburg A, editors. Nyhus and Condon's hernia. Philadelphia: Lippincott Williams & Wilkins; 2002. p. 435–51.
4. Lao OB, Fitzgibbons RJ Jr, Cusick RA. Pediatric inguinal hernias, hydroceles, and undescended testicles. Surg Clin North Am 2012;92(3):487–504.
5. Shrock P. The precessus vaginalis and gubernaculums. Their raison d'etre redefined. Surg Clin North Am 1971;51(6):1263–8.
6. Kawaguchi AL, Shaul DB. Inguinal hernias can be accurately diagnosed using the parent's digital photographs when the physical examination is nondiagnostic. J Pediatr Surg 2009;44:2327–9.
7. Luo CC, Chao HC. Prevention of unnecessary contralateral exploration using the silk glove sign (SGS) in pediatric patients with unilateral inguinal hernia. Eur J Pediatr 2007;166(7):667–9.
8. Grosfelf JL. Current concepts in inguinal hernia in infants and children. World J Surg 1989;13(5):506–15.
9. Stylianos S, Jacir NN, Harris BH. Incarceration of inguinal hernia in infants prior to elective repair. J Pediatr Surg 1993;28(4):582–3.
10. Erez I, Rathause V, Vacian I, et al. Preoperative ultrasound and intraoperative findings of inguinal hernias in children: a prospective study of 642 children. J Pediatr Surg 2002;37(6):865–8.
11. Chen KC, Chu CC, Chou TY, et al. Ultrasonography for inguinal hernias in boys. J Pediatr Surg 1998;33(12):1784–7.
12. Rajput A, Gauderer MW, Hack M. Inguinal hernias in very low birth weight infants: incidence and timing of repair. J Pediatr Surg 1992;27(10):1322–4.
13. Gonzalez Santacruz M, Mira Navarro J, Encinas Goeenechea A, et al. Low prevalence of complications of delayed herniotomy in the extremely premature infant. Acta Paediatr 2004;93(1):94–8.
14. Misra D. Inguinal hernias in premature babies: wait or operate? Acta Paediatr 2001;90(4):370–1.

15. Uemura S, Woodward AA, Amerena R, et al. Early repair of inguinal hernia in premature babies. Pediatr Surg Int 1999;15(1):36–9.
16. Flick RP, Katusic SK, Colligan RC, et al. Cognitive and behavioral outcomes after early exposure to anesthesia and surgery. Pediatrics 2011;128(5): e1053–61.
17. van Wessem KJ, Simons MP, Plaisier PW, et al. The etiology of indirect inguinal hernias: congenital and/or acquired? Hernia 2003;7(2):76–9.
18. van Veen RN, van Wessem KJ, Halm JA, et al. Patent processus vaginalis in the adult as a risk factor for the occurrence of indirect inguinal hernia. Surg Endosc 2007;21(2):202–5.
19. Rothenberg RE, Barnett T. Bilateral herniotomy in infants and children. Surgery 1955;37(6):947–50.
20. Ein SH, Njere I, Ein A. Six thousand three hundred sixty-one pediatric inguinal hernias: a 35 year review. J Pediatr Surg 2006;41(5):980–6.
21. Le Coultre C, Cuendet A, Richon J. Frequency of testicular atrophy following incarcerated hernia. Z Kinderchir 1983;38(Suppl):39–41.
22. Slomann JG, Mylius RE. Testicular infarction in infancy: its association with irreducible inguinal hernia. Med J Aust 1958;45:242–4.
23. Wiklander O. Incarcerated inguinal hernia in childhood. Acta Chir Scand 1951; 101:303–11.
24. Tackett LD, Breuer CK, Luks FI, et al. Incidence of contralateral inguinal hernia: a prospective analysis. J Pediatr Surg 1999;34(5):684–7.
25. Fenig DM, Snyder HM 3rd, Wu HY, et al. The histopathology of iatrogenic cryptorchid testis: an insight into etiology. J Urol 2001;165(4):1258–61.
26. Patrick DA, Bensard DD, Karrer FM, et al. Is routine pathological evaluation of pediatric hernia sacs justified? J Pediatr Surg 1998;33(7):1090–2.
27. Steigman CK, Sotelo-Avila C, Weber TR. The incidence of spermatic cord structures in inguinal hernia sacs from male children. Am J Surg Pathol 1999;23(8): 880–5.
28. Spurbeck WW, Prasad R, Lobe TE. Two-year experience with minimally invasive herniorrhaphy in children. Surg Endosc 2005;19(4):551–3.
29. Montupet P, Esposito C. Laparoscopic treatment of congenital inguinal hernia in children. J Pediatr Surg 1999;34(3):420–3.
30. Schier F. Laparoscopic surgery of inguinal hernias in children: initial experience. J Pediatr Surg 2000;35(9):1331–5.
31. Gorsler CM, Schier F. Laparoscopic herniorrhaphy in children. Surg Endosc 2003;17(4):571–3.
32. Schier F. Laparoscopic inguinal hernia repair—a prospective personal series of 542 children. J Pediatr Surg 2006;41(6):1081–4.
33. Riquelme M, Aranda A, Riquelme- QM. Laparoscopic pediatric inguinal hernia repair: no ligation, just resection. J Laparoendosc Adv Surg Tech A 2010; 20(1):77–80.
34. Harrison MR, Lee H, Albanese CT, et al. Subcutaneous endoscopically assisted ligation (SEAL) of the internal ring for repair of inguinal hernias in children: a novel technique. J Pediatr Surg 2005;40(7):1177–80.
35. Patkowski D, Czernik J, Chrzan R, et al. Percutaneous internal ring suturing: a simple minimally invasive technique for inguinal hernia repair in children. J Laparoendosc Adv Surg Tech A 2006;16(5):513–7.
36. Takehara H, Yakabe S, Kameoka K. Laparoscopic percutaneous extraperitoneal closure for inguinal hernia in children: clinical outcome of 972 repairs done in 3 pediatric surgical institutions. J Pediatr Surg 2006;41(12):1999–2003.

37. Dutta S, Albanese C. Transcutaneous laparoscopic hernia repair in children: a prospective review of 275 hernia repairs with minimum 2-year follow-up. Surg Endosc 2009;23(1):103–7.

38. Parelkar SV, Oak S, Gupta R, et al. Laparoscopic inguinal hernia repair in the pediatric age group-experience with 437 children. J Pediatr Surg 2010;45(4): 789–92.

39. Montupet P, Esposito C. Fifteen years experience in laparoscopic inguinal hernia repair in pediatric patients. Results and considerations on a debated procedure. Surg Endosc 2011;25(2):450–3.

40. Yang C, Zhang H, Pu J, et al. Laparoscopic vs open herniorrhaphy in the management of pediatric inguinal hernia: a systemic review and meta-analysis. J Pediatr Surg 2011;46(9):1824–34.

41. Schier F, Klizaite J. Rare inguinal hernia forms in children. Pediatr Surg Int 2004; 20(10):748–52.

42. Maciel LC, Glina S, Palma PC, et al. Histopathological alterations of the vas deferens in rats exposed to polypropylene mesh. BJU Int 2007;100(1):187–90.

43. Peiper C, Junge K, Klinge U, et al. Is there a risk of infertility after inguinal mesh repair? Experimental studies in the pig and the rabbit. Hernia 2006; 10(1):7–12.

44. Shin D, Lipshultz LI, Goldstein M, et al. Herniorrhaphy with polypropylene mesh causing inguinal vassal obstruction: a preventable cause of obstructive azoospermia. Ann Surg 2005;241(4):553–8.

45. Al-Shanafey S, Giacomantonio M. Femoral hernia in children. J Pediatr Surg 1999;34(7):1104–6.

46. Lee SL, DuBois JJ. Laparoscopic diagnosis and repair of pediatric femoral hernia: initial experience of four cases. Surg Endosc 2000;14(12):1110–3.

47. Cilley R. Disorders of the umbilicus. In: Grosfeld JL, O'Neill J, Coran A, et al, editors. Pediatric surgery. Philadelphia: Elsevier; 2006. p. 1143–56.

48. Meier DE, OlaOlorun DA, Omolele RA, et al. Incidence of umbilical hernia in African children: redefinition of "normal" and reevaluation of indications for repair. World J Surg 2001;25(5):1665–8.

49. Kokoska E, Weber T. Umbilical and supraumbilical disease. In: Ziegler M, Azizkhan R, Weber T, editors. Operative pediatric surgery. New York: McGraw-Hill; 2003. p. 543–54.

50. Zendejas B, Kuchena A, Onkendi EO, et al. Fifty-three-year experience with pediatric umbilical hernia repairs. J Pediatr Surg 2011;46(11):2151–6.

51. Ikeda H, Yamamoto H, Fujino J, et al. Umbilicoplasty for large protruding umbilicus accompanying umbilical hernia: a simple and effective technique. Pediatr Surg Int 2004;20(2):105–7.

52. Coats RD, Helikson MA, Burd RS. Presentation and management of epigastric hernias in children. J Pediatr Surg 2000;35(12):1754–6.

53. Sharma A, Pandey A, Rawat J, et al. Congenital lumbar hernia: 20 years' single centre experience. J Paediatr Child Health 2012;48(11):1001–3.

54. Karmani S, Ember T, Davenport R. Congenital lumbar hernias: a case report. J Pediatr Surg 2009;37:921–2.

55. Stamatiou D, Skandalakis JE, Skandalakis LJ, et al. Lumbar hernia: surgical anatomy, embryology, and technique of repair. Am Surg 2009;75:202–7.

56. Losanoff JE, Richman BW, Jones JW. Spigelian hernia in a child: case report and review of the literature. Hernia 2002;6(4):191–3.

57. Alvarez SM, Burd RS. Increasing prevalence of gastroschisis repairs in the United States: 1996-2003. J Pediatr Surg 2007;42:943–6.

58. Calzolari E, Bianchi F, Dolk H, et al. Omphalocele and gastroschisis in Europe: a survey of 3 million births 1980-1990. EUROCAT Working Group. Am J Med Genet 1995;58:187–94.

59. Tan KH, Kilby MD, Whittle MJ, et al. Congenital anterior abdominal wall defects in England and Wales 1987-93: retrospective analysis of OPCS data. BMJ 1996; 313:903–6.

60. Frolov P, Alali J, Klein MD. Clinical risk factors for gastroschisis and omphalocele in humans: a review of the literature. Pediatr Surg Int 2010;26:1135–48.

61. Hoyme HE, Higginbottom MC, Jones KL. The vascular pathogenesis of gastroschisis: intrauterine interruption of the omphalomesenteric artery. J Pediatr 1981;98:228–31.

62. Sandler A, Lawrence J, Meehan J, et al. "Plastic" sutureless abdominal wall closure in gastroschisis. J Pediatr Surg 2004;39(5):738–41.

63. Ledbetter DJ. Gastroschisis and omphalocele. Surg Clin North Am 2006;86: 249–60, vii.

Laparoscopic Versus Open Inguinal Hernia Repair

Leandro Totti Cavazzola, MD, PhD[a],*, Michael J. Rosen, MD[b]

KEYWORDS

- Inguinal • Hernia surgery • Laparoscopic • Endoscopic • Mesh

KEY POINTS

- The laparoscopic approach to inguinal hernia surgery is a safe and reliable method with a similar recurrence rate as the open tension-free mesh repair.
- Because the laparoscopic approach shows clear advantages with regard to less chronic postoperative pain and numbness, fast return to normal activities, and a decrease in the incidence of wound infection and hematoma, it should be considered an appropriate approach for inguinal hernia surgery.
- The choice between the transabdominal preperitoneal (TAPP) procedure and the totally extraperitoneal (TEP) procedure should be based on patient and surgeon characteristics, because there is no evidence of superiority between either techniques.
- The use of lightweight mesh, with glue fixation (in TAPP procedures) or nonfixation (in TEP procedures), can achieve excellent results in the setting of a proficient surgeon.

Surgery has reached such a level of improvement that nothing more can be expected.
—Jean Nicholas Marjolin, 1828

Since the last publication, in 2008, of the *Surgical Clinics of North America* hernia edition, many important guidelines and meta-analyses concerning inguinal hernia surgery have been published.[1] One important contribution came from the European Hernia Society, when they published their guidelines for inguinal hernia repair in 2009,[2] followed by the International Endohernia Society in 2011.[3] Several prominent governmental agencies, including the Agency for Healthcare Research and Quality in the United States,[4] have recently reported evidence-based medicine guidelines dealing with the problem of hernia surgery and management.[5]

Disclosures: The authors have nothing to disclose.
[a] Department of Surgery, Universidade Federal do Rio Grande do Sul, Avenida Montenegro 163, Apartment 802, Bairro Petrópolis, Porto Alegre, Rio Grande do Sul 90460-160, Brazil; [b] Division of GI and General Surgery, Department of Surgery, Case Comprehensive Hernia Center, University Hospitals Case Medical Center, 11100 Euclid Avenue, Cleveland, OH 44106, USA
* Corresponding author.
E-mail address: cavazzola@gmail.com

Surg Clin N Am 93 (2013) 1269–1279
http://dx.doi.org/10.1016/j.suc.2013.06.013
0039-6109/13/$ – see front matter © 2013 Elsevier Inc. All rights reserved.

Why has hernia surgery continued to be such a vexing problem for surgeons across the world? Although it is a common disease, with approximately 1 million procedures performed annually in the United States and close to 20 million repairs worldwide, achieving excellent long-term results with a low recurrence rate and avoidance of chronic groin pain remains difficult when closely studied.[2,3,6–10] The lack of consensus in the literature as to the optimum repair technique or prosthetic mesh to insure a long-term durable result is also surprising.[2–4]

Although Marjolin thought that surgery had reached its ideal state in 1828, it is likely true that in groin surgery there will always be improvements in techniques and materials that address the changing spectrum of this disease. Even with the significant effort of evidence-based medicine to provide clear guidelines, it is conceivable that one answer will never suffice for all of groin surgery. This article focuses on common questions related to inguinal hernia surgery and tries to provide answers based on available published literature.

SHOULD ALL HERNIAS BE REPAIRED?

Since the conflicting results from the reports of watchful waiting from Fitzgibbons and colleagues[11] and O'Dwyer and colleagues in 2006,[12] there have been mounting data that not all hernias must be repaired promptly. There are data supporting that mildly symptomatic or asymptomatic men can be observed in a safe way without having major complications. With long-term follow-up, however, most of the patients during observation develop symptoms and likely require surgery if waiting long enough.[13,14] Their outcomes are not worse than those undergoing immediate repair.

Some groups of patients can be observed safely with a low probability of developing symptoms and necessity for repair.[15] A recent review of patients from the watchful waiting trial[16] showed that there are some risk factors that can help predict which patients will develop symptoms during observation and will ask for surgery. These patients probably should be considered early in their disease for surgical treatment. Factors identified include patients who have pain with strenuous activities, chronic constipation, or prostatism; married patients; and healthy individuals (American Society of Anesthesiologists class 1 vs class 2).

What is clear since the early results from O'Dwyer and colleagues and Fitzgibbons and colleagues is that what should drive the timing for surgery is not the risk of incarceration or strangulation (what is a common sense for surgeons in the past that should be considered as the main indication for surgery in hernia patients) but rather the change in quality of life that the presence of a hernia brings to a patient.[11,12] In an effectiveness review conducted by the Agency for Healthcare Research and Quality,[4] the long-term quality of life was better in patients repaired versus watchful waiting patients.

The authors' groups have used these results to manage patients as follows. Elderly patients with minimally symptomatic hernias are observed on an annual basis until symptoms develop. If they remain asymptomatic, surgery is not offered. In younger patients with asymptomatic or minimally symptomatic hernias, clear instructions as to the symptoms of incarceration are delineated, and often elective repair is encouraged.

DO ALL PATIENTS NEED A MESH REPAIR?

The concept of a tension-free hernia repair is widely accepted in inguinal hernia surgery, and the use of mesh is considered standard of care. Many studies have documented a 50% to 75% reduction in recurrence rates with the addition of mesh to an inguinal hernia repair. With the use of a mesh, most studies report recurrence rates in the 2% to 5% range with long-term follow-up. There is also evidence of quicker re-turn to work (overall hazard ratio of 0.81, 95% CI 0.73–0.91, P<0.001) and of lower rates of persisting pain (overall odd ratio of 0.36, 95% CI 0.29–0.46; P<0.001), after mesh repair.[17–21]

ARE ALL OPEN HERNIA REPAIRS EQUAL?

The European Union Trialists Collaboration did not find differences in recurrence or persistent pain for open mesh hernia repair based on mesh placement technique.[19] These results recently were consolidated by several investigators,[22–25] showing similar results for all open repairs regarding recurrence rates and postoperative com-plications when performed in experienced hands.

ARE ALL LAPAROSCOPIC INGUINAL HERNIA REPAIRS SIMILAR?

The individual merits of a laparoscopic TEP approach versus a TAPP approach are heavily debated. In both approaches, the operative site remains the same: the perper-itoneal space. In TAPP, the space is accessed intraperitoneally. In TEP, the space is accessed at the umbilicus in the retrorectus location. This space can be created by a special device (for example, a balloon dissector) or with blunt dissection.

Despite the general belief that the TAPP procedure is easier to teach and learn, there is no level 1 evidence in the literature to support this contention.[3,26,27] One of the inherent advantages of a TAPP procedure is to obtain in intraperitoneal view to ease anatomic structure identification.

A Cochrane review in 2005 stated that at that time there were insufficient data to allow conclusions to be drawn about the relative effectiveness of TEP approaches compared with TAPP approaches.[28] Almost 10 years later,[4] even with a multitude of articles dealing with this issue, there seems to be no definitive answer for this ques-tion.[2–4] Both procedures have similar results in quality of life, short-term and long-term pain, and recurrences.[4,29] Like most surgical procedures, in experienced hands, they are equally effective.

One of the major concerns of laparoscopic inguinal hernia repair is cost. In 2005, there was a health assessment analysis of a large randomized controlled trial, which reported that a TEP procedure is less costly (in the range of hundreds of dollars) than a TAPP procedure, but both are more expensive than an open repair. One of the most important points of this article was that the investigators not only considered direct costs (in which the laparoscopic approach was more expensive) but also eval-uated societal costs, such as productivity. With that analysis and because many lapa-roscopic patients returned to activity faster and with less chronic pain, the societal costs were equivalent.[30] One of the most important conclusions of this systematic re-view is that for bilateral inguinal hernias, the laparoscopic approach is more cost effec-tive and has better outcomes regarding quality of life than open surgery.

There are small specific concerns that varies between randomized clinical trials and meta-analyses regarding the incidence of minor complications,[31] such as seroma formation (at 7 days 32.5 % in TEP × 16.2 % in TAPP, p<0.001) and cord edema 7 days 12.6 % in TEP ×29.6 % in TAPP.[32,33] In a recent population based-study with more than 4500 patients, there were more complications in the TEP group (intraoper-ative complications - TEP 1.9% vs TAPP 0.9%, p=0.029 and postoperative complica-tions - TEP 2.3% vs TAPP 0.8%, p=0.003).[34] In a small subset of patients, a TEP procedure can be performed under regional anesthesia, and this can be an advantage in some clinical settings.[3] Another concern is that a TEP procedure can always be con-verted to a TAPP procedure before a definitive transition to open surgery is necessary, when some complications occur during surgery.[3] Major injuries to intrabdominal organs that were reported with early experience of TEP surgery are more related to laparoscopic surgery issues and not the laparoscopic repair of inguinal hernias.[35]

The authors' conclusion is that a laparoscopic repair of an inguinal hernia can be repaired with either a TAPP or a TEP approach, and this decision is likely made based on surgeon preference and expertise rather than evidenced-based medicine.[3,35]

IS THE LAPAROSCOPIC APPROACH BETTER THAN OPEN SURGERY FOR PRIMARY INGUINAL HERNIA REPAIR?

Early studies comparing both approaches had the bias of including tension-free laparoscopic repairs, with sutured tension repairs in the open group; thus, the better results achieved with laparoscopic approach could be attributed to the presence of mesh, not to the laparoscopic approach.[36]

The first meta-analysis where open repairs were stratified based on mesh and suture repair was the Cochrane review in 2003[37]; this article showed that laparoscopic repair was associated with major complications that were unusual with the open repair (bowel perforation and iliac vessel injury) but consistently showed an earlier return to daily activities, a lower incidence of chronic pain and paresthesia, and a recurrence rate better than open surgery with tension but equal to tension-free open surgery. Operative time was slightly higher in the laparoscopic group.

One of the most important articles recently questioning the benefit of a laparoscopic approach is the Veterans Affair Cooperative Study.[38] Despite exhibiting less postoperative pain and return to work on average a day earlier, the laparoscopy group patients had worse outcomes than the conventional open group regarding morbidity and recurrence. In this level 1A study, after comparing patients with primary hernias, the results showed that recurrence in patients undergoing laparoscopic surgery was higher (10.1%) than in the conventional group (4.9%); complications were also significantly higher in the laparoscopic group (39% × 33.4%). When examined critically, some important factors should be taken into account when using this information in clinical practice. For example, when stratified by surgeons who had performed more than 250 laparoscopic hernia procedures, the results become similar, reinforcing the need that laparoscopic hernia surgeons should perform it on a regular basis, not just intermittently. Another important aspect of this article is that the complication and recurrence rates for both procedures were higher than in other series in the literature. This series likely represents, however, real-life results, when all of these procedures are performed outside high-volume centers. This article highlights that a laparoscopic inguinal hernia repair can be a technically demanding procedure; however, if surgeons are committed to ascending the learning curve, excellent results can be obtained.

There is no doubt that the endoscopic approach is safe and feasible,[39] and it seems that recurrence and complication rates are associated with the learning curve of the procedure.[3,26,40] In most of the available literature, the laparoscopic procedure shows a small decrease in length of stay[8,41,42] although this is not universal.[43–45] Chronic pain and numbness are significantly reduced by the endoscopic approach,[8,32,34,41,46–50] and quality of life is higher in all groups tested.[29,50] Wound infection rates and the occurrence of seroma and hematoma have all been consistently less common with the endoscopic approach.[4,8,29,32,34,41,46–50]

Laparoscopic procedures were associated with a longer operative time[29,51] and major complications, such as great vessels or bowel injuries. These major complications are attributable, however, to the learning phase of this procedure.[3,29]

One adjuvant factor supporting the decision to perform a laparoscopic repair is the possibility of evaluating the contralateral side for occult hernias. In addition, the laparoscopic approach affords surgeons the ability to use an appropriately sized prosthetic to cover the entire myopectineal orifice.[52] Nevertheless, the potential advantages of treating occult hernias have never been evaluated in prospective randomized trials.

It is important to raise again the issue of costs. There are several series that have shown that despite higher direct costs, the laparoscopic repair seems cost effective from a societal perspective due to early return to normal activities and low incidence or recurrence of groin pain, even for a unilateral inguinal hernia repair.[42,47,51,53,54] Nevertheless, cost is a limitation for full acceptance of this procedure as routine.[41,55–57]

For bilateral inguinal hernia, there have been sufficient data since 2005 to choose the procedure as the first option in this setting.[2,3,29]

SHOULD LAPAROSCOPIC SURGERY BE DENIED TO ELDERLY PATIENTS?

Some surgeons deny the opportunity of the laparoscopic approach in older patients because of the fear of general anesthesia and potential complications in this age group. Evidence shows that the laparoscopic procedure is safe, with similar outcomes to open tension-free mesh repair in older adults, even with the addition of general anesthesia.[58] Some articles report that laparoscopic inguinal hernia repair confers a significantly shorter duration of pain and recovery time, with no increase in complications in this subset.[59,60] For elderly patients, laparoscopy is a viable alternative to open repair. There is some evidence that complications are slightly higher in nonagenarians and careful preoperative work-up should be done in these patients when a laparoscopic approach is used.[61] Therefore, in healthy elderly patients who can tolerate general anesthesia, the authors' groups offer laparoscopic repair.

ARE RECURRENCES BETTER TREATED WITH THE LAPAROSCOPIC APPROACH?

The European Hernia Society states in their guidelines that the endoscopic approach should be preferable in a recurrence when an anterior approach was done prior.[2]

More recent studies confirm that statement, showing that the results for laparoscopic repair in terms of chronic pain and recurrence are superior.[62–66] Some meta-analyses have challenged this statement,[67–69] specifically when comparing open preperitoneal inguinal repair with the laparoscopic approach.

Perhaps the most reasonable approach to repairing a recurrent inguinal hernia is to use the space that has not been violated in the past. This concept is based on the assumption that a surgeon is competent in both repair techniques.[2,3]

WHICH MESH SHOULD BE USED FOR THE LAPAROSCOPIC PROCEDURE?

There are a wide variety of prosthetic materials available to hernia surgeons to repair an inguinal hernia. In the authors' opinion, each product has its own unique advantages and disadvantages, and one product will never address the wide spectrum of inguinal hernia disease. One of the most basic classification systems for mesh material is the weight of the material. There remain conflicting results as to whether heavyweight material versus lightweight material provides any clinically measurable advantage. Several meta-analyses have been performed and have failed to provide a clear advantage to the lightweight products.[70]

When evaluating only open surgery, the evidence suggests that there is no risk for increased recurrence and that there is a significant reduction in the incidence of chronic groin pain as well as risk of developing other groin symptoms, like foreign body sensation,[71,72] particularly in the short-term postoperative period.[73,74]

For laparoscopic surgery, although recurrence rates have been similar with both types of mesh, differences regarding other outcomes are not easily demonstrated. The results are conflicting, with some investigators showing similar long-term and short-term postoperative outcomes,[75] whereas others show improved results for lightweight mesh obtained with open surgery,[76] in terms of reducing the incidence of chronic groin pain, groin stiffness, and foreign body sensations.[77] Based on this analysis, the authors routinely use lightweight mesh in young, healthy, and thin active adults to avoid groin pain and foreign body sensation; however, in obese elderly patients, heavyweight options are considered.

IS MESH FIXATION NECESSARY?

There are reasonably high-quality data that indicate mechanical fixation is not necessary in the TEP procedure[78] and that the number of tackers can be associated with an increasing incidence of pain.[43] In a recent meta-analysis, without increasing the risk of early hernia recurrence, the nonfixation of mesh in TEP seems a safe alternative that is associated with fewer costs and shorter operative time and hospital stay for selected patients.[79,80] Surgeons should consider nonfixation on a case-by-case basis; likely, those patients with large direct hernias should have some form of fixation, whereas those with small indirect defects likely do not require fixation if a large piece of mesh is used.

The use of glue for mesh fixation is comparable with tacker mesh fixation in terms of operative time, postoperative pain, postoperative complications, length of hospital stay, and risk for hernia recurrence. It also has been shown to reduce the risk for developing chronic groin pain.[77,81–83]

Self-adhesive meshes specially designed for laparoscopic use are appearing on the market and have shown promising results in terms of reducing pain without changing recurrence patterns.[84,85]

SUMMARY

The laparoscopic approach to inguinal hernia surgery is a safe and reliable method. In this extensive literature review, it seems that the laparoscopic approach has a similar recurrence rate compared with open tension-free mesh repair and that other outcomes should guide surgeons in choosing the most appropriate approach. Some of these important aspects include the incidence of chronic pain and numbness. Because the laparoscopic approach has shown clear advantages regarding less chronic postoperative pain and numbness, fast return to normal activities, and a decrease in the incidence of wound infection and hematoma, it should be considered an appropriate approach for inguinal hernia surgery. These results can only be achieved if a surgeon is proficient in the technique, has a clear understanding of the anatomy, and performs it on a regular basis. It is also important to consider the volume of laparoscopic repairs likely necessary to become proficient. If the laparoscopic approach is used only for recurrent or bilateral repairs, it is unlikely that the learning curve will be overcome. The choice between the TAPP or TEP procedure should be based on patient and surgeon characteristics, because there is no evidence of superiority between either technique. The use of lightweight mesh, with glue fixation (in TAPP procedures) or nonfixation (in TEP procedures) can achieve excellent results in the setting of a proficient surgeon.

REFERENCES

1. Goud J. Laparoscopic versus open inguinal hernia repair. Surg Clin North Am 2008;88:1073–81.
2. Simons MP, Aufenacker ET, Bay-Nielsen M, et al. European Hernia Society guidelines on the treatment of inguinal hernia in adult patients. Hernia 2009; 13:343–403.
3. Bittner R, Arregui ME, Bisgaard T, et al. Guidelines for laparoscopic (TAPP) and endoscopic (TEP) treatment of inguinal Hernia [International Endohernia Society (IEHS)]. Surg Endosc 2011;25:2773–843.
4. Treadwell J, Tipton K, Oyesanmi O, et al. Surgical options for inguinal hernia: comparative effectiveness review. Comparative effectiveness review No. 70 (Prepared by the ECRI Institute evidence-based Practice Center under Contract No. 290-2007-10063.) AHRQ publication No. 12-EHC091-EF. Rockville (MD): Agency for Healthcare Research and Quality; 2012. Available at:. www. effectivehealthcare.ahrq.gov/reports/final.cfm. Accessed August, 2012.
5. Rosenberg J, Bisgaard T, Kehlet H, et al, Danish Hernia Database. Danish Hernia Database recommendations for the management of inguinal and femoral hernia in adults. Dan Med Bull 2011;58(2):C4243.
6. Smink DS, Paquette IM, Finlayson SR. Utilization of laparoscopic and open inguinal hernia repair: a population-based analysis. J Laparoendosc Adv Surg Tech A 2009;19(6):745–8.
7. Burcharth J, Pedersen M, Bisgaard T, et al. Nationwide prevalence of groin hernia repair. PLoS One 2013;8(1):e54367.
8. Bittner R, Schwarz J. Inguinal hernia repair: current surgical techniques. Langenbecks Arch Surg 2012;397(2):271–82.
9. Zendejas B, Ramirez T, Jones T, et al. Trends in the utilization of inguinal hernia repair techniques: a population-based study. Am J Surg 2012;203(3):313–7.
10. Zendejas B, Ramirez T, Jones T, et al. Incidence of inguinal hernia repairs in Olmsted County, MN: a population-based study. Ann Surg 2013;257(3): 520–6.
11. Fitzgibbons RJ Jr, Giobbie-Hurder A, Gibbs JO, et al. Watchful waiting vs repair of inguinal hernia in minimally symptomatic men: a randomized clinical trial. JAMA 2006;295(3):285–92.
12. O'Dwyer PJ, Norrie J, Alani A, et al. Observation or operation for patients with an asymptomatic inguinal hernia: a randomized clinical trial. Ann Surg 2006;244(2): 167–73.
13. Chung L, Norrie J, O'Dwyer PJ. Long-term follow-up of patients with a painless inguinal hernia from a randomized clinical trial. Br J Surg 2011;98(4):596–9.
14. Mizrahi H, Parker MC. Management of asymptomatic inguinal hernia: a systematic review of the evidence. Arch Surg 2012;147(3):277–81.
15. van den Heuvel B, Dwars BJ, Klassen DR, et al. Is surgical repair of an asymptomatic groin hernia appropriate? A review. Hernia 2011;15(3):251–9.
16. Sarosi GA, Wei Y, Gibbs JO, et al. A clinician's guide to patient selection for watchful waiting management of inguinal hernia. Ann Surg 2011;253(3):605–10.
17. EU Hernia Trialists Collaboration. Mesh compared with non-mesh methods of open groin hernia repair: systematic review of randomized controlled trials. Br J Surg 2000;87(7):854–9.
18. Scott NW, McCormack K, Graham P, et al. Open mesh versus non-mesh for repair of femoral and inguinal hernia. Cochrane Database Syst Rev 2002;(4): CD002197.

19. EU Hernia Trialists Collaboration. Repair of groin hernia with synthetic mesh: meta-analysis of randomized controlled trials. Ann Surg 2002;235(3):322–32.

20. Amato B, Moja L, Panico S, et al. Shouldice technique versus other open techniques for inguinal hernia repair. Cochrane Database Syst Rev 2012;(4): CD001543.

21. Grant AM, EU Hernia Trialists Collaboration. Open mesh versus non-mesh repair of groin hernia: meta-analysis of randomised trials based on individual patient data. Hernia 2002;6(3):130–6.

22. Nienhuijs SW, van Oort I, Keemers-Gels ME, et al. Randomized trial comparing the Prolene Hernia System, mesh plug repair and Lichtenstein method for open inguinal hernia repair. Br J Surg 2005;92(1):33–8.

23. Dalenbäck J, Andersson C, Anesten B, et al. Prolene Hernia System, Lichtenstein mesh and plug-and-patch for primary inguinal hernia repair: 3-year outcome of a prospective randomised controlled trial. The BOOP study: bi-layer and connector, on-lay, and on-lay with plug for inguinal hernia repair. Hernia 2009; 13(2):121–9.

24. Zhao G, Gao P, Ma B, et al. Open mesh techniques for inguinal hernia repair: a meta-analysis of randomized controlled trials. Ann Surg 2009;250(1):35–42.

25. Sanjay P, Watt DG, Ogston SA, et al. Meta-analysis of Prolene Hernia System mesh versus Lichtenstein mesh in open inguinal hernia repair. Surgeon 2012; 10(5):283–9.

26. Bökeler U, Schwarz J, Bittner R, et al. Teaching and training in laparoscopic inguinal hernia repair (TAPP): impact of the learning curve on patient outcome. Surg Endosc 2013;27(8):2886–93.

27. Choi YY, Kim Z, Hur KY. Learning curve for laparoscopic totally extraperitoneal repair of inguinal hernia. Can J Surg 2012;55(1):33–6.

28. Wake BL, McCormack K, Fraser C, et al. Transabdominal pre-peritoneal (TAPP) vs totally extraperitoneal (TEP) laparoscopic techniques for inguinal hernia repair. Cochrane Database Syst Rev 2005;(1):CD004703.

29. McCormack K, Wake BL, Fraser C, et al. Transabdominal pre-peritoneal (TAPP) versus totally extraperitoneal (TEP) laparoscopic techniques for inguinal hernia repair: a systematic review. Hernia 2005;9(2):109–14.

30. McCormack K, Wake B, Perez J, et al. Laparoscopic surgery for inguinal hernia repair: systematic review of effectiveness and economic evaluation. Health Technol Assess 2005;9(14):1–203, iii–iv.

31. Tolver MA, Rosenberg J, Bisgaard T. Early pain after laparoscopic inguinal hernia repair. A qualitative systematic review. Acta Anaesthesiol Scand 2012;56(5): 549–57.

32. Krishna A, Misra MC, Bansal VK, et al. Laparoscopic inguinal hernia repair: transabdominal preperitoneal (TAPP) versus totally extraperitoneal (TEP) approach: a prospective randomized controlled trial. Surg Endosc 2012;26(3):639–49.

33. Bansal VK, Misra MC, Babu D, et al. A prospective, randomized comparison of long-term outcomes: chronic groin pain and quality of life following totally extraperitoneal (TEP) and transabdominal preperitoneal (TAPP) laparoscopic inguinal hernia repair. Surg Endosc 2013;27(7):2373–82.

34. Gass M, Banz VM, Rosella L, et al. TAPP or TEP? Population-based analysis of prospective data on 4,552 patients undergoing endoscopic inguinal hernia repair. World J Surg 2012;36(12):2782–6.

35. Bracale U, Melillo P, Pignata G, et al. Which is the best laparoscopic approach for inguinal hernia repair: TEP or TAPP? A systematic review of the literature with a network meta-analysis. Surg Endosc 2012;26(12):3355–66.

36. Liem MS, van Duyn EB, van der Graaf Y, et al, Coala Trial Group. Recurrences after conventional anterior and laparoscopic inguinal hernia repair: a randomized comparison. Ann Surg 2003;237(1):136–41.

37. McCormack K, Scott NW, Go PM, et al, EU Hernia Trialists Collaboration. Laparoscopic techniques versus open techniques for inguinal hernia repair. Cochrane Database Syst Rev 2003;(1):CD001785.

38. Neumayer L, Giobbie-Harder A, Jonasson O, et al, Veterans Affairs Cooperative Studies Program 456 Investigators. Open mesh versus laparoscopic mesh repair of inguinal hernia. N Engl J Med 2004;350(18):1819–27.

39. Wang WJ, Chen JZ, Fang Q, et al. Comparison of the effects of laparoscopic hernia repair and lichtenstein tension-free hernia repair. J Laparoendosc Adv Surg Tech A 2013;23(4):301–5.

40. El-Dhuwaib Y, Corless D, Emmett C, et al. Slavin Laparoscopic versus open repair of inguinal hernia: a longitudinal cohort study. Surg Endosc 2012;27(3): 936–45.

41. Gong K, Zhang N, Lu Y, et al. Comparison of the open tension-free mesh-plug, transabdominal preperitoneal (TAPP), and totally extraperitoneal (TEP) laparoscopic techniques for primary unilateral inguinal hernia repair: a prospective randomized controlled trial. Surg Endosc 2011;25(1):234–9.

42. Wittenbecher F, Scheller-Kreinsen D, Röttger J, et al. Comparison of hospital costs and length of stay associated with open-mesh, totally extraperitoneal inguinal hernia repair, and transabdominal preperitoneal inguinal hernia repair: an analysis of observational data using propensity score matching. Surg Endosc 2013;27(4):1326–33.

43. Belyansky I, Tsirline VB, Klima DA, et al. Prospective, comparative study of postoperative quality of life in TEP, TAPP, and modified Lichtenstein repairs. Ann Surg 2011;254(5):709–14.

44. Patel M, Garcea G, Fairhurst K, et al. Patient perception of laparoscopic versus open mesh repair of inguinal hernia, the hard sell. Hernia 2012;16(4):411–5.

45. Koning GG, Wetterslev J, van Laarhoven CJ, et al. The totally extraperitoneal method versus Lichtenstein's technique for inguinal hernia repair: a systematic review with meta-analyses and trial sequential analyses of randomized clinical trials. PLoS One 2013;8(1):e52599.

46. Nienhuijs S, Staal E, Strobbe L, et al. Chronic pain after mesh repair of inguinal hernia: a systematic review. Am J Surg 2007;194(3):394–400.

47. Langeveld HR, van't Riet M, Weidema WF, et al. Total extraperitoneal inguinal hernia repair compared with Lichtenstein (the LEVEL-Trial): a randomized controlled trial. Ann Surg 2010;251(5):819–24.

48. Eklund A, Montgomery A, Bergkvist L, et al, Swedish Multicentre Trial of Inguinal Hernia Repair by Laparoscopy (SMIL) study group. Chronic pain 5 years after randomized comparison of laparoscopic and Lichtenstein inguinal hernia repair. Br J Surg 2010;97(4):600–8.

49. O'Reilly EA, Burke JP, O'Connell PR. A meta-analysis of surgical morbidity and recurrence after laparoscopic and open repair of primary unilateral inguinal hernia. Ann Surg 2012;255(5):846–53.

50. Abbas AE, Abd Ellatif ME, Noaman N, et al. Patient-perspective quality of life after laparoscopic and open hernia repair: a controlled randomized trial. Surg Endosc 2012;26(9):2465–70.

51. Kuhry E, van Veen RN, Langeveld HR, et al. Open or endoscopic total extraperitoneal inguinal hernia repair? A systematic review. Surg Endosc 2007;21(2): 161–6.

52. Castorina S, Luca T, Privitera G, et al. An evidence-based approach for laparoscopic inguinal hernia repair: lessons learned from over 1,000 repairs. Clin Anat 2012;25(6):687–96.

53. Gholghesaei M, Langeveld HR, Veldkamp R, et al. Costs and quality of life after endoscopic repair of inguinal hernia vs open tension-free repair: a review. Surg Endosc 2005;19(6):816–21.

54. Eker HH, Langeveld HR, Klitsie PJ, et al. Randomized clinical trial of total extraperitoneal inguinal hernioplasty vs Lichtenstein repair: a long-term follow-up study. Arch Surg 2012;147(3):256–60.

55. Eklund A, Carlsson P, Rosenblad A, et al, Swedish Multicentre Trial of Inguinal Hernia Repair by Laparoscopy (SMIL) study group. Long-term cost-minimization analysis comparing laparoscopic with open (Lichtenstein) inguinal hernia repair. Br J Surg 2010;97(5):765–71.

56. Smart P, Castles L. Quantifying the cost of laparoscopic inguinal hernia repair. ANZ J Surg 2012;82(11):809–12.

57. Stylopoulos N, Gazelle GS, Rattner DW. A cost–utility analysis of treatment options for inguinal hernia in 1,513,008 adult patients. Surg Endosc 2003; 17(2):180–9.

58. Hope WW, Bools L, Menon A, et al. Comparing laparoscopic and open inguinal hernia repair in octogenarians. Hernia 2012. [Epub ahead of print].

59. Hernandez-Rosa J, Lo CC, Choi JJ, et al. Laparoscopic versus open inguinal hernia repair in octogenarians. Hernia 2011;15(6):655–8.

60. Dallas KB, Froylich D, Choi JJ, et al. Laparoscopic versus open inguinal hernia repair in octogenarians: a follow-up study. Geriatr Gerontol Int 2013;13(2): 329–33.

61. Pallati PK, Gupta PK, Bichala S, et al. Short-term outcomes of inguinal hernia repair in octogenarians and nonagenarians. Hernia 2013. [Epub ahead of print].

62. Shah NR, Mikami DJ, Cook C, et al. A comparison of outcomes between open and laparoscopic surgical repair of recurrent inguinal hernias. Surg Endosc 2011;25(7):2330–7.

63. Sevonius D, Gunnarsson U, Nordin P, et al. Recurrent groin hernia surgery. Br J Surg 2011;98(10):1489–94.

64. Bignell M, Partridge G, Mahon D, et al. Prospective randomized trial of laparoscopic (transabdominal preperitoneal-TAPP) versus open (mesh) repair for bilateral and recurrent inguinal hernia: incidence of chronic groin pain and impact on quality of life: results of 10 year follow-up. Hernia 2012;16(6): 635–40.

65. Gopal SV, Warrier A. Recurrence after groin hernia repair-revisited. Int J Surg 2013;11(5):374–7.

66. Yang J, Tong da N, Yao J, et al. Laparoscopic or lichtenstein repair for recurrent inguinal hernia: a meta-analysis of randomized controlled trials. ANZ J Surg 2013;83(5):312–8.

67. Karthikesalingam A, Markar SR, Holt PJ, et al. Meta-analysis of randomized controlled trials comparing laparoscopic with open mesh repair of recurrent inguinal hernia. Br J Surg 2010;97(1):4–11.

68. Sgourakis G, Dedemadi G, Gockel I, et al. Laparoscopic totally extraperitoneal versus open preperitoneal mesh repair for inguinal hernia recurrence: a decision analysis based on net health benefits. Surg Endosc 2013;27(7):2526–41.

69. Dedemadi G, Sgourakis G, Radtke A, et al. Laparoscopic versus open mesh repair for recurrent inguinal hernia: a meta-analysis of outcomes. Am J Surg 2010;200(2):291–7.

70. Li J, Ji Z, Cheng T. Lightweight versus heavyweight in inguinal hernia repair: a meta-analysis. Hernia 2012;16(5):529–39.
71. Sajid MS, Leaver C, Baig MK, et al. Systematic review and meta-analysis of the use of lightweight versus heavyweight mesh in open inguinal hernia repair. Br J Surg 2012;99(1):29–37.
72. Uzzaman MM, Ratnasingham K, Ashraf N. Meta-analysis of randomized controlled trials comparing lightweight and heavyweight mesh for Lichtenstein inguinal hernia repair. Hernia 2012;16(5):505–18.
73. Śmietański M, Śmietańska IA, Modrzejewski A, et al. Systematic review and meta-analysis on heavy and lightweight polypropylene mesh in Lichtenstein inguinal hernioplasty. Hernia 2012;16(5):519–28.
74. Bury K, Śmietański M, Polish Hernia Study Group. Five-year results of a randomized clinical trial comparing a polypropylene mesh with a poliglecaprone and polypropylene composite mesh for inguinal hernioplasty. Hernia 2012;16(5): 549–53.
75. Currie A, Andrew H, Tonsi A, et al. Lightweight versus heavyweight mesh in laparoscopic inguinal hernia repair: a meta-analysis. Surg Endosc 2012;26(8): 2126–33.
76. Schopf S, von Ahnen T, von Ahnen M, et al. Chronic pain after laparoscopic transabdominal preperitoneal hernia repair: a randomized comparison of light and extralight titanized polypropylene mesh. World J Surg 2011;35(2):302–10.
77. Sajid MS, Kalra L, Parampalli U, et al. A systematic review and meta-analysis evaluating the effectiveness of lightweight mesh against heavyweight mesh in influencing the incidence of chronic groin pain following laparoscopic inguinal hernia repair. Am J Surg 2013;205(6):726–36.
78. Sajid MS, Ladwa N, Kalra L, et al. A meta-analysis examining the use of tacker mesh fixation versus glue mesh fixation in laparoscopic inguinal hernia repair. Am J Surg 2013;206(1):103–11.
79. Teng YJ, Pan SM, Liu YL, et al. A meta-analysis of randomized controlled trials of fixation versus nonfixation of mesh in laparoscopic total extraperitoneal inguinal hernia repair. Surg Endosc 2011;25(9):2849–58.
80. Sajid MS, Ladwa N, Kalra L, et al. A meta-analysis examining the use of tacker fixation versus no-fixation of mesh in laparoscopic inguinal hernia repair. Int J Surg 2012;10(5):224–31.
81. Tolver MA, Rosenberg J, Juul P, et al. Randomized clinical trial of fibrin glue versus tacked fixation in laparoscopic groin hernia repair. Surg Endosc 2013; 27(8):2727–33.
82. Kaul A, Hutfless S, Le H, et al. Staple versus fibrin glue fixation in laparoscopic total extraperitoneal repair of inguinal hernia: a systematic review and meta-analysis. Surg Endosc 2012;26(5):1269–78.
83. Fortelny RH, Petter-Puchner AH, Glaser KS, et al. Use of fibrin sealant (Tisseel/Tissucol) in hernia repair: a systematic review. Surg Endosc 2012;26(7): 1803–12.
84. Birk D, Pardo CG. Self gripping Parietex Progrip™ Mesh in Laparoscopic Hernia Repair. Have we found the ideal implant? Surg Technol Int 2012. [Epub ahead of print].
85. Fumagalli Romario U, Puccetti F, Elmore U, et al. Self-gripping mesh versus staple fixation in laparoscopic inguinal hernia repair: a prospective comparison. Surg Endosc 2013;27(5):1798–802.

Index

Note: Page numbers of article titles are in **boldface** type.

A

Abdominal incisions
    choice of, 1028
    closure of, **1027–1040**
        introduction, 1027–1028
    wound healing, 1028–1037
        discussion, 1036–1037
        risk factors for wound dehiscence and incisional hernia, 1030–1031
        suture technique in relation to incisional hernia, 1033–1035
        suture technique in relation to surgical-site infection, 1029–1030, 1031–1032
        suture technique in relation to wound dehiscence, 1031–1033
Abdominal sepsis
    diagnosis and management of, 1166–1167
Abdominal wall
    adult
        anatomy of, 1059–1060
    embryology of, 1058–1059
Abdominal wall defects
    large contaminated
        reconstruction of, **1163–1183**. *See also* Enterocutaneous fistulas
    pediatric, **1255–1267**
        congenital, 1262–1264
        epigastric hernias, 1262
        femoral hernias, 1261
        inguinal hernias, 1255–1261. *See also* Inguinal hernias, pediatric
        introduction, 1255
        lumbar hernias, 1262
        Spigelian hernias, 1262
        umbilical hernias, 1261
Abdominal wall hernia
    repair of
        hospital costs related to, 1248–1249
Abdominal wall reconstruction
    economics of, **1241–1253**
        biological mesh, 1249–1251
        component separation procedures, 1247–1248
        cost-effectiveness of mesh for hernia repair, 1245–1246
        hernia prevention, 1246–1247
        hospital costs, 1248–1249
        introduction, 1241–1242
        laparoscopic hernia repair–related, 1246
        scope of problem, 1242–1245

Surg Clin N Am 93 (2013) 1281–1291
http://dx.doi.org/10.1016/S0039-6109(13)00121-7
0039-6109/13/$ – see front matter © 2013 Elsevier Inc. All rights reserved.

surgical.theclinics.com

Abdominal (*continued*)
    soft tissue coverage in, **1199–1209**
        flap donor site options in, 1203–1205
        free tissue transfer in, 1203
        introduction, 1199–1200
        local flap options in, 1200–1203
        recipient vessels in, 1205–1208
        regional flap options in, 1203
Abdominal wall transplantation, 1208–1209
Acute intestinal failure
    enterocutaneous fistulation and, 1164
Adolescent(s)
    inguinal hernias in, 1260–1261
Antibiotic(s)
    perioperative
        in preoperative risk reduction, 1045–1046
Ascites
    umbilical and epigastric hernia repair in patients with, 1083

B

Biological mesh(es)
    economics of, 1249–1251
    in hernia repair
        basic concepts, 1212
        biology of, **1211–1215**
            collagen cross-linking, 1212
            mesh migration and host reactions, 1212–1213
        clinical outcomes of, **1217–1225**
            cost analyses, 1222–1223
            FDA review, 1219–1220
            introduction, 1217–1218
            literature and systemic reviews, 1220–1222
        introduction, 1211–1212
        remodeling, 1213–1214
        types of, 1218–1219
Bleeding
    after laparoscopic ventral hernia repair, 1106
Blood glucose
    perioperative management of
        in preoperative risk reduction, 1046–1047

C

Children
    abdominal wall defects in, **1255–1267**. *See also* Abdominal wall defects, pediatric
Cirrhosis
    umbilical and epigastric hernia repair in patients with, 1083
Collagen cross-linking
    biological meshes in hernia repair and, 1212
Complex abdominal wall reconstruction, **1163–1183**. *See also* Enterocutaneous fistulas
    takedown of, 1163–1164

Component separation procedures
    economic impact of, 1247–1248

D

Diastasis recti
    in umbilical and epigastric hernia repair, 1082–1083
Direct inguinal hernias
    pediatric, 1260

E

Elderly
    inguinal hernias in
        laparoscopic repair of, 1273
Enterocutaneous fistulas, **1163–1183**
    abdominal sepsis and
        diagnosis and management of, 1166–1167
    acute intestinal failure related to, 1164–1180
    causes of, 1164–1166
    classification of, 1164–1166
    described, 1164
    takedown of, **1163–1183**
        definitive surgical reconstruction in
            principles of, 1169–1171
        introduction, 1163–1164
        nutritional support in, 1168
        operative technique, 1171–1180
            closure, 1174
            gaining entry to abdomen, 1171–1173
            immediate preoperative preparation, 1171
            for larger abdominal wall defects, 1177
            positioning, 1171
            reconstruction with autologous tissue, 1177–1178
            reconstruction with biological implants, 1178–1180
            restoration of gastrointestinal continuity, 1174
            single-stage *vs.* multiple-staged approaches, 1174–1177
        preoperative management in, 1166
        psychological support in, 1168–1169
        wound and fistula care in, 1167–1168
Epigastric hernias, **1057–1089**
    anatomy related to, 1058–1060
    causes of, 1060–1064
        acquired, 1061–1064
        congenital, 1060–1061
    classification of, 1066
    clinical presentation of, 1066
    epidemiology of, 1064–1066
    introduction, 1057–1058
    pediatric, 1262
    repair of

Epigastric (*continued*)
    acutely incarcerated hernia, 1081–1082
    in ascitic patients, 1083
    in cirrhotic patients, 1083
    complications of, 1081
    diastasis recti, 1082–1083
    immediate postoperative care and recovery, 1080–1081
    laparoscopic, 1079
    pain management in, 1079–1080
    during pregnancy, 1082
    preoperative planning in, 1066–1069
    special considerations in, 1081–1083
    surgical technique in, 1066–1079
        mesh repair *vs.* primary repair, 1070–1073
        open prosthetic repair, 1073–1079
        types of, 1070–1079

F

Femoral hernias
    pediatric, 1261
Fistula(s)
    enterocutaneous. *See* Enterocutaneous fistulas
Flank hernias
    repair of
        laparoscopic, 1104
        surgical techniques, 1149–1155
            laparoscopic approach, 1151–1155
            open approach, 1149–1151

G

Gastroschisis
    pediatric, 1262–1264

H

Hernia(s)
    abdominal wall
        repair of
            hospital costs related to, 1248–1249
    acutely strangulated
        emergent prosthetic repair of, 1231–1232
    atypical, **1135–1162**. *See also* specific types
        introduction, 1135–1136
        preoperative planning for, 1136
        repair of
            clinical results in literature, 1155–1159
            surgical techniques, 1136–1159
                flank hernia, 1149–1155
                subxiphoid hernia, 1144–1149
                suprapubic hernia, 1136–1144

described, 1057–1058
epigastric, **1057–1089**. *See also* Epigastric hernias
    pediatric, 1262
femoral
    pediatric, 1261
flank
    repair of
        laparoscopic, 1104
        surgical techniques, 1149–1155
incisional. *See* Incisional hernias
inguinal
    pediatric, 1255–1261. *See also* Inguinal hernias, pediatric
    repair of, **1269–1279**. *See also* Inguinal hernias, repair of
lumbar
    laparoscopic repair of, 1104
    pediatric, 1262
parastomal
    prevention of, 1193–1195
    prosthetic
        prevention of, 1232–1233
    repair of, **1185–1198**. *See also* Parastomal hernia repair
prevention of
    economic impact of, 1246–1247
recurrent
    laparoscopic repair of, 1105
repair of
    biological meshes in
        biology of, **1211–1215**. *See also* Biological mesh(es), in hernia repair
    laparoscopic
        economic impact of, 1246
    prosthetic
        in contaminated fields
            safety of, **1227–1239**. *See also* Prosthetic mesh hernia repair, in contaminated
                fields
Spigelian
    pediatric, 1262
subxiphoid. *See* Subxiphoid hernias
suprapubic. *See* Suprapubic hernias
umbilical, **1057–1089**. *See also* Umbilical hernias
    pediatric, 1261
ventral. *See* Ventral hernias

I

Incision(s)
    abdominal. *See* Abdominal incisions
Incisional hernias
    abdominal incisions and
        risk factors for, 1030–1031
    causes of, 1062–1064
    introduction, 1027–1028

Incisional (*continued*)
  prevention of, **1027–1040**
  suture technique in relation to, 1033–1035
Infection(s). *See also specific types*
  surgical site. *See* Surgical site infections (SSIs)
Inguinal hernias
  in adolescents, 1260–1261
  pediatric, 1255–1261
    anatomy of, 1256
    clinical presentation of, 1256
    contralateral groin assessment related to, 1257
    diagnostic imaging in, 1256
    direct inguinal hernias, 1260
    embryology of, 1256
    epidemiology of, 1255–1256
    examination of, 1256
    patent processus *vs.* hernia, 1257
    repair of
      extracorporeal ligation in, 1259
      intracorporeal, 1258–1259
      laparoscopic, 1258–1260
      open, 1257–1260
    risk of incarceration in, 1256
    surgery for
      timing of, 1257
  recurrence of
    repair of
      laparoscopic, 1273
  repair of
    equality of, 1271
    indications for, 1270
    introduction, 1269–1270
    laparoscopic
      in children, 1258–1260
      in the elderly, 1273
      mesh selection for, 1273–1274
      similarity among, 1271–1272
      vs. open, **1269–1279**
    open
      vs. laparoscopic, **1269–1279**
Intestinal failure
  acute
    enterocutaneous fistulation and, 1164
Intestinal injury
  after laparoscopic ventral hernia repair, 1106–1107

L

Laparoscopic hernia repair
  economic impact of, 1246
Laparoscopic ventral hernia repair, **1091–1110**

complications of, 1106–1108
for hernias in difficult locations, 1104–1105
indications for, 1092–1093
introduction, 1091–1092
patient selection for, 1092–1093
postoperative care, 1105–1106
preoperative planning for, 1093
of recurrent hernias, 1105
surgical technique, 1094–1104
    access, 1094
    closure, 1103–1104
    defect size measurement, 1097–1099
    lysis of adhesions, 1096
    management of inadvertent enterotomy, 1096–1097
    mesh fixation, 1101–1103
    mesh insertion, 1101
    mesh selection and preparation, 1099–1100
    patient positioning, 1094
    port layout, 1095–1096
    preparation, 1094
    providing clearance for mesh, 1097
    reduction of hernia contents, 1096
Laparoscopy
  in umbilical and epigastric hernia repair, 1079
Lumbar/flank hernias
  laparoscopic repair of, 1104
Lumbar hernias
  pediatric, 1262

M

Mesh(es)
  biological
    economics of, 1249–1251
    in hernia repair
      biology of, **1211–1215**. *See also* Biological mesh(es), in hernia repair, biology of
  for hernia repair
    cost-effectiveness of, 1245–1246
  lightweight
    in hernia repair in contaminated fields
      safety of, 1234–1235
Mesh infections
  after laparoscopic ventral hernia repair, 1107–1108
Metabolic control
  in preoperative risk reduction, 1043–1044

N

Nutritional support
  in enterocutaneous fistula management, 1168
  in preoperative risk reduction, 1043–1044

O

Obese patients
    operative risks associated with
        guidelines for reducing, 1047
Omphalocele(s)
    pediatric, 1262–1264
Open ventral hernia repair
    with component separation, **1111–1133**
        clinical anatomy related to, 1113–1114
        introduction, 1111–1112
        mesh selection in, 1114–1115
        outcomes of, 1126–1130
        postoperative care, 1124–1125
        postoperative complications, 1125–1126
        preoperative planning, 1113
        surgical techniques, 1114–1124
            anterior component separation, 1121–1124
                outcomes of, 1126–1128
            posterior component separation, 1114–1121
                outcomes of, 1128–1130
            PUPS method
                outcomes of, 1128

P

Pain
    persistent
        after laparoscopic ventral hernia repair, 1107
Pain management
    in umbilical and epigastric hernia repair, 1079–1080
Parastomal hernia
    prevention of, 1193–1195
    prosthetic
        prevention of, 1232–1233
    repair of, **1185–1198**. *See also* Parastomal hernia repair
Parastomal hernia repair, **1185–1198**
    introduction, 1185–1886
    laparoscopic repair, 1187
        mesh selection, 1193
        outcomes, 1190–1193
        technique, 1188–1190
    open repair, 1186–1187
Pregnancy
    umbilical and epigastric hernia repair during, 1082
Preoperative axial imaging
    in preoperative risk reduction, 1047
Preoperative risk reduction, **1041–1055**
    introduction, 1041–1042
    nutrition and metabolic control in, 1043–1044
    obesity complicating, 1047

perioperative antibiotics in, 1045–1046
perioperative blood glucose management in, 1046–1047
preoperative axial imaging in, 1047
skin preparation and decolonization protocols in, 1048
smoking cessation in, 1042–1043
Primary ventral hernia
   epigastric
      causes of, 1062
   umbilical
      causes of, 1061–1062
Prosthetic incisional hernia
   prevention of, 1232
Prosthetic mesh hernia repair
   in contaminated fields
      acutely strangulated hernias, 1231–1232
      described, 1230–1231
      safety of, **1227–1239**
         early experience, 1228–1229
         introduction, 1227–1228
         midterm experience, 1229–1230
         modern era and lightweight mesh, 1234–1235
         prosthetic incisional hernia prevention, 1232
         prosthetic parastomal hernia prevention, 1232–1233
         retrospective database outcomes related to, 1233–1234
Prosthetic parastomal hernia
   prevention of, 1232–1233
Psychological support
   in enterocutaneous fistula management, 1168–1169
PUPS method
   in open ventral hernia repair with component separation
      outcomes of, 1128

R

Rives-Stoppa-Wantz retrorectus repair
   described, 1112

S

Seroma(s)
   after laparoscopic ventral hernia repair, 1107
Skin preparation and decolonization protocols
   in preoperative risk reduction, 1048
Smoking cessation
   in preoperative risk reduction, 1042–1043
Soft tissue coverage
   in abdominal wall reconstruction, **1199–1209**. *See also* Abdominal wall reconstruction,
      soft tissue coverage in
Spigelian hernias
   pediatric, 1262
SSIs. *See* Surgical site infections (SSIs)

Subxiphoid hernias
    repair of
        laparoscopic, 1104
        surgical techniques, 1145–1149
            laparoscopic approach, 1146–1149
            open approach, 1145–1146
Suprapubic hernias
    repair of
        laparoscopic, 1104–1105
        surgical techniques
            laparoscopic approach, 1140–1144
            open approach, 1136–1140
Surgery(ies)
    preoperative metabolic preparation for, 1044–1045
Surgical site infections (SSIs), 1045

T

Transplantation
    abdominal wall, 1208–1209

U

Umbilical hernias, **1057–1089**
    anatomy related to, 1058–1060
    causes of, 1060–1064
        acquired, 1061–1064
        congenital, 1060–1061
    classification of, 1066
    clinical presentation of, 1066
    epidemiology of, 1064–1066
    introduction, 1057–1058
    pediatric, 1261
    repair of, **1057–1089**
        acutely incarcerated hernia, 1081–1082
        in ascitic patients, 1083
        in cirrhotic patients, 1083
        complications of, 1081
        diastasis recti, 1082–1083
        immediate postoperative care and recovery, 1080–1081
        laparoscopic, 1079
        pain management in, 1079–1080
        during pregnancy, 1082
        preoperative planning in, 1066–1069
        special considerations in, 1081–1083
        surgical techniques in, 1066–1079
            mesh repair *vs.* primary repair, 1070–1073
            open prosthetic repair, 1073–1079
            types of, 1070–1079

V

Ventral hernias
  recurrence of
    after laparoscopic ventral hernia repair, 1108
  repair of
    laparoscopic, **1091–1110**. *See also* Laparoscopic ventral hernia repair
    open
      with component separation, **1111–1133**. *See also* Open ventral hernia repair, with
        component separation

W

Wound dehiscence
  abdominal incisions and
    risk factors for, 1030–1031
Wound healing
  of abdominal incisions, 1028–1037. *See also* Abdominal incisions, wound healing
Wound infections
  after laparoscopic ventral hernia repair, 1107–1108

United States Postal Service

Statement of Ownership, Management, and Circulation
(All Periodicals Publications Except Requestor Publications)

1. Publication Title	2. Publication Number	3. Filing Date
Surgical Clinics of North America	5 2 9 - 8 0 0 0	9/14/13

4. Issue Frequency	5. Number of Issues Published Annually	6. Annual Subscription Price
Feb, Apr, Jun, Aug, Oct, Dec	6	$353.00

7. Complete Mailing Address of Known Office of Publication (Not printer) (Street, city, county, state, and ZIP+4®)

Elsevier Inc.
360 Park Avenue South
New York, NY 10010-1710

Contact Person
Stephen Bushing

Telephone: (Include area codes)
215-239-3688

8. Complete Mailing Address of Headquarters or General Business Office of Publisher (Not printer)

Elsevier Inc., 360 Park Avenue South, New York, NY 10010-1710

9. Full Names and Complete Mailing Addresses of Publisher, Editor, and Managing Editor (Do not leave blank)

Publisher (Name and complete mailing address)

Linda Belfus, Elsevier, Inc., 1600 John F. Kennedy Blvd. Suite 1800, Philadelphia, PA 19103-2899

Editor (Name and complete mailing address)

John Vassallo, Elsevier, Inc., 1600 John F. Kennedy Blvd. Suite 1800, Philadelphia, PA 19103-2899

Managing Editor (Name and complete mailing address)

Adrianne Brigido, Elsevier, Inc., 1600 John F. Kennedy Blvd. Suite 1800, Philadelphia, PA 19103-2899

10. Owner (Do not leave blank. If the publication is owned by a corporation, give the name and address of the corporation immediately followed by the names and addresses of all stockholders owning or holding 1 percent or more of the total amount of stock. If not owned by a corporation, give the names and addresses of the individual owners. If owned by a partnership or other unincorporated firm, give its name and address as well as those of each individual owner. If the publication is published by a nonprofit organization, give its name and address.)

Full Name	Complete Mailing Address
Wholly owned subsidiary of	1600 John F. Kennedy Blvd., Ste. 1800
Reed/Elsevier, US holdings	Philadelphia, PA 19103-2899

11. Known Bondholders, Mortgagees, and Other Security Holders Owning or Holding 1 Percent or More of Total Amount of Bonds, Mortgages, or Other Securities. If none, check box ☐ None

Full Name	Complete Mailing Address
N/A	

12. Tax Status (For completion by nonprofit organizations authorized to mail at nonprofit rates) (Check one)
The purpose, function, and nonprofit status of this organization and the exempt status for federal income tax purposes:
☐ Has Not Changed During Preceding 12 Months
☐ Has Changed During Preceding 12 Months (Publisher must submit explanation of change with this statement)

PS Form 3526, September 2007 (Page 1 of 3 (Instructions Page 3)) PSN 7530-01-000-9931 PRIVACY NOTICE: See our Privacy policy in www.usps.com

---

13. Publication Title	14. Issue Date for Circulation Data Below
Surgical Clinics of North America	June 2013

15. Extent and Nature of Circulation

		Average No. Copies Each Issue During Preceding 12 Months	No. Copies of Single Issue Published Nearest to Filing Date
a. Total Number of Copies (Net press run)		1990	1771
b. Paid Circulation (By Mail and Outside the Mail)	(1) Mailed Outside-County Paid Subscriptions Stated on PS Form 3541. (Include paid distribution above nominal rate, advertiser's proof copies, and exchange copies)	818	714
	(2) Mailed In-County Paid Subscriptions Stated on PS Form 3541 (Include paid distribution above nominal rate, advertiser's proof copies, and exchange copies)		
	(3) Paid Distribution Outside the Mails Including Sales Through Dealers and Carriers, Street Vendors, Counter Sales, and Other Paid Distribution Outside USPS®	634	498
	(4) Paid Distribution by Other Classes Mailed Through the USPS (e.g. First-Class Mail®)		
c. Total Paid Distribution (Sum of 15a (1), (2), (3), and (4))	►	1452	1212
d. Free or Nominal Rate Distribution (By Mail and Outside the Mail)	(1) Free or Nominal Rate Outside-County Copies Included on PS Form 3541	92	114
	(2) Free or Nominal Rate In-County Copies Included on PS Form 3541		
	(3) Free or Nominal Rate Copies Mailed at Other Classes Through the USPS (e.g. First-Class Mail)		
	(4) Free or Nominal Rate Distribution Outside the Mail (Carriers or other means)		
e. Total Free or Nominal Rate Distribution (Sum of 15d (1), (2), (3) and (4))	►	92	114
f. Total Distribution (Sum of 15c and 15e)	►	1544	1326
g. Copies not Distributed (See instructions to publishers #4 (page #3))	►	446	445
h. Total (Sum of 15f and g)	►	1990	1771
i. Percent Paid (15c divided by 15f times 100)		94.04%	91.40%

16. Publication of Statement of Ownership
☐ If the publication is a general publication, publication of this statement is required. Will be printed in the October 2013 issue of this publication.
☐ Publication not required.

17. Signature and Title of Editor, Publisher, Business Manager, or Owner	Date
[signature] Stephen R. Bushing –Inventory/Distribution Coordinator	September 14, 2013

I certify that all information furnished on this form is true and complete. I understand that anyone who furnishes false or misleading information on this form or who omits material or information requested on the form may be subject to criminal sanctions (including fines and imprisonment) and/or civil sanctions (including civil penalties).

PS Form 3526, September 2007 (Page 2 of 3)

Moving?

Make sure your subscription moves with you!

To notify us of your new address, find your **Clinics Account Number** (located on your mailing label above your name), and contact customer service at:

Email: journalscustomerservice-usa@elsevier.com

800-654-2452 (subscribers in the U.S. & Canada)
314-447-8871 (subscribers outside of the U.S. & Canada)

Fax number: 314-447-8029

Elsevier Health Sciences Division
Subscription Customer Service
3251 Riverport Lane
Maryland Heights, MO 63043

*To ensure uninterrupted delivery of your subscription, please notify us at least 4 weeks in advance of move.

Printed and bound by CPI Group (UK) Ltd, Croydon, CR0 4YY

03/10/2024

01040493-0009